Small Animal Anesthesia Techniques

Small Animal Anesthesia Techniques

Second Edition

Edited by

Amanda M. Shelby, BSc, RVT, VTS (Anesthesia & Analgesia)

Jurox, Inc.
North Kansas City, Missouri, USA

Carolyn M. McKune, DVM, DACVAA

Mythos Veterinary LLC
Gainesville, Florida, USA

WILEY Blackwell

Registered Office
John Wiley & Sons, Inc., 111 River Street, Hoboken, NJ 07030, USA

Editorial Office
111 River Street, Hoboken, NJ 07030, USA

For details of our global editorial offices, customer services, and more information about Wiley products visit us at www.wiley.com.

Wiley also publishes its books in a variety of electronic formats and by print-on-demand. Some content that appears in standard print versions of this book may not be available in other formats.

Library of Congress Cataloging-in-Publication Data
Names: Shelby, Amanda M., editor. | McKune, Carolyn M., editor. | Shelby,
    Amanda M. Small animal anesthesia techniques.
Title: Small animal anesthesia techniques / [edited by] Amanda M. Shelby,
    Carolyn M. McKune.
Description: Second edition. | Hoboken, NJ : Wiley, 2023. | Preceded by
    Small animal anesthesia techniques / Amanda M. Shelby, Carolyn M.
    McKune. Ames, Iowa : Wiley/Blackwell, 2014. | Includes bibliographical
    references and index.
Identifiers: LCCN 2022023687 (print) | LCCN 2022023688 (ebook) | ISBN
    9781119710820 (paperback) | ISBN 9781119710844 (adobe pdf) | ISBN
    9781119710851 (epub)
Subjects: MESH: Anesthesia–methods | Anesthesia–veterinary | Cats | Dogs
    | Pets | Handbook
Classification: LCC SF914 (print) | LCC SF914 (ebook) | NLM SF 914 | DDC
    636.089/796–dc23/eng/20220727
LC record available at https://lccn.loc.gov/2022023687
LC ebook record available at https://lccn.loc.gov/2022023688

Cover Design: Wiley
Cover Images: Courtesy of Carolyn M. McKune,
Courtesy of Michael J. Dark, Courtesy of Laurel Housden Photography

Set in 10/12.5 pt and TimesLTStd by Straive, Chennai, India
SKY10036884_101722

Contents

Section II: Drug formulary   277
Dario A. Floriano and Amanda M. Shelby

List of Contributors

Angela Borchers, DVM, DACVIM, DACVECC
Department of Pathobiological Sciences
School of Veterinary Medicine, University of Wisconsin-Madison
Madison, Wisconsin, USA

Stephen Cital, RVT, SRA, RLAT, CVPP, VTS-LAM (Res. Anesthesia)
Stanford University
San Jose, California, USA

Dario A. Floriano, DMV
University of Pennsylvania
Philadelphia, Pennsylvania, USA

Yishai Y. Kushnir, DVM, DACVAA
Department of Anaesthesia and Pain Management
Koret School of Veterinary Medicine-Veterinary Teaching Hospital
The Hebrew University of Jerusalem, Israel

Carolyn M. McKune, DVM, DACVAA
Mythos Veterinary LLC
Gainesville, Florida, USA

Vaidehi V. Paranjape, BVSc, MVSc, MS, Diplomate ACVAA
Anesthesiology and Pain Management
Virginia-Maryland College of Veterinary Medicine
Blacksburg, Virginia, USA

Jennifer K. Sager, BS, CVT, VTS (Anesthesia & Analgesia, ECC)
University of Florida Veterinary Hospitals and Midmark Animal Health
Gainesville, Florida, USA

Amanda M. Shelby, BSc, RVT, VTS (Anesthesia & Analgesia)
Jurox, Inc.
North Kansas City, Missouri, USA

Sharon Tenenbaum Shih, DVM, DACVAA
Veterinary Referral Associates
Gaithersburg, Maryland, USA

Preface

The purpose of the second edition of this book is to broaden this easily accessible guide, which is focused on developing a balanced anesthesia protocol and appropriate multimodal analgesia, through including a diverse set of authors who are experts in their field. As the field of veterinary anesthesia evolves and becomes more complex, the role of the anesthetist as the patient's advocate remains critical as ever. It is the authors' intention to provide evidence-based information to assist with the anesthetic process, patient protocols, and anticipating and managing potential anesthetic complications. However, this work is also reflective of the authors' personal preferences and experiences. Our hope is that this will provide a useful tool with which to manage anesthesia in a variety of situations, for a variety of anesthetists who serve as the guardians of their patients.

Amanda M. Shelby
Carolyn M. McKune

Acknowledgments

While it is my sincere hope that the reader will enjoy this work, the finished product cannot convey the minutes, hours, days, weeks, and months that turned into years of effort to create the second edition of *Small Animal Anesthesia Techniques*. This work was written during a time of remarkable worldwide struggle as a pandemic raged (and still does rage at the time of authorship) through our nations. This pandemic put many things in perspective. Science moved at lightning speed to create safe vaccinations to curb an insatiable virus, while ignorance also moved at lightning speed to create fissure lines along the most fragile parts of society: our bonds with each other. As my own home became a residence, school, gym, and workplace, I would like to acknowledge the "village" that was indispensable for allowing me the precious time to complete this work (namely, the women that cared lovingly for my children). As a professional and a mother, I have accepted that the crux of contributing to one's profession resides in one's children being well cared for, which is challenging under normal circumstances but even more so in a pandemic. This book would not have been possible without Sofia Tabi, Magalia Garcia, and Nerea Martin Gonzalez. Thank you for taking care of my three most precious gifts, so I could share my knowledge.

My greatest strength continues to be my husband, Dr Michael J. Dark, who selflessly provides support to all of our family, who makes me laugh even when I don't want to, and is truly my better half. This work is only possible with his love and support.

Carolyn M. McKune

It is also my sincere hope that readers value the collective thoughts and expertise of the contributors who faced these unique and globally impacting times. The effect on the veterinary profession as a whole, with excessive wait times, limited accessibility to pet care due to staff shortages and the overwhelming need of pets, has placed demands beyond measure on both our expertise and our mental and emotional health. As Dr McKune mentioned above, the global pandemic left many of us isolated or with limited contact outside our profession and our immediate family. This balance of personal and professional needs is hard to achieve even in "normal" times. Therefore, without a doubt, my greatest strength is the support of loved ones – support by helping with the household and children's needs and allowance for time and dedication to this work. My husband, the scientist Daniel E. Shelby, for recognizing the importance of sharing knowledge and allowing me the time to focus on this work. Where would we be as a profession if we didn't share what we have learned? Readers, I hope you find this helpful in your daily endeavors and use the information shared by our contributors to improve your anesthetic practices and the lives of pets.

Amanda M. Shelby

About the companion website

This book is accompanied by a companion website:

www.wiley.com/go/shelby/anesthesia2

The website includes:

* Videos
* Figures from the book as downloadable PPTs
* Supplementary material as downloadable PDFs
* Appendices from the book as downloadable PDFs

Section I: General topics in anesthesia and analgesia

Chapter 1

Anesthetic process

Yishai Kushnir and Carolyn M. McKune

Anesthesia is the technical process of causing a temporary loss of consciousness, most commonly in order to facilitate a medical or surgical procedure. Anesthesia aims to achieve loss of consciousness, inhibition of reflexes, muscle relaxation, amnesia, and analgesia. However, it also depresses homeostatic processes, which leads to morbidity and mortality. The role of the anesthetist is to maintain adequate anesthetic depth, in order to perform the intended procedure, while supporting normal physiologic function. However, there is now universal acceptance that "'anesthesia' is not limited to the period when the patient is unconscious but is a continuum of care that begins before the patient leaves home and ends when the patient is returned home with appropriate physiologic function and absent or minimal pain levels" [1]. This more holistic approach to anesthetic care begins with understanding the anesthetic process and the role of the anesthetist in achieving these goals.

I. Preanesthetic workup

"By failing to prepare, you are preparing to fail"

(Benjamin Franklin)

Evaluating, stabilizing and preparing the patient for anesthesia is a vital first step to provide safe anesthesia. This includes a thorough patient workup, with a focus on the patient's history, physical examination, and necessary diagnostic tests, as well as assessing and treating abnormal findings. This is also a suitable time to determine whether sedation alone may be sufficient to meet the needs of the patient. Procedures of a short duration (30–60 min), that are minimally invasive and/or patients with compromised health may benefit from sedation as opposed to general anesthesia. However, it is advisable for the anesthetist to be prepared to convert from sedation to general anesthesia if necessary. It is equally as important in sedated patients that they are monitored and supported (e.g., supplemental oxygenation, fluid therapy, etc.) as well as they would be if general anesthesia were elected.

　　The veterinary profession as a whole is now recognizing the importance of asking critical questions about whether or not the veterinary team is in a position to safely anesthetize the

Small Animal Anesthesia Techniques, Second Edition. Edited by Amanda M. Shelby and Carolyn M. McKune.
© 2023 John Wiley & Sons, Inc. Published 2023 by John Wiley & Sons, Inc.
Companion website: www.wiley.com/go/shelby/anesthesia2

patient. For example, the time of day for the procedure or experience level of the staff may alter the safety of the anesthesia. Please see Chapter 3 for more information.

A. Patient workup

1. History

As for any veterinary procedure, a thorough history is taken prior to anesthesia. This consists of identifying the chief complaint and obtaining the signalment, current and chronic medical history, allergies or known sensitivities, and drugs and supplements administered. Information obtained from the history will influence the choice of analgesics, fluid therapy, anesthetic drugs, support, and the monitoring parameters.

Breed-specific sensitivity to anesthesia is rarely reported. Greyhounds demonstrate prolonged and exaggerated responses to several anesthetic drugs, such as barbiturates [2, 3]. However, for most other breeds, sensitivities are associated with comorbidities common for the breed. These may include upper respiratory (brachycephalic or toy breeds), cardiac (Cavalier King Charles spaniels, Dobermans, Maine Coon), coagulopathies (Doberman), A1B1 mutation (Collies), for example. Physiologic function varies from normal in neonatal and geriatric patients, and is further disrupted by anesthesia, and extreme age has been associated with increased perianesthetic morbidity [4, 5]. This is explored further as its own topic (see Chapter 5).

Sex differences in response to pain and analgesia have been demonstrated in humans and laboratory animals [6]. Although the importance of these findings in companion animals has not been studied, sex and neutering status may also affect the perianesthetic period.

A thorough history of drugs and supplements (including nutraceuticals) administered to the patient must be taken, so the anesthetist may advise on drugs to be avoided or included perianesthetically. Drugs for administration prior to anesthesia include medications such as pimobendan, furosemide, maropitant, thyroid supplementation, steroids, and gabapentin. Patients requiring sedation should definitely receive it prior to presentation. Conversely, other medications, such as antihypertensive medication, aspirin or other anticoagulants, and drugs that increase the risk of serotonin syndrome (trazadone or selegiline), may be withheld, at the practitioner's discretion.

A preanesthetic history also includes questions regarding previous anesthesia episodes. Problems observed in previous anesthesia may be avoided or reduced in impact by changing the anesthetic protocol or increasing awareness of complications.

Fasting suggestions have gradually changed over time. The American Animal Hospital Association has created guidelines for appropriate fasting depending on the particular patient. Recommended fasting periods in cats and dogs vary from 4–6 to 6–12 hours prior to elective anesthesia. Fundamentally, most of the concern regarding appropriate fasting is due to the potential for reflux or regurgitation, which may lead to esophagitis, esophageal stricture or aspiration pneumonia. It is advised that whatever fasting standards a practitioner uses are predictable and consistent, so it is easy for staff to ensure that these guidelines are followed. One guideline most anesthesiologists agree on is that shorter fasting times, up to 2 hours, are recommended for cats and dogs under 8 weeks old or weighing less than 2 kg (see Chapter 5 for anesthetic management of neonates, p.185). Drinking water should be available until premedication [1]. Fasting in diabetic animals should be tailored specifically to the patient, the type and duration of procedure, and clinic practices (such as the time of day, with most anesthesiologists advising taking diabetic patients for anesthesia early in the day, so they may recover by the time of their evening meal). AAHA guidelines suggest one option: a soft food/ paté type meal 2–4 hours prior to the procedure, administering half of the dose of insulin and trying to schedule the case for the first thing in the morning [1]. Anesthesia of diabetic patients is further discussed in Chapter 5.

2. Physical examination

A complete physical exam is performed by the primary clinician, prior to anesthesia. The anesthetist must perform a physical exam emphasizing, but not limited to, the aspects of the exam that are important for anesthesia.

The exam begins with general observation. The patient's level of consciousness and temperament are assessed, as these will influence choice of premedication. Abnormal gait, posture, abdominal distention, and skin conditions that may indicate systemic or regional disease may require evaluation prior to anesthesia. The rate and pattern of breathing are assessed to recognize respiratory pathologies. The anesthetist is also aware of behavioral signs of pain as these may influence perioperative pain management.

Obtaining a baseline pain assessment in an animal prior to an anesthetic procedure will help guide the anesthetic plan as well as familiarize the anesthetist with the patient's demeanor, which plays a major role postoperatively in evaluating the results of therapeutic interventions for pain management.

Pain is defined as "an unpleasant sensory and emotional experience associated with, or resembling that associated with, actual or potential tissue damage" [7]. Thus, a complex variety of experiences can result in pain, and the first step to successful treatment is to effectively assess the animal. Several tools may aid the anesthetist in assessing pain; see Appendix A. Different pain assessment tools are used for acute or chronic pain and vary in their complexity of use and flexibility. Simpler pain scales are often less flexible and may not fit your patient's specific behavior. A list of tools available online for acute pain evaluation is provided in the companion website provided with this book, and pain assessment is further discussed in the appendices.

Parameters monitored during anesthesia are evaluated prior to premedication to provide baseline measurements, for the same reason pain scores are assigned prior to premedication. These anesthesia parameters include eye position and palpebral reflexes; an oral examination to rule out loose teeth or masses which may impede intubation; mucous membranes and capillary refill time; palpation of the neck for abnormalities, and to assess tracheal size; skin tenting; chest auscultation; abdominal palpation; palpation of peripheral pulses for pulse rate, rhythm, and strength; body temperature; body weight and body condition score (BCS). Abnormal findings in the evaluation stage are addressed and treated prior to anesthesia, to the best of our ability. Findings that may indicate a disease process such as a heart murmur, azotemia, or elevated liver enzymes are investigated in order to determine the nature and severity of the disease. Dehydration and hypovolemia should be corrected with adequate fluid therapy. Further diagnosis and treatment may lead to postponing elective procedures, based on the perceived increased risk for the patient, the procedure and other case-specific factors. For emergency cases, the time necessary for further investigation and therapy with its associated potential benefit is weighed against the harm caused by postponing the procedure.

3. Diagnostics

The minimal blood tests required prior to elective anesthesia include a packed cell volume (PCV), total solids (TS), blood glucose and renal status (i.e., Azo-Stick®, creatinine, or SDMA) taken within 24 hours. Prior to major operations, in patients with ASA ≥III, patients with previous blood work abnormalities, and geriatric patients, a complete blood count (CBC) and chemistry with electrolytes are performed within a relevant time period (approximately 2–4 weeks is usually acceptable if no change occurred in the patient's condition). Further diagnostic tests, e.g., coagulation tests or blood gases, are performed if necessary, based on the patient or the planned procedure. Animals with low albumin (<2 g/dL), acute anemia (PCV <20%) or hyperkalemia (K+ >6.0 mEq/L) that impair physiologic function are corrected prior to anesthesia induction; see Chapter 3. Reference ranges for blood tests and blood gases are available on the companion website provided with this book.

II. Factors involved in creating an anesthetic plan

When creating an anesthesia plan, the anesthetist anticipates the *potential* problems associated with the event of general anesthesia. These may stem from the patient's species, the specific patient itself, the use of inhalant, and the planned procedure; see Table 1.2. Predicting these problems guides the anesthetist in choosing anesthetic drugs and monitoring devices, and preparing for potential complications. This is also a good time to communicate with the patient's owners about the animal's level of anesthetic risk and additional necessary steps (including working up or treating a newly identified disease process) to improve the safety of anesthesia for the patient.

The protocol itself includes emergency drug calculations, premedication, induction and maintenance drugs, monitoring, medication and techniques for support (fluid therapy, antinausea medication, warming, etc.), and perioperative pain management. It is generally advantageous for anesthesia drugs to be given intravenously when possible, as this assures optimal bioavailability of the drug.

All the elements for anesthesia are prepared prior to induction, when possible. This includes an anesthetic record sheet (and if this record is electronic, a hard copy of this sheet in case the computer system fails) to record all events during anesthesia. Various designs of anesthesia records are available, and they may be electronic or recorded on paper; see this chapter's online supplementary material for hyperlinks to anesthesia record templates, and Table 1.1 for hard text. The anesthesia machine and equipment should undergo a routine check prior to use (see Chapter 2), in order to detect malfunctions. Using a documented standard operating procedure, or a shortened anesthesia machine checklist with only the necessary points, ensures that all the necessary elements are checked. An example of an anesthesia machine checklist is available in the companion website provided with this book. Missing or malfunctioning elements are repaired or replaced; inability to resolve equipment issues may result in cancelation of the procedure.

Table 1.1   Resources for anesthesia record templates.

Anesthesia record provider	Website
American Animal Hospital Association (fee payable)	https://ams.aaha.org/eweb/DynamicPage.aspx?site=store&Action=Add&ObjectKeyFrom=1A83491A-9853-4C87-86A4-F7D95601C2E2&WebCode=ProdDetailAdd&DoNotSave=yes&ParentObject=CentralizedOrderEntry&ParentDataObject=Invoice%20Detail&ivd_formkey=69202792-63d7-4ba2-bf4e-a0da41270555&ivd_cst_key=&ivd_cst_ship_key=&ivd_prc_prd_key=0f20d049-90cc-44af-87dc-39a77417c7c9
Association of Veterinary Anaesthetists (High ASA score)	https://ava.eu.com/wp-content/uploads/2015/11/AVA-ASA-Hi-Electronic.pdf
Association of Veterinary Anaesthetists (Low ASA score)	https://ava.eu.com/wp-content/uploads/2017/10/AVA-ASA-Low-Electronic-UK.pdf
Jurox	http://thinkanesthesia.education/sites/default/files/2019-05/US%20-%20Multidose-MonitoringChart%20V2.05%20-%20WEB_0.pdf

A. Patient species problem list

Different species have different anesthetic risks (Table 1.2). For example, cats are more sensitive to errors in fluid therapy, tracheal trauma, and laryngospasm [8]. Rabbits are difficult to intubate and gain intravenous access to, and are prone to laryngospasm and gastrointestinal complications. Understandably, rabbits are also at high risk of anesthetic death compared to dogs and cats [9].

B. Specific patient problem list

Signalment, chronic and acute conditions, abnormal diagnostic findings, and concurrent medications influence the response to anesthesia, and anesthesia may adversely affect underlying conditions.

C. Inhaled anesthesia and drug-induced problem list

Inhalants will result in hypotension, hypothermia, and hypoventilation for every patient anesthetized; bradycardia in most species is often secondary to the essential administration of opioids.

D. Procedure-driven problem list

Breaking down the procedure into its basic steps will help to assess the adverse events associated with the procedure itself, positioning, or ancillary procedures, and allow adequate preparation.

Table 1.2   Theoretical anesthesia problem list examples.

Problem list group	Example 1: A geriatric cat for a dental prophylaxis	Example 2: A 6-month-old bulldog for an ovariohysterectomy
Species	Hyperthyroidism, cardiac disease, renal failure, laryngospasm, tracheal tear from intubation, fluid sensitivity, relative increase in mortality secondary to anesthesia as compared to canine patients	Brachycephalic airway concerns (hypoplastic trachea, elongated soft palate, prolong extubation, pre-oxygenate, regurtitation)
Specific patient	Geriatric	Brachycephalic airway syndrome (stenotic nares, elongated soft palate, everted laryngeal saccules, hypoplastic trachea), high resting vagal tone (author's experience), prolonged recovery
Inhaled anesthesia and drug induced	Hypotension, hypoventilation, hypothermia, bradycardia	Hypotension, hypoventilation, hypothermia, bradycardia
Procedure	Prolonged if extensive dental disease is present, patient will cool rapidly, aspiration of exogenous fluids used to lavage mouth, may require airway packing, pain/noxious stimuli if dental extractions. Gag associated post anesthetic blindness	Noxious stimuli/pain, hemorrhage fluid and heat loss
Total problems anesthetist prepares for	17	9

Protocols for invasive procedures are always multimodal in nature; that is, there should be a diverse range of methods for addressing pain and noxious stimuli (see Chapter 3 for additional information on differentiation of the two). Adequate pain prevention and management is not only ethically important for animals in both the short and long term, but will also facilitate a decrease in drugs required to maintain the patient under anesthesia, and therefore reduce negative side-effects associated with these drugs (such as hypotension and hypoventilation) or the negative side-effects associated with noxious stimuli under anesthesia (such as the patient becoming abruptly light, hypertensive, and tachypnea). The drug formulary (Section II) provides a dedicated review of a multimodal analgesic plan.

E. Anesthetic morbidity and mortality

The anesthetist incorporates information from the comprehensive anesthesia problem list to assess the patient's anesthetic risk. The American Society of Anesthesiologists (ASA) physical status is a risk score based on the patient's perceived health (Table 1.3). This methodology allows anesthetic risk to be stratified, with patients in ASA 1–2 being considered at less anesthetic risk than patients who are assigned an ASA 3–5. Higher ASA scores are

Table 1.3   American Society of Anesthesiologists (ASA) Physical Status Classification.

ASA physical status	Description
1	A normal healthy patient
2	A patient with mild systemic disease which is not a threat to life
3	A patient with severe systemic disease which is not a threat to life
4	A patient with severe systemic disease that is a constant threat to life
5	A moribund patient who is not expected to survive without the operation
E (added to score)	Emergency surgery: defined as existing when delay in treatment of the patient would lead to a significant increase in the threat to life or body part

associated with longer intensive care hospitalization and increased risk for hypothermia, acute kidney injury (AKI), and mortality [10, 11]. Indeed, stabilization to reduce the assigned ASA category in ASA 3–5 patients demonstrated a reduction in anesthetic-related morbidity and mortality [12]. Please see Anesthetic morbidity and mortality in Chapter 3 for more information.

One of the most remarkable differences between human and domestic animal anesthesia is the perianesthetic mortality rate, with human anesthesia being up to 100-fold less risky than that of our veterinary patients [13]. When evaluating a morbidity and mortality study, it is imperative to ensure that the study has significant case enrollment, as subtle details are often difficult to discern, even when several thousand patients are enrolled. To date, the largest study involved almost 98 000 dogs and approximately 78 000 cats [4, 8, 9, 14, 15]. This study, performed by Brodbelt and colleagues, is arguably the largest study performed in veterinary medicine and strongly powered. The overall risk of mortality under anesthesia is 0.17% in canine patients and when stratified for ASA 1–2 (healthy) canines is about 0.05%. For those who prefer these numbers in a user-friendly fashion, 1 in 2000 dogs (classified as healthy) have an anesthetic-related mortality. In cats, overall sedation- and general anesthetic-related mortality is 0.24%; again, when one includes only healthy ASA 1–2 cats, the mortality rate is 0.11%, which translates into 1 in 900 "healthy" cats dying as a result of anesthesia. Mortality in other pet species including rabbits (1.4–4.8%) [16], guinea pigs (3.8%) and avian species (up to 16%) [17] is even higher [9].

Mortality rates are decreasing over the years in healthy patients, and newer studies demonstrate lower rates. This may be due to advances in knowledge, training, equipment safety, and monitoring [9,18,19]. In a recent study investigating healthy animals undergoing anesthesia for neutering, fewer than 1/10 000 dogs and 1/2000 cats died [18].

New work on the horizon by Redondo and colleagues is not as reassuring. Initial abstracts released at the World Congress of Veterinary Anesthesia in 2018 incorporated data from multiple countries all over the world, enrolling just over 10 000 dogs. Overall mortality rate in the canine was a shocking 0.76%, with the bulk of mortality occurring in patients with an ASA score of 3 or greater (ASA 1 0.18%, ASA 2 0.30%, ASA 3 1.11%, ASA 4–5 13.05%) [20]. Likewise, Redondo presented data on feline mortality rate of 0.74%, again with the bulk of mortality in patients with an ASA score of 3 or greater (ASA 1 0.14%, ASA 2 0.00%, ASA 3 3.32%, ASA 4–5 7.05%) [21]. In summary, things have improved for young and healthy animals consistently over the years, but clearly, veterinary medicine has a significant way to go to rival our human colleagues for all animals.

Increasing ASA status is associated with risk of death in every species examined. In dogs, cats, and rabbits, an ASA score ≥3 is associated with a 3.3-fold, 4.8-fold, and 11.3-fold increase in risk of death compared to ASA score <3 [10]. Mortality is higher in emergency procedures and in procedures performed after hours [4, 10]. Mortality is also affected by procedure type, and may be as high as 5–7% for thoracic or cervical spinal surgery [22, 23].

Death is not the only possible negative outcome; many other complications that occur perioperatively may lead to increased morbidity, prolonged hospitalization, and suffering. These include hypothermia, nausea, pain, hypotension, AKI, pneumonia, and others. A common misconception is that the improved morbidity and mortality rates in human anesthesia reflect a greater infusion of financial dollars into the personnel, drugs, and equipment used for human anesthesia. However, evidence-based literature reinforces that simple things, such as the use of checklists, documenting that these checklists were performed, and performing surgeries within normal hours of operation (when possible) [24], will reduce anesthetic mortality [9, 25]. Morbidity and mortality may also be decreased by continuous monitoring of heart rate and oxygen saturation (SpO_2), and by the presence of a dedicated veterinary technician during anesthesia [8, 19]. These are simple strategies that every veterinarian can use.

F. Anesthesia checklist

Modern anesthesia is a complex process, involving numerous drugs, equipment, and personnel. Errors may arise from any of these parts or their interactions. Using a checklist is a simple way for the anesthetist to assure that all parts in this complex endeavor are in place. A checklist is a tool that aids the anesthetist to simplify work in a complex environment and improves patient safety. Using a checklist leads to a 60% or higher decrease in peri- and postoperative complications, and wound infections [25, 26].

The checklist is simple to use and minimally time consuming but must incorporate the potential failure points (Figure 1.1); this differentiates the checklist from its close relative, the standard operating procedure (SOP). An SOP is intended to be thorough so no detail is overlooked, whereas a checklist is meant to be quick and cover only the commonly overlooked points. An excellent baseline for an initial checklist is the World Health Organization's Surgical Safety Checklist (www.who.int/patientsafety/safesurgery/checklist/en/). This checklist is then modified and tailored, after use, to each hospital's specific needs.

A separate checklist, or SOP if preferred, can be designed for preanesthetic testing of anesthesia equipment and monitors, which should be turned on, evaluated and determined to be functional prior to induction. Please see Chapter 2 on essential equipment and necessary safety checks, as well as the critical role trained staff play in anesthesia safety. Other useful visual aids in the clinic are a table of emergency drug doses and volumes (see Appendix B) and a table of constant rate infusion doses and rates. Please refer to the companion website for printable tables with this information.

Surgical safety checklist

Sign in (before induction of anesthesia)

- ☐ Confirm identity of the animal and presence of the correct medical file
- ☐ Confirm procedure, brief plan and surgery site Confirm that required pre-operative imaging has been performed and is available in the OR
- ☐ Check completeness of anesthesia machine, monitoring equipment, and drugs
- ☐ Any special anesthetic concerns yes/no
- ☐ Preoperative blood work has been viewed and abnormalities have been addressed
- ☐ Preoperative analgesia, antimicrobial
- ☐ Risk of bleeding yes/no blood or blood donor available yes/no
- ☐ Confirm that required equipment in the surgery room is working (suction, cautery, battery for drill) Confirm that if required diagnostic imaging is set up in the surgery suite
- ☐ Confirm that informed owner consent to the procedure, post-op therapy and cost has been received

Time out (before surgery is initiated)

- ☐ All team members, name and role
- ☐ Confirm procedure and place and side (R/L, fore/rear) of incision, name all the procedures to be performed under this anesthesia
- ☐ The surgeon: Critical part of the procedure and estimated time
- ☐ Confirm sterility of the equipment and sterile scrub in the correct location
- ☐ Confirm that all required instruments are available
- ☐ OR tech state any equipment concerns / missing equipment in sets
- ☐ Confirm appropriate anesthetic depth, and state if there are any anesthetic concerns

Sign out (before recovery, at the end of the surgical procedure)

- ☐ Is the correct procedure performed and are all planned events performed
- ☐ Are all samples labelled and has one responsible person for submission
- ☐ Any issues regarding the anesthesia/monitoring or surgical instruments
- ☐ Any abnormalities that should be addressed for the recovery.
- ☐ Read out blood gas prior to moving to recovery.
- ☐ State the recovery sedation and analgesia plan.
- ☐ Confirm that the recovery room is prepared.
- ☐ Confirm that bladder has been voided, that bandages are placed where necessary, and that unnecessary catheters / tubes/ tourniquets have been removed.

Figure 1.1   Surgical safety checklist example.

III. Patient preparation

Common-sense preparation begins at home, with appropriate fasting for the patient prior to anesthesia, as well as ensuring any necessary drugs such as pimobendan or thyroxine (drugs which do not have an injectable equivalent) are administered; please see the section entitled

"History" in this chapter for more details (p.4). Other important drugs may include anxiolytic drugs, such as trazadone and gabapentin, which help with reduced stress for the patient and easier handling for the staff. The administration (or withholding) of these drugs is shared with the anesthetist, and can be conveyed either verbally by the owner or via completion of a patient dropoff form with short, pertinent questions such as this. At the time of dropoff, an accurate weight is obtained on the day of surgical procedure, and drug dosages are based on the animal's lean body weight [1].

IV. Premedication

The aims of premedication are to decrease stress, provide preemptive analgesia, decrease the dose of anesthetic drugs, and improve the quality of anesthesia and recovery. Traditionally, premedication drugs are administered by the hospital staff in close proximity to anesthesia. However, at least some of these drugs may be administered orally at home by the owner before arrival to the hospital. Premedication is usually administered intramuscularly (IM) or intravenously (IV) if a catheter is present. The epaxial muscles near the lumbar spine are commonly used for IM injection but other extensor muscles (such as the quadriceps, the dorsal muscles of the neck or supraspinatus muscle above the shoulder) are alternative sites. A list of drugs commonly used for premedication is provided in Table 1.4 and further discussed in the drug formulary (Section II). When selecting premedications, one must take into account the goals for both the patient (such as additional analgesia) and the veterinary staff (such as reversibility or desired level of patient hand ability).

During the premedication phase, an IV catheter is placed (if not already in place), ideally after peak sedation is achieved. The IV catheter is located where it will be easily accessible during the procedure. For example, for procedures involving the head, the catheter is ideally placed in a hindlimb and for abdominal procedures, in the forelimb. Other patient monitoring and support is initiated during this phase as well. In order to decrease hypoxemia and desaturation during induction and intubation, the patient is preoxygenated (Figure 1.2) for 3–5 minutes with a mask connected to a source of 100% oxygen prior to induction [27]. Thermal support is often warranted in the premedicated patient, as many drugs used for premedication also result in central thermal dysregulation.

To achieve the most benefit out of a premedication, certain nonpharmacologic options are considered. This includes things like separate areas for dogs and cats post premedication, the use of a quiet, dark room with minimal stimulation for patients receiving dexmedetomidine, and pheromones in holding areas. These interventions often reduce patient stress, allowing for a greater premedication effect.

V. Induction

During induction, the patient transitions from a state of consciousness to unconsciousness. General anesthesia is composed of several stages that appear in sequence (Tables 1.5 and 1.6). During the initial stages, the patient may exhibit increased motion, muscle rigidity, and

Table 1.4 Commonly used premedication drugs in cats and dogs; see the drug formulary for details of dosage, route, and effects.

Drug	Benefits	Disadvantages
Acepromazine	Antiemetic Antihistamine High margin of safety	Vasodilation Hypotension No reversal Not antianxiety [30]
Alfaxalone	Useful for fractious animals Minimal cardiovascular effects Off-label use: IM administration	Large volume Shivering/twitching and muscle rigidity on recovery
Buprenorphine	Minimal cardiovascular effects Analgesia Reversible Available in a variety of concentrations for varying durations of effect	Mild reduction in inhalant requirements in dogs (minimal in cats) Outcompetes other opioids for the same receptor
Butorphanol	Minimal cardiovascular effects Analgesia Reversible	Antagonizes mu agonist opioids Short-acting in canines
Dexmedetomidine	Reversible Synergistic with opioids Can be used as an oral gel at home 1 h prior to visit as an anxiolytic	Decreased cardiac output due to bradycardia Emesis
Diazepam	Muscle relaxation Minimal cardiopulmonary effects Reversible	Unreliable in healthy patients as it may cause excitement Although labeled for IM, this is discouraged
Gabapentin	Analgesia Can be given orally at home as an anxiolytic 1–2 h prior to visit Often used in combination with melatonin and trazadone for patients who are difficult to handle due to fear or anxiety	Too much drug can result in profound sedation and obtundation, with hypothermia and possible state of shock Not reversible
Hydromorphone	Minimal cardiovascular effects Analgesia Reversible	High incidence (almost 40%) of postoperative hyperthermia in cats May cause vomiting
Ketamine	Useful for fractious animals Increases sympathetic tone	Muscle rigidity Pain on injection Dysphoric recoveries especially in cats
Melatonin	Promotes sleep Can be given orally at home as an anxiolytic 1–2 h prior to visit Often used in combination with gabapentin and trazadone for patients who are difficult to handle due to fear or anxiety	May not provide appreciable sedation when used alone

(Continued)

Table 1.4   (*Continued*)

Drug	Benefits	Disadvantages
Meperidine	No vomiting Minimal cardiovascular effects Analgesia Reversible	Unreliable in cats Short-acting Histamine release
Methadone	No vomiting Minimal cardiovascular effects Analgesia Reversible	Bradycardia
Midazolam	Muscle relaxation Minimal cardiopulmonary effects Reversible	Unreliable in healthy patients as it may cause excitement
Morphine	Minimal cardiovascular effects Analgesia Reversible	Vomiting Histamine release
Trazadone	Used to promote sleep in people, and for cage rest in animals Can be given orally at home as an anxiolytic 1–2 h prior to visit Often used in combination with gabapentin and melatonin for patients who are difficult to handle due to fear or anxiety	No analgesia Not reversible

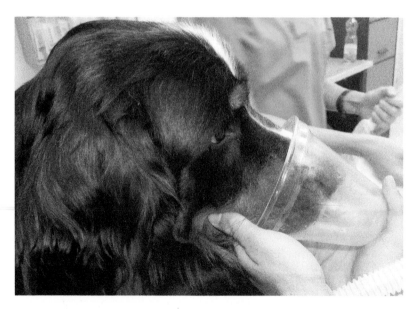

Figure 1.2   Preoxygenation (canine).

Table 1.5   Guedel's stages of anesthesia.

Stage	Name	Description
I	Analgesia or disorientation	Amnesia and decreased sensitivity to pain, still conscious
II	Excitement or delirium	Loss of consciousness, irregular breathing, may struggle or vomit
III	Surgical anesthesia[a]	Loss of motion, decreased response to stimulus and reflex activity
IV	Medullary paralysis or coma	Respiratory arrest, vasomotor collapse, lack of reflexes

[a]Divided into planes (see Table 1.6).

Table 1.6   Planes within stage III of anesthesia (surgical anesthesia).

Plane	Name	Eye position	Palpebral reflex	Jaw muscle tone	Cough and swallow
I	Light	Central to rotated	Present	Strong	May be present
II	Moderate	Rotated ventromedial	Relaxed to absent	Relaxed	Absent
III	Deep	Rotated to central	Reduced to absent	Relaxed	Absent
IV	Very deep	Central	Absent	Flaccid	Absent

delirium. Modern anesthetics induce rapid anesthesia that shortens these stages and decreases excitement.

Preoxygenation is standard of care. Effectively preoxygenating a patient for 3–5 minutes prior to induction allows the anesthetist 3–5 minutes of increased oxygen in the blood (PaO_2) [27], which is critical for patients with any type of respiratory compromise, including but not limited to brachycephalic airway syndrome, pregnancy, lower airway disease or thoracic trauma. In the case of pregnant animals, the fetus as well as the mother benefits from this increased oxygenation. The authors emphasize *effective* oxygen delivery; oxygen delivered by a well-fitting mask provides more effective oxygenation than attempting flow-by oxygen delivery via the end of the anesthetic circuit (i.e., circle or nonrebreathing hose), which does not provide a high concentration of oxygen. Sedating a patient either during the premedication phase or with an initial quarter dose of induction drug increases an animal's tolerance to an oxygen facemask.

Induction is typically achieved with injectable drugs administered IV (Table 1.7). The drug formulary reviews induction drugs in greater depth. Although anesthesia may be induced with an inhalant, this is a longer process (during which the patient has an unsecure airway), often involves a state of excitement and disinhibition, and is associated with a six-fold increase in mortality [4]. Furthermore, inhalant inductions increase the exposure of staff to inhalant anesthetics that are considered a work hazard by the United States Department of Labor, which has strict regulations on work practices surrounding waste anesthetic gases. An IM induction with

Table 1.7   Commonly used induction drugs in cats and dogs; see the drug formulary for details such as route and dosage.

Drug	Advantages	Disadvantages
Alfaxalone	Minimal cardiovascular depression, smooth induction, can be given IM (off-label)	Apnea and oxygen desaturation; preoxygenate, myoclonus and poor recoveries for short procedures
Etomidate	Minimal cardiovascular and respiratory depression	If not well premedicated may display vomiting, salivation, and strong laryngeal tone; adrenocortical suppression
Fentanyl + midazolam/diazepam	Minimal cardiovascular effects, large therapeutic index	May cause dysphoria in healthy patients. Not a reliable induction technique in cats
Ketamine	Short-acting, minimal respiratory depression, increases HR and BP, antihyperalgesia, analgesic properties, high therapeutic index, can be given IM	Muscle rigidity when used alone (tip: administer with benzodiazepine or an alpha-2-agonist), does not depress cough and swallow reflex, poor recoveries in cats
Propofol	Fast onset, short-acting, excellent recoveries, smooth induction	Apnea, oxygen desaturation (tip: preoxygenate), vasodilation, relatively narrow therapeutic index
Thiopental[a]	Decreases intracranial and intraocular pressure, minimal effect on laryngeal motion, smooth induction	May cause sloughing if injected subcutaneously, vasodilation and arrhythmias, respiratory depression
Tiletamine/zolazepam (Zoletil®, Virbac; Telazol®, Zoetis)	Fast onset, increases HR and BP, antihyperalgesia, longer lasting than ketamine, small volume, can be given IM, effective immobilization in fractious patients	Burns on injection when administered IM, poor recoveries, seizures at high doses, requires reconstitution, has limited shelf-life after reconstitution
Isoflurane	No IV access required, minimal contact with fractious animals with chamber induction	Dose-dependent cardiovascular and respiratory depression, prolonged excitement phase, may irritate respiratory tract, increases environmental and personnel exposure, increases risk of morbidity and mortality for patients when used alone (i.e., without premedicating)
Sevoflurane	No IV access required, minimal contact with fractious animals with chamber induction, faster and less irritation than isoflurane	Dose-dependent cardiovascular and respiratory depression, prolonged excitement phase, increases environmental and personnel exposure, expensive, increases morbidity and mortality for patients when used alone (i.e., without premedication)

[a]Currently unavailable in USA.
BP, blood pressure; HR, heart rate; IM, intramuscular; IV, intravenous.

combinations that include ketamine or alfaxalone, in addition to opioids and sedatives, is a useful tool in small patients undergoing a short procedure (such as a cat neuter) or in aggressive or fearful animals. As with an inhalant induction, there is no secure airway using this methodology, although a well-fitting facemask can provide oxygen supplementation once the patient is induced. Careful monitoring and observation are necessary for any patient who is induced without a secure airway.

The total induction dose is calculated based on the patient's clinical state, ideal body weight, and response to premedication administered. Geriatric, neonatal, deeply sedated, and sick patients require lower induction doses. Induction agents are titrated to effect, with one-quarter to one-third of the calculated dose administered every 30–60 seconds until patient depth is sufficient for intubation.

The transition from wakefulness to an anesthetized state is not without risk. Of deaths occurring within 48 hours of anesthesia, 1% occur during induction; this number is quite high considering induction lasts less than 0.2% of this period [9].

A. Intubation

Placing an endotracheal tube (ETT) or supraglottic device such as the v-gel® enables administration of oxygen, inhalant anesthetics, emergency and aerosolized drugs, and positive pressure ventilation, and protects the lungs and airways from aspiration.

The largest ETT which comfortably fits the patient's trachea is used, to decrease resistance to respiration and therefore work of breathing. Palpating the trachea allows for an estimate of the ETT, which the anesthetist uses to select two or three tubes which might be suitable. Visualizing the space between the arytenoids after induction allows selection of the most appropriate of those tubes. Other described methods (based on weight, the distance between the nares, etc.) are less reliable. Compared to dogs of a similar size, brachycephalic dogs need smaller ETTs, and sight hounds and dachshunds need larger ETTs. A 3.5–4.5 mm internal diameter (ID) ETT tube fits most cats. The length required is measured externally from the tip of the nose to the thoracic inlet. Longer tubes are shortened (i.e., cut) to decrease airway resistance, dead space, and risk of endobronchial intubation. Ideally, the distal tip of the ETT sits just outside the thoracic inlet, and the connection to the Y-piece is within a couple of centimeters of the mouth. Measuring and cutting the ET tube prior to intubation will save stress for the anesthetist. The steps for endotracheal intubation are described in Table 1.8.

1. Difficult intubation

Patients with upper airway pathology (such as masticatory muscle disease, trauma, or anatomic abnormalities) may be difficult to intubate, due to an obstructed view or path to the larynx. For these cases, the anesthetist prepares the necessary equipment (Figure 1.7) and a plan of action in order to secure the airway (Figure 1.8). The patient should be preoxygenated (under sedation if necessary to tolerate the mask), and SpO_2 monitored. A retrograde intubation may prove useful in these cases; see Table 1.9 for steps and materials for a retrograde intubation. If at any stage there is a threat to the patient's life, a tracheostomy tube is placed, and the discontinuation of anesthesia is considered.

Table 1.8 Intubation.

Materials: Laryngoscope, 3 ETTs, lubricant, tie to secure ETT, 4 × 4 gauze square to hold the tongue, stylet and lidocaine (cats)

Techniques:

1. Induction agent is appropriately administered until jaw and tongue are lax.
2. The patient is placed in sternal recumbency, although large dogs can be placed in lateral recumbency. The assistant opens the mouth of the patient by placing one hand over the snout, holding behind the maxillary canine teeth and extending the tongue between the mandibular canine teeth with the other hand. Extension of the head and neck helps the anesthetist visualize the larynx (see Figures 1.3, 1.4).
3. The anesthetist places the laryngoscope blade on the base of the tongue under the epiglottis. Placing the tip of the blade on the epiglottis may damage this sensitive tissue, and may contribute to airway obstruction at extubation. Applying pressure on the base of the tongue will help displace the epiglottis and allow visualization and brief examination of the larynx (see Figure 1.5).
4. Lubricate the ETT at the distal end with lubricant. In cats, a drop of lidocaine is placed on each arytenoid to minimize laryngeal spasm. Wait 60 seconds for this to take effect.
5. Once the anesthetist visualizes the larynx, the ETT is advanced between the arytenoids.
   (a) In dogs, when resistance is encountered, a slight twist of the ETT helps facilitate advancement. In brachycephalic patients, an elongated soft palate often obstructs visualization of the arytenoids. The tip of the ETT is used to displace the soft palate.
   (b) For cats, position the end of the ETT over the arytenoids, *be patient*, and wait for the patient to take a breath. At inspiration, the arytenoids will open slightly. With a gentle, determined motion, insert the ETT between the arytenoids. Slight rotation may help facilitate intubation if resistance is encountered. However, feline laryngeal tissue is easily damaged and therefore, applying any force during intubation is highly discouraged.
6. Once the patient is intubated, the anesthetist visually confirms proper intubation and the ETT is tied over the muzzle or behind the ears.
7. The ETT is then attached to the breathing circuit with an appropriate flow rate of 100% oxygen. The ETT cuff is inflated to 20–25 cmH$_2$O, or by performing a leak test: while the anesthetist attempts to "hold" a 20–25 cmH$_2$O breath, the cuff is inflated until there is no leak. Higher pressures may lead to tracheal necrosis and rupture, especially in cats. A cuff inflation syringe (see Figure 1.6) helps with objectively knowing how much air was used to inflate the cuff.
8. Once the cuff is sealed, inhalant anesthetics are initiated.

VI. Anesthetic maintenance

Once intubation is complete, anesthetic monitoring equipment is appropriately placed (see Chapter 2), eyes are lubricated, and the patient is supported with intermittent manual ventilation. A common misconception in veterinary anesthesia is that the patient is allowed to initiate breathing on their own after induction, and so it is best not to breathe for the patient. This scenario often leads to a patient getting acutely light, in that the inhalant is not being effectively taken up (due to the hypoventilation brought on by the injectable induction agent), and yet the effects of the injectable agent are fading as the drug is redistributed or metabolized. Thus, it is the recommendation of the authors to supplement ventilation immediately post induction, until the patient begins ventilating on their own. Oxygen support is provided to the patient at all times, regardless of maintenance anesthesia choice.

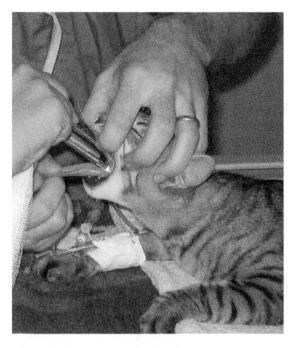

Figure 1.3   Sternal positioning for intubation (feline).

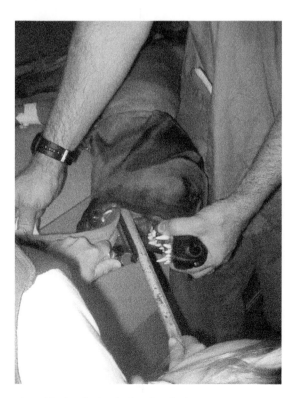

Figure 1.4   Lateral positioning for intubation (canine).

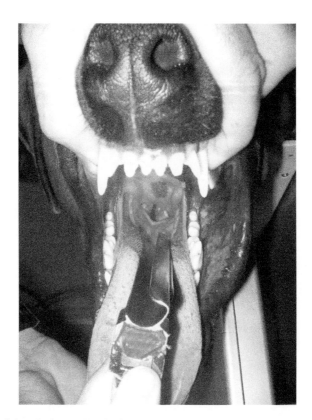

Figure 1.5   Visualizing the larynx (canine).

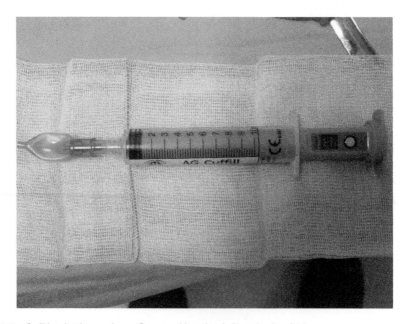

Figure 1.6   Cuff intubation syringe. *Source:* Hospitech Respiration Ltd.

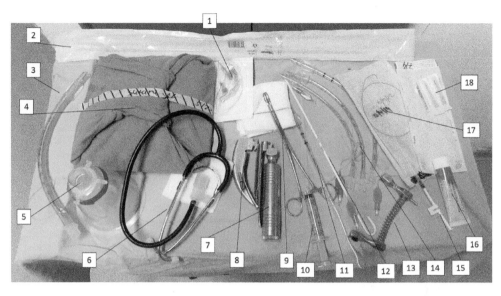

Figure 1.7 Difficult intubation tray. When difficult intubation is anticipated, the necessary equipment is arranged in advance. These are some items which may aid in this situation. 1. Tracheostomy tube of appropriate size, 2. Insemination tubes (potential guide for endotracheal [ET] tubes), 3. Large ET tube to block esophagus, 4. Surgical set for tracheostomy placement, 5. Facemask for preoxygenation, 6. Stethoscope connected to an airway adaptor, 7. Laryngoscope with a straight (Miller) blade, 8. Alternative curved blade (MacIntosh), 9. Gauze forceps and gauze pads to swab secretions, 10. Cuff inflation syringe, 11. ET tube of appropriate size with a stylet in place, 12. Stylet for ET tube, 13. Spring-loaded mouth gag, 14. ET tubes of various smaller sizes, 15. Local anesthetic connected to a tom cat catheter for local anesthesia atomization on the larynx, 16. Local anesthesia gel for cuff lubrication, 17. Guidewire for retrograde intubation, 18. 18 G needles for transcutaneous retrograde intubation or emergency oxygen insufflation.

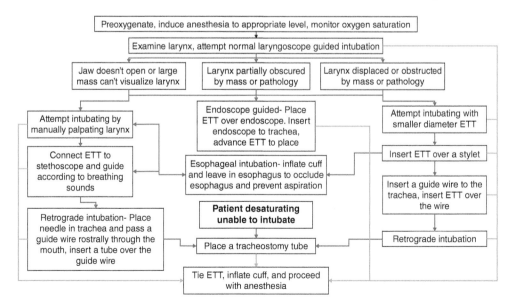

Figure 1.8 Difficult intubation algorithm.

Table 1.9 Retrograde intubation.

Materials: Laryngoscope, 3 ETTs, lubricant, tie to secure ETT, 4 × 4 gauze square to hold the tongue, guidewire tested to fit through an 18 G needle, 18 G needle and local anesthetic

Techniques:

1. Induction agent is appropriately administered until jaw and tongue are lax.
2. The patient is placed in sternal or dorsal recumbency, after the skin over the trachea is clipped and aseptically prepped from the caudal edge of the mandible to thoracic inlet. The assistant elevates the head and is prepared to hold the mouth as if for intubation (see Table 1.8).
3. The trachea is palpated and at the midpoint, an 18 G needle is rostrally passed through the trachealis muscle, between the hyaline cartilage rings.
4. A guidewire is passed through the needle, and rostrally, while the assistant holds the mouth appropriately for intubation. The guidewire should be visualized as it passes between the arytenoids and exits the mouth. Enough guidewire should be present to accommodate the whole length of the tube, and an additional 3–4 cm for the anesthetist to grasp. The guidewire must fully exit the tube or it will not be possible to pass the tube effectively.
5. Lubricate the ETT at the distal end with lubricant. In cats, a drop of lidocaine is placed on each arytenoid if possible to minimize laryngeal spasm.
6. The tube is fed over the guidewire and blindly but gently between the arytenoids. Several small sizes of tubes should be available as it may not be possible to fit an appropriate sized ETT past the obstruction.
7. Once the anesthetist has felt the tube pass between the arytenoids, the guidewire and needle are removed from the trachea, and the tube is seated just rostral to the thoracic inlet.
8. Once intubated, the anesthetist only has $EtCO_2$ as confirmation that the tube is appropriately placed. This monitoring device should be connected and several hand breaths given to confirm the ETT is appropriately placed. .
9. The ETT is then attached to the breathing circuit with an appropriate flow rate of 100% oxygen. The ETT cuff is inflated to 20–25 cmH_2O, or by performing a leak test: while the anesthetist attempts to "hold" a 20–25 cmH_2O breath, the cuff is inflated until there is no leak. Higher pressures may lead to tracheal necrosis and rupture, especially in cats.
10. Once the cuff is sealed, inhalant anesthetics are initiated.

A. Options for anesthetic maintenance

Anesthesia is typically maintained with inhalant anesthetics. However, other options for maintenance include total IV anesthesia (TIVA), a combination of inhalants and injectable drugs (balanced anesthesia; partial IV anesthesia [PIVA]), or, in the case of short procedures, injectable drugs administered IM [PIMA]) (Table 1.10). During this period, the patient's vital signs and depth of anesthesia are monitored and adjusted continuously. Planes I or II of anesthesia are appropriate for diagnostic procedures, and planes II or III are appropriate for surgical procedures (see Table 1.6). The anesthetist must support all homeostatic requirements for the patient at this stage, such as maintaining normal blood pressure, pulse, ventilation, and temperature. Continuous monitoring of vital signs during maintenance is a simple tool to decrease mortality 8, 19]. Any interventions or treatments are based on the anesthetist's observations of the patient as well as information supplied by multiparameter monitoring. Monitoring for the anesthetized patient is the subject of Chapter 2.

Table 1.10 Commonly used maintenance drugs; see the drug formulary for details such as route and dosage.

Drug	Advantages	Disadvantages
Isoflurane	Easily titratable, no IV access required (although it is recommended), inexpensive	Dose-dependent cardiovascular and respiratory depression, noxious smell
Sevoflurane	Easily titratable, no IV access required (although it is recommended), less noxious smell, statistically faster recovery times	Dose-dependent cardiovascular and respiratory depression, expensive, recovery times (while statistically faster) are not clinically different from isoflurane
Alfaxalone	No ETT is required but recommended, not dependent on pulmonary function, IM administration option if no IV access is present, cardiovascular friendly	Apnea, muscle rigidity, shivering, opisthotonos and hypermetria on recovery
Ketamine	No ETT is required but recommended, not dependent on pulmonary function, has analgesic properties, quarter doses can be given IV as a top up as opposed to a CRI, wide margin of safety, IM option if IV access is not present	Muscle rigidity, increased heart rate [31], poor recovery in cats
Propofol	No ETT is required but recommended, not dependent on pulmonary function	Apnea, vasodilation, prolonged recovery after long anesthesia

ETT, endotracheal tube; CRI, constant-rate infusion; IM, intramuscular; IV, intravenous.

B. Fluid therapy

Fluid therapy is an essential part of perianesthetic support. Hydration status is evaluated prior to anesthesia and corrected if necessary. Fluid requirements are dynamic during anesthesia. Anesthetic agents and changes in hormone excretion may affect renal fluid excretion. Losses may be increased due to evaporation from the respiratory tract or surgical site. Fluid requirement may increase due to vasodilation and decreased cardiac stroke volume. Crystalloid solutions are administered at a rate of 5 mL/kg/h for anesthetized dogs and 3 mL/kg/h for cats. Fluid rates may be higher for dehydrated, neonatal, and hypovolemic patients, or for patients undergoing laparotomy or thoracotomy. Rates are decreased in geriatric patients and those susceptible to volume overload, such as patients with cardiac disease. Extreme care is required to maintain fluid balance in anesthetized patients with renal or cardiac disease.

In certain patients, necessary fluids for the procedure may not be crystalloids; for example, patients with severe hemorrhage may require a blood transfusion or patients with a protein-losing enteropathy may require colloidal support. Please see Chapter 5 for more information.

VII. Recovery from anesthesia in the clinical setting

Recovery begins when the maintenance anesthetic is discontinued and continues until all effects of the anesthetics wear off and homeostasis returns. Before the anesthetic is discontinued, confirm that all planned procedures have been performed and examine the oral cavity for regurgitation or other foreign material. Additional analgesia and sedation are administered if necessary, and a plan for further pain management is formed. Use of a checklist at this stage decreases the risk of omission. The recovery location, while often predetermined, should be evaluated for its level of noise, lighting, and general demeanor before a patient is located there. Recovering a patient who may be physiologically challenging in the OR or in another minimally trafficked area, such as a relatively unused radiology suite, may facilitate a smoother recovery. All necessary monitoring must be on hand, however.

The patient is extubated when a strong swallow or cough reflex is observed, at which point the ETT cuff is deflated. In cases where there may be risk of fluid in the trachea (e.g., a patient who underwent a dental procedure or was known to have regurgitated), the ETT cuff may be left partially inflated to help draw out some of that material. Brachycephalic dogs and patients with upper airway disease are extubated only when they are able to maintain a patent airway (see Chapter 4). Normal airflow through the nares is confirmed after extubation in order to rule out laryngospasm.

Recovery is the most dangerous period of anesthesia. In large-scale work, approximately 47–60% of perioperative deaths occur in this period, most of which occur in the first 3 hours [9]. Newer research is even more disturbing, with up to 90% of canine mortality and approximately 74% of feline mortality occurring postoperatively [20, 21]. It is wise to leave an IV catheter in place throughout the entire recovery period in case of adverse events requiring injectable medication, and to lubricate the eyes during the recovery as necessary. Patient monitoring by vigilant staff as well as support of the patient continues until the patient's protective reflexes have fully recovered, vital signs are within normal limits and stable, and the patient is fully awake and ambulatory. Often times, recovery includes monitoring equipment that is easy to remove (such as a capnograph or pulse oximeter) to ensure a normal return of respiratory function. For young animals, periodic blood glucose monitoring is important during recovery. Prolonged recoveries may be observed in obese and hypothermic animals; however, these lengthy recoveries may have other rule-outs, including hypoglycemia or decreased drug metabolism due to hepatic, renal, cardiopulmonary or hormonal dysfunction [1]. Patients with delayed recovery are adequately supported and these causes are ruled out.

Please see Chapter 3 for more information on problems that may occur during recovery.

A. Timeline and signs of recovery at home

Animals recovering from anesthesia may display a variety of abnormal behaviors, including drowsiness, sedation, decreased appetite, pain-associated behaviors or clinical manifestations of anesthesia-associated complications (e.g. coughing from tracheitis, or signs of nausea due to esophagitis) [1]. Signs of drowsiness and sedation should show a trend of improvement over the 24–48 hours following anesthesia, and pain should decrease over time depending on the procedure performed and the efficacy of the postoperative pain management plan.

B. Communications about returning home

Owners are informed as to what they should expect during the first days of recovery and what signs necessitate contacting the clinic or an emergency center. Since oral communication during stressful situations is less effective, these points are stated on the patient's discharge form; separate anesthesia-focused discharge instructions may assist with this. Such forms are available online, at no cost [28]. Abnormal behaviors presented by their beloved pets may distress owners, and this may be exacerbated by concerns regarding the medical procedure or economic issues. Availability and good communication skills are important at this stage to improve outcome of the interactions, and owner satisfaction [29].

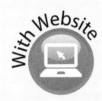

www.wiley.com/go/shelby/anesthesia2

Please go to the companion website for access to videos relating to the book

References

1. Grubb T, Sager J, Gaynor JS et al. 2020 AAHA Anesthesia and Monitoring Guidelines for Dogs and Cats. J Am Anim Hosp Assoc. 2020;56(2):59–82.
2. Robinson EP, Sams RA, Muir WW. Barbiturate anesthesia in greyhound and mixed-breed dogs: comparative cardiopulmonary effects, anesthetic effects, and recovery rates. Am J Vet Res. 1986;47(10):2105–12.
3. Sams RA, Muir WW, Detra RL, Robinson EP. Comparative pharmacokinetics and anesthetic effects of methohexital, pentobarbital, thiamylal, and thiopental in Greyhound dogs and non-Greyhound, mixed-breed dogs. Am J Vet Res. 1985;46(8):1677–83.
4. Brodbelt D, Pfeiffer D, Young L, Wood J. Results of the confidential enquiry into perioperative small animal fatalities regarding risk factors for anesthetic-related death in dogs. J Am Vet Med Assoc. 2008;233(7):1096–104.
5. Matthews NS, Mohn TJ, Yang M et al. Factors associated with anesthetic-related death in dogs and cats in primary care veterinary hospitals. J Am Vet Med Assoc. 2017;250(6):655–65.
6. Mogil JS. Qualitative sex differences in pain processing: emerging evidence of a biased literature. Nat Rev Neurosci. 2020;21(7):353–65.

7. IASP. Part III: Pain Terms, A Current List with Definitions and Notes on Usage. www.iasp-pain. org/resources/terminology/

8. Brodbelt D, Pfeiffer D, Young L, Wood J. Risk factors for anaesthetic-related death in cats: results from the confidential enquiry into perioperative small animal fatalities (CEPSAF). Br J Anaesth. 2007;99(5):617–23.

9. Brodbelt D, Blissitt K, Hammond R et al. The risk of death: the confidential enquiry into perioperative small animal fatalities. Vet Anaesth Analg. 2008;35(5):365–73.

10. Portier K, Ida KK. The ASA Physical Status Classification: what is the evidence for recommending its use in veterinary anesthesia? A systematic review. Front Vet Sci. 2018;5:204.

11. Kavkovsky A, Avital Y, Aroch I, Segev G, Shipov A. Perioperative urinary heat shock protein 72 as an early marker of acute kidney injury in dogs. Vet Anaesth Analg. 2020;47(1):53–60.

12. Bille C, Auvigne V, Bomassi E, Durieux P, Libermann S, Rattez E. An evidence-based medicine approach to small animal anaesthetic mortality in a referral practice: the influence of initiating three recommendations on subsequent anaesthetic deaths. Vet Anaesth Analg. 2014;41(3):249–58.

13. Carter J, Story DA. Veterinary and human anaesthesia: an overview of some parallels and contrasts. Anaesth Intensive Care. 2013;41(6):710–18.

14. Brodbelt D. Perioperative mortality in small animal anaesthesia. Vet J. 2009;182(2):152–61.

15. Brodbelt D, Hammond R, Tuminaro D, Pfeiffer D, Wood J. Risk factors for anaesthetic-related death in referred dogs. Vet Rec. 2006;158(16):563–4.

16. Lee HW, Machin H, Adami C. Peri-anaesthetic mortality and nonfatal gastrointestinal complications in pet rabbits: a retrospective study on 210 cases. Vet Anaesth Analg. 2018;45(4):520–8.

17. Seamon AB, Hofmeister EH, Divers SJ. Outcome following inhalation anesthesia in birds at a veterinary referral hospital: 352 cases (2004–2014). J Am Vet Med Assoc. 2017;251(7):814–17.

18. Levy JK, Bard KM, Tucker SJ, Diskant PD, Dingman PA. Perioperative mortality in cats and dogs undergoing spay or castration at a high-volume clinic. Vet J. 2017;224:11–15.

19. Dyson DH, Maxie MG, Schnurr D. Morbidity and mortality associated with anesthetic management in small animal veterinary practice in Ontario. J Am Anim Hosp Assoc. 1998;34(4):325–35.

20. Redondo JI. Perianaesthetic mortality in dogs: preliminary data of a worldwide multicentric study. [Abstract]. Presented at the 13th World Congress of Veterinary Anaesthesiology, Venice, Italy 2018.

21. Redondo JI. Perianaesthetic mortality in cats:preliminary data of a worldwide multicentric study. [Abstract]. Presented at the 13th World Congress of Veterinary Anaesthesiology, Venice, Italy 2018.

22. Posner LP, Mariani CL, Swanson C, Asakawa M, Campbell N, King AS. Perianesthetic morbidity and mortality in dogs undergoing cervical and thoracolumbar spinal surgery. Vet Anaesth Analg. 2014;41(2):137–44.

23. Robinson R, Chang YM, Seymour CJ, Pelligand L. Predictors of outcome in dogs undergoing thoracic surgery (2002–2011). Vet Anaesth Analg. 2014;41(3):259–68.

24. Stefani LC, Gamermann PW, Backof A et al. Perioperative mortality related to anesthesia within 48h and up to 30 days following surgery: a retrospective cohort study of 11,562 anesthetic procedures. J Clin Anesth. 2018;49:79–86.

25. Hofmeister EH, Quandt J, Braun C, Shepard M. Development, implementation and impact of simple patient safety interventions in a university teaching hospital. Vet Anaesth Analg. 2014;41(3):243–8.

26. Bergstrom A, Dimopoulou M, Eldh M. Reduction of surgical complications in dogs and cats by the use of a surgical safety checklist. Vet Surg. 2016;45(5):571–6.

27. McNally E, Robertson S, Pablo L. Comparison of time to desaturation between preoxygenated and nonpreoxygenated dogs following sedation with acepromazine maleate and morphine and induction of anesthesia with propofol. Am J Vet Res. 2009;70(11):1333–8.

28. American Animal Hospital Association. Anesthesia Discharge Template. www.aaha.org/aaha-guidelines/2020-aaha-anesthesia-and-monitoring-guidelines-for-dogs-and-cats/anesthesia-discharge-template/
29. Bonvicini KA, Cornell K. Are clients truly informed? Communiation tools and risk reduction. Compend Contin Educ Vet. 2008;30(11):572–6.
30. Bergeron R, Scott SL, Emond JP, Mercier F, Cook NJ, Schaefer AL. Physiology and behavior of dogs during air transport. Can J Vet Res. 2002;66(3):211–16.
31. Sumikura H, Andersen OK, Drewes AM, Arendt-Nielsen L. Spatial and temporal profiles of flare and hyperalgesia after intradermal capsaicin. Pain. 2003;105(1-2):285–91.

Chapter 1

Chapter 2

Anesthesia equipment and monitoring

Jennifer Sager and Carolyn M. McKune

This chapter details common small animal anesthesia equipment, and how to properly and safely set up an anesthetic machine [1]. Descriptions of monitoring equipment, equipment use, advantages and disadvantages of the devices, and how to properly place equipment on the patient are provided. In addition, the chapter outlines tools to assist the anesthetist in monitoring patient vital signs and anesthetic depth, with normal waveforms and referenced parameter ranges.

I. Gas pressures in a hospital system

While most people are familiar with the anesthesia machine as a critical piece of equipment producing a gas mixture with variable composition of precisely selected gases [2], many are not familiar with the gas pressures in a system that ultimately results in gas flow to a patient. The gas originates and then moves through three systems: high-pressure system, intermediate-pressure system, and low-pressure system (Boxes 2.1–2.4).

Box 2.1 High-pressure system

- Receives gases at cylinder pressure and then decreases that pressure and makes it constant. Before beginning an anesthetic procedure, it is important to ensure adequate psi in the high-pressure system (above 200–500 psi).
- Yoke or yoke block connects the machine to the compressed gas source (pipeline or cylinder).
- Pressure regulator reduces pressure (which fluctuates with temperature and content) to 50 psi and maintains constant flow of compressed gas to the anesthetic system.

Box 2.2 Intermediate-pressure system

- Receives gases from the regulator or pipeline, which are made constant. From there, gases pass to the flowmeter and oxygen flush valve (separately).
- Pipeline inlet allows access to a hospital pipeline system, if present.

Small Animal Anesthesia Techniques, Second Edition. Edited by Amanda M. Shelby and Carolyn M. McKune.
© 2023 John Wiley & Sons, Inc. Published 2023 by John Wiley & Sons, Inc.
Companion website: www.wiley.com/go/shelby/anesthesia2

- An oxygen pressure failure device attempts to protect the patient in case of delivery of a hypoxic gas mixture, and will either alarm or cut off nonoxygen gases, should supply of oxygen pressure drop considerably.
- The flowmeter assembly controls and measures the amount of gas flow in liters per minute (L/min). Gas flow is measured at the largest point on the indicator (e.g., if a ball is used, it is measured at the center of the ball). Each flowmeter will depict where an indicator is read on the flowmeter.

Chapter 2

Box 2.3 Low-pressure system (Figure 2.1).

- The low pressure system encompasses gases from the flowmeter, moving forward.
- The vaporizer, a device uniquely customized for each anesthetic agent, converts an agent from liquid to vapor form. Ensure the vaporizer is filled at the beginning of the procedure.
- The common gas outlet is where all gases from the machine arrive. Depending on the machine, a separate common gas outlet for a rebreathing (RC) system and nonrebreathing (NRC) system may be present.

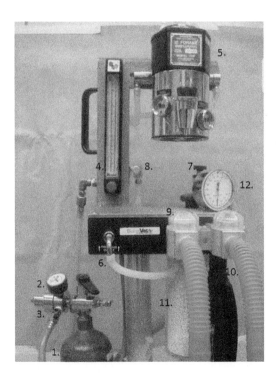

Figure 2.1 Anesthesia machine with circle system labeled: 1. oxygen "E" cylinder; 2. cylinder pressure gauge; 3. pressure regulator; 4. oxygen flowmeter; 5. vaporizer; 6. common gas outlet; 7. APL or "pop-off" valve; 8. oxygen flush valve; 9. unidirectional valves; 10. reservoir bag connection; 11. CO_2-absorbent canister; 12. pressure manometer.

Box 2.4 Other critical components of the anesthesia machine

- Adjustable pressure-limiting (APL) valve (or "pop-off" valve) limits or allows gas to remain or exit the breathing circuit, depending on its degree of closure.
- A temporary occlusion device should be placed within the circuit to allow for momentary closure during hand ventilation, without closing the APL valve (see section on preventing barotrauma).
- An oxygen flush button connects the oxygen flush valve to the anesthesia system, and rapidly delivers oxygen into the circuit (bypassing the vaporizer). Never depress this button when the breathing circuit is attached to patient, as this could cause barotrauma.
- An in-circuit manometer indicates circuit pressure within the circuit. This is useful during intermittent positive pressure ventilation (IPPV).
- The cylinder pressure gauge uses a bourdon tube to indicate how much pressure the remaining compressed gas in the tank exerts, as an indicator of how much supply is available. Equation 2.1 shows how this translates to minutes of oxygen available for the procedure.

Equation 2.1

E tank:

Time until cylinder is empty = [0.3 × (Tank pressure in PSI − 200)]/ flow rate in L/minute

H tank:

Time until cylinder is empty = [3.1 × (Tank pressure in PSI − 200)]/ flow rate in L/minute

*Note, 200 is subtracted from the PSI as that is the minimum amount in the tank before the tank should be switched.

Example:

An E tank with 500 PSI being run at 1 L/min
Time until cylinder is empty = [0.3 × (500 − 200)]/1
Time until cylinder is empty = 90 minutes

- Modern vaporizers with safety features are agent specific, precision, out of circuit and temperature compensated. These vaporizers should be calibrated every 12 months for accuracy, as well as any time the vaporizer is tipped or possibly damaged.
- Addition of a heat and moisture exchange (HME) device can help with humidification and temperature regulation of inspired and expired gases.
- All machines should be equipped with either active or passive scavenge devices to reduce waste anesthetic gas (WAG) exposure.

II. Setting up the anesthesia machine

A. Selecting a breathing system

Its important to recognize that common nomenclature is misleading. The fresh gas flow rate dictates the nature (i.e., rebreathing or nonrebreathing) of the circuit (Box 2.5). The Mapleson systems are used as nonrebreathing systems with oxygen flow rates at 200 mL/kg/min or greater and therefore avoid any rebreathing of expired gases. Circle systems are traditionally employed at lower fresh gas flow rates and called rebreathing circuits as they allow for some degree of rebreathing of expired gases, after using CO_2 absorbent to remove CO_2 from the system. Another important feature of rebreathing circuits is the functional inspiratory and expiratory valves which keep flow unidirectional.

Box 2.5　Breathing circuits

- Rebreathing circuits (RCs), commonly referred to as circle systems (Figure 2.2), are typically selected for patients more than 5–7 kg. Recommended oxygen flow rates are 10–30 mL/kg/min (Table 2.1). Pediatric circle systems reduce the dead space in the system, while providing the advantages of the circle system (see Table 2.1). Ensure that the CO_2 absorbent has less than 8 hours of use time or replace the absorbent if there is a question about its use time. It is also important to ensure the unidirectional valves are functional.
- Nonrebreathing circuits (NRCs), typically classified according to the Mapleson system, are typically reserved for patients less than 7 kg. The most common circuits in practice are the modified Bain circuit (Figure 2.3) and the modified Jackson–Rees. Required oxygen flow rates are 200–300 mL/kg/min with a minimum acceptable flow of 0.5 L/min, and an inspired CO_2 of 5 mmHg or less.

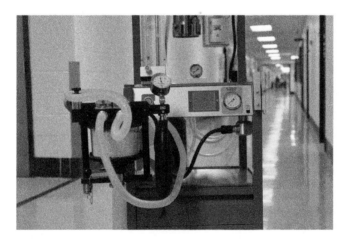

Figure 2.2　Circle system connected to anesthesia machine. *Source:* Courtesy of Anderson da Cunha.

Table 2.1　Comparison of breathing systems.

Nonrebreathing system (i.e., Mapleson circuits >200 mL/kg/min)		Rebreathing system (i.e., circle systems at <30 mL/kg/min)	
Advantages	Disadvantages	Advantages	Disadvantages
Minimal resistance Less dead space Light weight High oxygen flow rates allow rapid change in inspired anesthetic concentration	High oxygen flows lead to heat loss, water loss, more expense If oxygen flow is too low, patient will rebreathe expired gases	Low oxygen flow rates, less expense Less body heat loss Closed circuit is performed if desired Rebreathing of expired carbon dioxide difficult if all components are functional	Increased resistance in circuit (unidirectional valves and carbon dioxide absorber) More components of anesthetic machine lead to risk of malfunction "Y" piece adds dead space Large volume of breathing circuit requiring longer time between changes in inspired anesthetic concentration More maintenance (changing CO_2 absorbent) Bulkier system

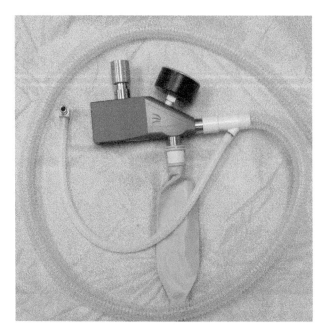

Figure 2.3   Modified Bain circuit.

B. Reservoir bag

The reservoir bag allows manually assisted ventilation by the anesthetist (Box 2.6). To deliver a breath, close the APL, compress the reservoir bag to desired size breath by watching the manometer (less than 20 cmH$_2$O in dogs and cats), and do not forget to open the APL valve after. Alternatively, a temporary occlusion device allows the anesthetist to forgo closing the APL and instead press the spring-loaded temporary occluder button to deliver a breath.

Pressure checking the anesthesia machine

Table 2.2 details a common method for pressure checking both the RC and NRC systems. However, this method of pressure checking the breathing system does not check the integrity of the inspiratory tube of a modified Bain system.

Box 2.6 Reservoir bag selection

The reservoir bag is equal to or larger than the calculated size:

Equation 2.2

Weight (kg) × minute volume × V$_t$ = bag size

Example: 20 kg × 6 ×10 = 1200 mL (use a 2 L bag)

Typical ranges for minute volume and tidal volume are 3–6 L/min and 10–20 mL/kg, respectively. The example shows that a 20 kg patient would require a 2 L reservoir bag.

Table 2.2   Pressure checking the anesthesia machine.

1. Turn on oxygen tank or connect to oxygen source.
2. Connect the breathing circuit appropriate for the patient. Ensure the fresh gas outlet is connected.
3. Connect the reservoir bag.
4. Close the pop-off valve or APL valve.
5. Occlude the patient end of the breathing circuit.
6. Turn on the oxygen flowmeter and fill the breathing circuit with oxygen until the manometer reaches 30 cmH$_2$O. Turn off the flowmeter.
7. Hold this pressure for 10–20 seconds.[a]
8. *Open the APL valve to relieve pressure from the circuit.*

[a]If the pressure doesn't hold, leaks are present. See "Troubleshooting Leaks."

Safety note: In an effort to ensure a system does not have a leak (preventing effective gas containment), this system requires a pressure check. In order to effectively pressure check a system, this system must be fully closed off to possible means of venting the gas to outside system. In circumstances where the adjustable pressure-limiting valve is not reopened, pressure can build in the system and result in pulmonary barotrauma when the patient is connected. See section on reducing the possibility of barotrauma through equipment features in this chapter.

C. Troubleshooting leaks (Box 2.7)

Box 2.7 Identifying leaks
• Ensure the pop-off valve is closed completely.
• Replace the breathing circuit and/or reservoir bag.
• If using a circle system, check the sodasorb canister and unidirectional valves for proper placement or cracks. Please note that one of the most common sites of equipment leakage, when the circuit and bag have already been replaced, is granular dust from the sodasorb preventing the sodasorb canister from making an adequate seal.
• Ensure fresh gas outlet is connected to the circuit in use.

III. Barotrauma

Pulmonary, or lung, barotrauma is damage to the lungs due to excessive pressure buildup, occurring over a short span of time. The lungs are unable to accommodate this rapid pressure increase, causing damage to the lung tissue. Depending on the species in question, the alveoli can endure up to 36 cmH$_2$O before there is possible barotrauma.

Barotrauma secondary to excessive positive pressure is almost exclusively the result of a mechanical error, as most mammals breathe using negative pressure (i.e., they inhale air from their environment by moving musculature and entraining that air down to the alveoli, where gases are exchanged). Under certain circumstances, such as a patient under general anesthesia or supported with mechanical ventilation due to a critical respiratory illness, *positive* pressure is used to artificially introduce gases to a patient's lungs. During general anesthesia, positive pressure is provided by hand or via a mechanical ventilator, both of which require temporarily occluding the APL, or "pop off" valve.

The APL valve is also closed to ensure an anesthesia system does not have a leak (preventing effective gas containment) while pressure checking the machine. In circumstances where the APL valve is not reopened, pressure can build in the system and result in pulmonary barotrauma.

In order to prevent pulmonary barotrauma, there are two broad strategies: anesthesia machines with built-in features, and aftermarket add-ons. In machines which have built-in features, pulmonary barotrauma is prevented by integrating features which preclude the necessity of a human performing a leak test. These include features such as the machine electronically leak checking itself or automatically switching from manual to mechanical ventilation without closing the APL valve (generally by flipping a switch). Many anesthesia machines targeted for human patients integrate these technologies along with automated preuse self-checks. Few veterinary anesthesia workstations offer all these features.

Most veterinary market machines will include aftermarket add-ons. Two key pieces of equipment are used to accomplish barotrauma safety.

A. Temporary occlusion device (Figure 2.4)

This device has a button which is depressed when the anesthetist gives a breath, in lieu of closing the APL valve. While this prevents barotrauma as a result of APL valve occlusion when giving a breath, it is only a partial solution as it does not prevent pressure buildup from leak testing a machine. It is advisable to couple this valve with a pressure relief valve.

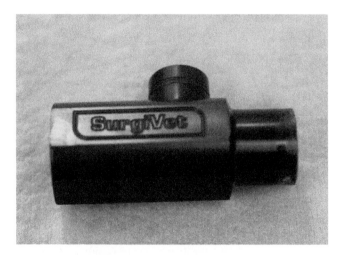

Figure 2.4   Temporary occluder device.

B. Pressure relief valves (Table 2.3, Figure 2.5)

These valves are intended for postmanufacture additions and are adaptable to most veterinary anesthesia machine. These valves are retrofitted to most present-day anesthesia machines and will automatically vent the system as that pressure exceeds a preset safety limit (usually >25 cmH$_2$O). Please note that many also require additional gas scavenging to prevent vented waste gas from accumulating in the operating room.

Table 2.3   Examples of postmanufacture pressure relief valves

Valve	Advantages	Disadvantages
Supera safety pop-off valve (www.superavet.com/safety)	Even when the valve is closed, it prevents buildup of excessive pressure and will thus still open if excess pressure builds in the system. The Supera safety pop-off valve vents at any pressure above zero regardless of the dial position. It must be manually depressed to generate pressure within the system. Anesthetic gas is automatically vented to scavenge system (no additional modification needed). Removal from circuit is *not* required to perform proper machine leak check, which reduces risk of barotrauma secondary to pressure checking machine, and leaving APL closed. Functions as its own pop-off temporary occlusion device. This is a replacement for the adjustable pressure-limiting valve so it is similar in appearance to the way most anesthesia machines are already equipped, reducing the change management hurdle	The user must manually depress and hold the valve closed to perform a leak test. Requires purchase of a cap for use with a mechanical ventilator (in order to overcome the pressure relief safety features to ventilate). If the cap is *not* removed after removal of the ventilator from the circuit, this device can cause barotrauma
Essential Medical Devices (EMD) valve (www.essentialmedicaldevices.com/products/emd-safety-valve)	Valves open at approximately 26 cmH$_2$O, vent to the environment, and allow for flow up to 4 L/min when open. The system comes with a means to scavenge waste anesthetic gases. Ventilator compatible	In addition to the valve itself, a temporary occlusion device is also indicated to fully reduce the risk of barotrauma. Waste gas is vented to the environment without use of the scavenge adaptation. The valve and scavenge system must be removed to properly leak test the machine to 30 cmH$_2$O, which creates barotrauma risk from incorrect disconnection and set up with pressure check

(Continued)

Table 2.3 *(Continued)*

Valve	Advantages	Disadvantages
JD Medical safety pressure relief valve (http://jdmedical.com/veterinary-anesthesia-machines-products/anesthesia-accessories/safety-pressure-relief-valve/)	Two different valves are available, which vent at either 20 or 30 cmH$_2$O. Ventilator compatible. Vents directly into scavenger system	In addition to the valve itself, a temporary occlusion device is also indicated to fully reduce the risk of barotrauma. The valve and scavenge system must be removed to properly leak test the machine to 30 cmH$_2$O, which creates barotrauma risk from incorrect disconnection and set up with each pressure check
Hallowell relief valve (combination of a Run Tee piece and a PEEP valve) (www.hallowell.com/index.php?pr=z242A1407)	Inexpensive. Adaptable to any machine	This valve must be removed to properly leak test the machine to 30 cmH$_2$O, which creates barotrauma risk from incorrect disconnection and set up with each pressure check. Requires an F-air to scavenge waste gases. Fatigues over time; authors advise assessing PEEP valve for replacement every 6 months. An additional pop-off temporary occlusion device is also indicated to fully reduce the risk of barotrauma

Note: Review and follow manufacturer guidelines on appropriate scavenging for these valves, if necessary.
APL, adjustable pressure limiting; PEEP, positive end-expiratory pressure.

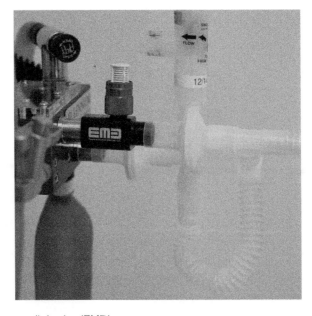

Figure 2.5 Pressure relief valve (EMD).

IV. Mechanical ventilation (MV) or intermittent positive pressure ventilation (IPPV)

Mechanical ventilation is useful in cases where the patient is not ventilating adequately due to respiratory depression, disease, or paralysis (e.g., use of neuromuscular blockers). MV exerts positive pressure and, while useful, it is important to recognize that IPPV has negative effects on cardiac output (CO) by decreasing venous return to the heart, decreasing CO_2, and increasing delivery of inhalant anesthetic. Only experienced personnel should operate a mechanical ventilator; caution is exercised in patients with hypovolemia and cardiopulmonary disease. Basic concepts of commercial ventilators are similar in function; however, the terminology or labeling may vary. It is important to understand how adjustments to the ventilator settings will affect ventilation before using the ventilator for the patient. Thorough review of the manufacturer's operation manual prior to using a ventilator is advised to ensure proper and safe use. Table 2.4 provides a general overview of how to set up a mechanical ventilator.

A. Classification of ventilators

There are three basic characteristics of ventilators: the mechanism by which they are controlled, the mechanism by which they are cycled from inspiration to expiration, and the mechanism that triggers the ventilator to begin a breath (Boxes 2.8 and 2.9). Ventilators are further classified as having ascending or descending bellows. Ascending bellows, which are most commonly used, compress down during inspiration and ascend during expiration. Leaks are easily detected in these ventilators because the bellows fall when a leak is present (a distinct advantage). Descending bellows compress upward during inspiration and descend during expiration.

Table 2.4   General setup of a mechanical ventilator.

1. Connect the ventilator's driving gas to source. While any pressurized gas will drive the ventilator, typically the driving gas is oxygen.
2. If the ventilator requires electrical power, plug in to outlet.
3. Ensure ventilator settings are set appropriately or turned to the lowest delivery pressure to avoid barotrauma when turned on. Depending on the make and model of the ventilator, this involves reducing the inspiratory time, inspiratory flow, or volume controls.
4. Evacuate the reservoir bag on the anesthetic machine to avoid personnel exposure to waste anesthetics.
5. Replace the reservoir bag with the breathing line from the ventilator.
6. Close the pop-off (APL) valve on the anesthetic machine.
7. Connect the ventilator's scavenging hose to a scavenging system.
8. To inflate the bellows, increase the oxygen flow on the flowmeter. Reduce flow to appropriate rate for patient and breathing circuit when bellows are full.
9. Turn on ventilator; watch the patient's V_T, PIP, and $EtCO_2$. Adjust to ensure adequate ventilation.

Box 2.8 Classification of ventilators

- *Control* refers to how the ventilator delivers its flow.
  - *Volume control*: flow is administered to a certain volume, regardless of the amount of pressure delivered.
  - *Pressure control*: flow is administered to a certain pressure, regardless of how much volume is administered. As the reader can deduce, pressure-controlled ventilation is likely to result in less barotrauma.
- *Cycle* is the mechanism by which the ventilator moves from inspiration to expiration.
  - *Time-cycled ventilation*: inspiration occurs for a set period of time (e.g., 1.5 seconds are spent in inspiration before the ventilator moves to expiration). Time-cycled ventilation is how the vast majority of veterinary anesthesia ventilators function.
  - *Volume-cycled ventilation*: achieving a target volume moves the ventilator from inspiration to expiration.
  - *Pressure-cycled ventilation*: achieving a target pressure moves the ventilator from inspiration to expiration.
- *Trigger* is what tells the ventilator to begin inspiration.
  - *Time-triggered ventilation*: uses time to initiate a cycle based on the respiratory rate the anesthetist has selected; this is the way most veterinary anesthesia mechanical ventilators function.
  - *Pressure-triggered ventilation*: waits for feedback from the patient (usually in the form of an attempted breath) to trigger the beginning of a cycle, a feature important in critically ill patients a clinician is trying to wean from the ventilator but often impractical in anesthetized animals.

Box 2.9 Terminology and adjustable parameters of ventilators

- *Inspiratory time to expiratory time (I: E) ratio*: the relationship between time of inspiration and expiration. Normal I:E ratios range from 1:2 to 1:3.5. Increasing the I:E ratio (i.e., 1:5) decreases inspiratory time, whereas decreasing the ratio (i.e., 1:1) gives the patient longer inspiratory times.
- *Peak inspiratory pressure (PIP)*: the maximum pressure during the inspiratory phase or breath. In healthy small animal patients, PIP of 12–20 cmH_2O is enough to provide a "normal" breath for adequate ventilation. Rarely is a PIP greater than 20 cmH_2O needed or recommended for the small animal patient.
- *Tidal volume (V_T)*: the volume of breath the patient receives. Normal V_T is between 10 and 20 mL/kg. Graduations typically located on the bellow casing allow the anesthetist to estimate V_T; however, these graduations may be inaccurate. A spirometer is an accurate reflection of tidal volume, if available.
- *Respiratory rate (RR)*: the number of breaths per minute the patient receives. Normal RR for anesthetized canine patients is between 6 and 12; for feline patients, between 8 and 16.
- *Inspiratory flow rate*: the speed of flow of air during the inspiratory phase or breath, expressed in milliliters per second. Adjustments in inspiratory flow on many ventilators will linearly influence the V_T and PIP.
- *Inspiratory time*: the length of time a breath is given during the inspiratory phase. Increasing inspiratory time may increase the V_T and PIP.
- *Expiratory time*: the time allowed between inspirations. Some ventilators use expiratory time as a means to set the RR. Expiratory time is inversely related to the RR, meaning an increase in expiratory time decreases RR.

B. Optional ventilator features

A pressure relief valve is not present on all ventilators as an adjustable feature; however, this allows the release of excessive pressure or sets off an alarm to notify the anesthetist that the maximum PIP has been exceeded. It is recommended that this valve is set to 5 cmH$_2$O over the maximum PIP.

A peak end-expiratory pressure (PEEP) valve is not present on all ventilators but allows the anesthetist to hold positive pressure at the end of the expiratory phase. This technique is used for specific situations where the patient may experience severe atelectasis. PEEP over 10 cmH$_2$O is typically not recommended. PEEP valves of fixed pressures are available for application to an anesthetic machine or ventilator. The anesthetist observes the manometer to ensure the PEEP valve is functional. It is worth noting that although not all ventilators have a PEEP valve feature, most have an inherent PEEP of 2–4 cmH$_2$O.

Inspiratory hold (breath hold) is not present on all ventilators; however, this feature allows the anesthetist to hold a breath with the lungs inflated to a desired PIP.

C. Troubleshooting common problems of a mechanical ventilator

The mechanical ventilator has several common areas for failure that the anesthetist may need to address (Box 2.10).

Box 2.10 Common problems when ventilating a patient

Leaks: An ascending bellow that will not fill or gradually loses volume indicates the presence of a leak.

- Check to ensure that the drive gas source is connected.
- Ensure the breathing circuit did not become disconnected from the patient and that connection of ventilator is secure.
- Ensure the bellow casing is secured and no tears are present in the bellow.
- Ensure adequate oxygen flow from the anesthetic machine.
- Make sure the pop-off (APL) valve is closed.

Hypoventilation: adjustment of these following parameters may address hypoventilation (i.e., they will decrease EtCO$_2$). Additionally, several of these maneuvers increase oxygenation.

- Increasing inspiratory time (affects V$_T$)
- Increasing PIP (affects V$_T$)
- Increasing inspiratory flow (affects V$_T$)
- Increasing RR (or decreasing expiratory time)

Hyperventilation: adjustment of the following parameters may address hyperventilation (i.e., they will increase EtCO$_2$).

- Decreasing RR (increases expiratory time)
- Decreasing inspiratory time (affects V$_T$)
- Decreasing inspiratory flow (affects V$_T$)
- Decreasing PIP (affects V$_T$)
- V$_T$ can be decreased but is not typically decreased below 10 mL/kg

Sudden change in PIP or VT

- Changes in lung compliance or elasticity and resistance may be the result of possible anesthetic complications such as a spontaneous pneumothorax (see Chapter 3) or anaphylactic reaction (see Chapter 3).
- An airway or ET tube obstruction will cause an increase in PIP and decrease in VT.

V. Monitoring equipment

The most accurate determinant of anesthetic depth is the patient itself. Heart rate (HR), respiratory rate (RR), and blood pressure (BP) will change with anesthetic depth but are also influenced by other factors. Table 1.6 (p.15) lists clinical signs of anesthetic depth in dogs and cats at surgical anesthetic depth (Stage III), while Table 2.5 lists vital parameters to be monitored under anesthesia.

A. Circulatory system

1. Invasive blood pressure monitoring

Invasive blood pressure (IBP) monitoring via arterial line is useful in debilitated or critically ill patients (ASA III–V) because of its accuracy. Common arteries for catheterization include the dorsal pedal, auricular, deep lingual, radial, and coccygeal. A variety of equipment is used to measure arterial pressure. A simple aneroid manometer is used to measure mean arterial pressure (MAP) directly, or a transducer can give direct systolic, diastolic, and mean pressures (Figure 2.6). Regardless of the equipment used to measure direct arterial pressure, the arterial

Table 2.5   Normal vital parameters under anesthesia.

	Canine	Feline
Heart rate (bpm)	60–160	100–250
Respiratory rate (breaths/min)	6–12	8–16
Systolic arterial pressure (mmHg)	90–160	90–160
Diastolic arterial pressure (mmHg)	45–55	45–55
Mean arterial pressure (mmHg)	60–80	60–80
Temperature (F)	96–98	96–98
EtCO$_2$ (mmHg)	35–45	35–45
SpO$_2$ (%)	97–100	97–100

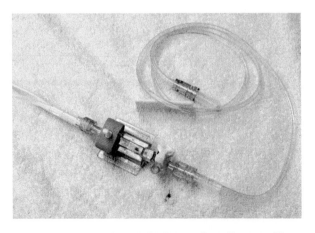

Figure 2.6   Arterial blood pressure continuous flush transducer for use with an automated system.

catheter is flushed periodically to avoid clotting and maintain patency. Placement of the fluid line connected to the aneroid manometer, or the pressure transducer, should be leveled with the apex of the heart to ensure accurate values. See Table 2.6 for directions on setup of IBP monitoring. If the aneroid manometer or pressure transducer is below the apex of the heart, values are falsely high. Conversely, if the transducer is above the heart, values are falsely low. An example of a classic arterial tracing is depicted in Figure 2.7.

(a) Advantages: IBP monitoring is accurate and provides continuous monitoring of arterial BP. Arterial pressure is truly measured (as opposed to calculated) and therefore serves as a reliable tool on which to base intraoperative management decisions. In patients anticipated to require a fair number of intraoperative adjustments (ASA III–V patients), having a direct arterial line provides a sound basis for alterations to the anesthetic plan. Additionally, a direct arterial line is useful for sampling: the arterial line is used to collect samples for blood gas assessment, electrolytes, packed cell volume/total solids (PCV/TS), blood glucose, and so on, which will also help with modifications of the intraoperative plan. The arterial waveform helps with assessment of volume status. Systolic arterial pressure (SAP) variations (changes

Table 2.6 Placement of arterial catheter and setup of methods to measure IBP.

Materials: Over-the-needle catheter, aseptic prep, noncompliant pressure tubing, transducer or aneroid manometer, tape, clippers, syringe of heparinized saline; optional: T-port[a] or injection cap, pressure bag with heparinized saline (1–2 units/mL) when using a continuous flush transducer

Techniques:

1. Palpate the artery. An artery that is not palpable is almost impossible to catheterize.
2. Clip and aseptically prepare site for catheterization.
3. Select size of catheter (often based on the size of the patient); for example, a medium-sized dog may take a 20 G catheter and a cat may take a 22 G catheter. In general, the arterial catheter in the dorsal pedal artery is typically one size smaller than the cephalic venous catheter. Catheters larger than 20 G (even for an animal as large as a horse!) are unnecessary.
4. The skin is either left intact or nicked at the chosen site of entrance (operator preference).
5. Insert the catheter at a 45° angle to the skin to begin; the catheter is inserted distal to where the pulse is palpated. It is helpful to continue to palpate the pulse as a guide while placing the catheter. Arteries spasm, clot quickly, and have thick vascular walls, which make them more difficult than veins to catheterize. Often, the anesthetist must be mildly aggressive to achieve success (this is a skill that takes several attempts to develop proficiency).
6. Once blood is present in the stylet, advance the over-the-needle catheter slightly farther into the artery and slide the catheter off the stylet. It is important to use the stylet as a guide, leaving it in place until the catheter is completely fed into the artery.
7. Remove the stylet. Arterial blood is bright red and should be pulsing. Place the T-port, injection cap, or pressure tubing on the catheter and secure with tape similar to techniques used for IV catheters.
8. Once the catheter is correctly placed, connect the transducer to the arterial catheter using noncompliant pressure tubing (tubing that has limited elasticity) filled with heparinized saline. If an injection cap is used on the arterial catheter, a needle of the same size as the catheter is used to connect pressure tubing. Alternatively, a three-way stopcock can be added to serve as a port for sampling.
9. The next step depends on whether an aneroid manometer or an automated system is used to determine IBP.

(Continued)

Table 2.6   *(Continued)*

Automated system	*Aneroid manometer*
The appropriate transducer (check manufacturer's specifications) is connected to the transducer cable. The catheter is zeroed to atmospheric pressure at the automated monitoring system. This is accomplished by turning the three-way stopcock *off* to the patient and open to room air. Once a baseline zero has registered, turn the stopcock off to the atmosphere, and an arterial BP appears along with a distinct waveform (see Figure 2.7). For an accurate pressure, the transducer is level with the apex of the heart.	With the stopcock *off* to the patient, disposable tubing (often an extension set) is connected to the aneroid manometer to prevent contamination of the manometer. This tubing is then connected to a stopcock and filled approximately halfway with heparinized saline. The meniscus of the waterline is placed at heart level and taped in place on a fixed object (e.g., an IV pole). The stopcock is then turned off to the atmosphere, and the waterline will reset itself in accordance with the animal's pressure. The gauge of manometer will register the MAP and moves with each heartbeat (i.e., the anesthetist can obtain HR as well from this device).

Note: Placing arterial lines is an advanced skill that requires practice.
[a]Luer-Lock T-ports, injection caps or pressure tubing should be used when attached to the arterial catheter to ensure that accidental loss of blood from the catheter does not occur. The use of T-ports, injection caps, or needles to connect the pressure tubing will cause dampening of the pressure waveform; however, they allow sampling access.

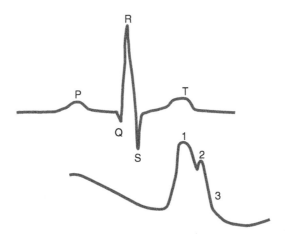

Figure 2.7   ECG with correlating arterial wave form. ECG waves are labeled P, Q, R, S, and T. 1. Systolic blood pressure. 2. Dicrotic notch. 3. Runoff during diastole.

in the arterial wave form secondary to IPPV) are correlated to states of hypovolemia [3]. In cases of cardiac arrest, observing pulse pressure waves tells the anesthetist the effectiveness of chest compressions as well as when it is necessary to rotate personnel performing compressions prior to the 2-minute personnel change.

(b) Disadvantages: IBP monitoring requires advanced skills; placement is more challenging than a peripheral catheter. Because the arterial line is often out of sight of the anesthetist,

dislodgment results in a significant amount of hemorrhage before it is noticed. Direct pressure applied for no less than 5–10 minutes is necessary once the arterial line is removed to prevent hematoma formation at the site of catheterization. Arterial lines, especially in the feline, are not intended for long-term use, as the semiocclusion of an artery by a catheter may result in poor limb perfusion. Although arterial lines do not require a tremendous amount of additional equipment, there is an initial investment of noncompliant tubing and a BP measurement device.

2. Noninvasive blood pressure (NIBP) monitoring

(a) Doppler, cuff, and sphygmomanometer: Using a Doppler, cuff, and sphygmomanometer allows continuous audible HR assessment, and obtains indirect SAP. The Doppler in tandem provides additional assurance that BP obtained with an oscillometric monitor is accurate (Table 2.7, Figures 2.8 and 2.9).

(b) Oscillometric BP monitoring: There are many oscillometric units available, but most operate under the same principles. A distensible cuff is inflated and obstructs blood flow through the artery. As the cuff deflates, the oscillations are detected and reported as systolic, diastolic, and mean BP (Figure 2.10). The methods with which these three pressures are derived vary from manufacturer to manufacturer, but it is safe to say that not every value is

Table 2.7 Obtaining an noninvasive blood pressure reading.

Materials: Clippers, Doppler, BP cuff, ultrasound gel, tape, sphygmomanometer or oscillometric unit

Techniques:

1. Clip area over artery (common areas include radial, dorsal pedal, or coccygeal artery).
2. Fill the crystal (concave side of the Doppler probe) with ultrasound gel; at this point, it is useful to test the Doppler on the anesthetist to ensure it is properly functioning prior to placing it on the patient.
3. Place the crystal over the artery and secure in place with tape. Turn on the Doppler to hear audible heartbeat. If audible heartbeat is not heard, feel for a pulse to confirm patient has heartbeat, and then slight manipulation of the probe under the tape may facilitate an audible sound.
4. Select a BP cuff with a width that is 30–40% of the circumference of the patient's limb and place on the limb proximal to the Doppler (see Figure 2.9).
5. For obtaining a BP using a sphygmomanometer, connect the sphygmomanometer to the BP cuff and inflate cuff until the arterial flow is obstructed (heart sounds are no longer audible on Doppler). Ideally, the inflation pressure is no less than 20–30 mmHg higher than anticipated BP. While watching the gauge, slowly release the sphygmomanometer's pressure until audible heart sounds (arterial flow) are heard. This value is the SAP.
6. For obtaining a BP using an oscillometric unit, following placement of the cuff on the patient's limb proximal to the Doppler, connect the oscillometric unit to the cuff. In some cases, only the cuff supplied by the manufacturer is compatible for use with the oscillometric device. Activate the oscillometric unit by pressing start or inflate. When the BP cuff is inflated, the Doppler noise should disappear, reappearing as pressure is released from the cuff. The complete occlusion of the artery, resulting in cessation of the Doppler heart sounds, is essential for accuracy in oscillometric units. Typically, the anesthetist has the option of selecting an interval (stat, every minute, every 3 minutes, etc.). An oscillometric unit reports systolic, diastolic, and mean arterial pressures.

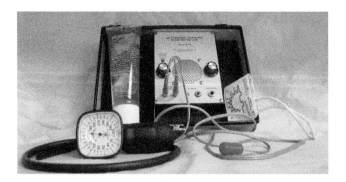

Figure 2.8   Doppler, sphygmomanometer, and blood pressure cuff for obtaining NIBP.

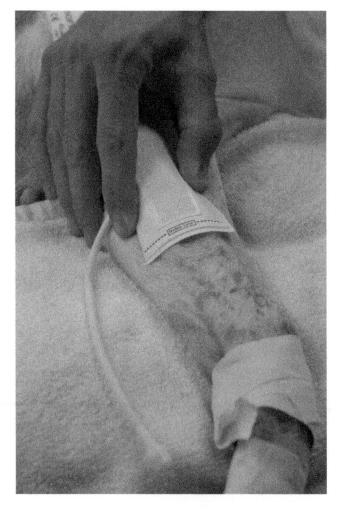

Figure 2.9   Patient with Doppler placed on front limb. The anesthetist is demonstrating how to properly size a BP cuff for the front limb of a canine patient.

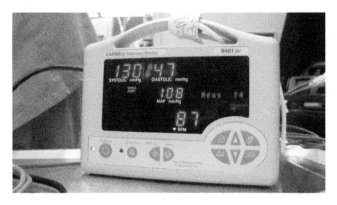

Figure 2.10   Cardell oscillometric BP monitor. *Source:* Midmark Corporation.

actually measured – some are calculated, increasing the room for error and inaccuracy. In general, MAP is usually measured and systolic/diastolic pressures are calculated with a proprietary algorithm.

3. Electrocardiography

Electrocardiography (ECG) allows evaluation of the heart's electrical activity and arrhythmia detection but does not assess structural function of the heart (see Table 2.8 and Figure 2.11 for lead placement). Additionally, the ECG allows the anesthetist to determine the patient's HR. First, the anesthetist must know the paper speed at which the ECG was run. At a 50 mm/s speed, 10 "big" boxes equal 1 second. At a 25 mm/s speed, five "big" boxes equal 1 second. The simple way to estimate HR is to take a standard pen and lay it across the ECG. At a 50 mm/s speed, one pen equals approximately 3 seconds; count the number of complexes that

Table 2.8   Placement of three-lead ECG.

Materials: ECG pads or leads with alligator clips, monitoring unit, conduction gel (ultrasound) or alcohol

Techniques:

1. White lead = right arm (RA)
   Black lead = left arm (LA)
   Red lead = left leg (LL)

2. RA and LA leads are placed at their respective locations on the leg or axial region of the front limb, and the LL is placed caudal to the apex of the heart or on the left hindlimb.

3. Leads need adequate contact with the skin. If electrode pads are used, they may be placed on the pad of the paws; otherwise, a section of hair is shaved and lead is applied. Alligator clips are used, but attention should be paid to placement to avoid traumatic damage to the patient's skin. A conductive gel or alcohol is used with alligator clips.

4. Lead II is the routinely evaluated lead (see Figure 2.11).

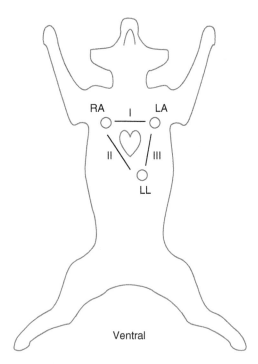

Figure 2.11   Diagram of patient showing electrode placement of a traditional ECG leads I, II, and III.

run the length of the pen and multiple by 20 to get the beats per minute. At a 25 mm/s speed, one pen equals 6 seconds. Count the number of complexes that run the length of the pen and multiple by 10 to calculate the number of beats per minute.

4. Esophageal stethoscope

An esophageal stethoscope is used to audibly quantitate the heartbeat and assess cardiac rhythm (Table 2.9 and Figure 2.12). This device is also useful to assess effective occlusion of a patent ductus arteriosus (PDA).

Table 2.9   Esophageal stethoscope placement.

Techniques:
1. Insert the esophageal stethoscope into the mouth of the anesthetized intubated patient. The stethoscope will pass into the esophagus smoothly if the tongue is pulled forward.
2. Use earpieces to auscultate for a heartbeat as the anesthetist continues to insert the esophageal probe. Continue to advance the probe until the strongest heart sounds are heard.
3. Secure the esophageal probe to the ET tube to avoid dislodgment. The HR and rhythm can be continuously monitored by wearing the earpiece or attaching it to an audio box (see Figure 2.12).

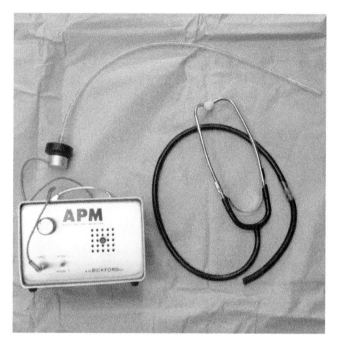

Figure 2.12 Esophageal stethoscope, audible box.

B. Ventilation

1. Capnograph and agent analysis

The capnograph allows evaluation of ventilation and circulation by a display of $EtCO_2$ (Figure 2.13) and assists with error identification, such as obstructions of the airway, leakage of the endotracheal (ET) tube cuff, and rebreathing of CO_2 secondary to equipment malfunctions (Figure 2.14). When $EtCO_2$ is compared with arterial CO_2 ($PaCO_2/PEtCO_2$ gradient), the anesthetist has information regarding alveolar perfusion, ventilation to perfusion (V/Q) mismatching, and venous admixture. Monitoring $EtCO_2$ is also useful in evaluating cardiopulmonary resuscitation (CPR) efforts. Often, one has the option to purchase an agent analyzer that commonly functions as a capnograph as well. The agent analyzer gives the anesthetist inspired and expired inhalant and oxygen concentrations. This assists in the fine-tuning of changes in the anesthetic plane based on expired inhalant concentrations which closely correspond to alveolar concentrations. This analysis also assesses the accuracy of the vaporizer. Table 2.10 compares the differences between mainstream and sidestream capnograph sampling.

2. Oxygenation

Pulse oximetry is commonly referred to as SpO_2. The pulse oximeter uses red and infrared light to measure oxygen saturation of hemoglobin (Hb). Pulse oximeters are available as convenient portable patient-side monitors or as part of a multiparameter monitoring system. Normal values are above 92%. Low readings indicate improper probe placement, hypoxemia, vasoconstriction,

Chapter 2

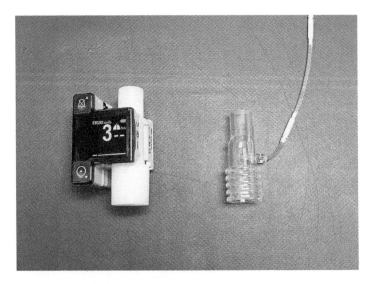

Figure 2.13   (a) Mainstream and (b) sidestream CO_2 analyzers.

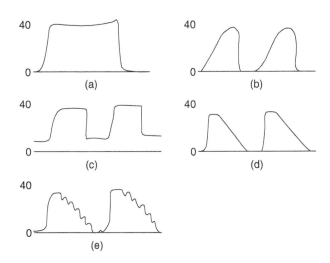

Figure 2.14   Normal (a) capnograph waveform and common abnormal capnograph waveforms, (b) obstructive waveform, (c) rebreathing CO_2, (d) leaks within the breathing circuit or ET tube, (e) cardiac oscillations.

methemoglobinemia, or extreme hypotension. It is also possible for the pulse oximeter to read within a normal range in a patient experiencing carbon monoxide poisoning, although the oxygen saturation is actually low. Readings are also affected by patient motion, external light sources, and prolonged placement of probe in one location. It is ideal to place the probe over nonpigmented skin. Typical areas used are the tongue, webbing between toes, lip, ear, vulva, or prepuce. Pulse oximeters with a plethysmograph display of the pulse amplitude allow the user to visualize the presence of a pulse, ensuring the oximeter is reading accurately.

Table 2.10   Comparison of mainstream and sidestream capnograph units.

Mainstream		Sidestream	
Advantages	**Disadvantages**	**Advantages**	**Disadvantages**
"Real" time Does not produce waste gas, does not require scavenging Easy to calibrate Respiratory secretions are not an issue due to the use of infrared technology measuring CO_2 levels	Bulky unit placed on the end of the ET tube Adaptor is expensive to replace Difficult to clean	Minimal bulk to the end of the ET tube Adaptor is inexpensive Submersible for easy cleaning	Delay in display secondary to sampling Increased possibility of sample contamination Requires scavenging of waste gas Difficult to calibrate in-house Requires respiratory secretions to be trapped in Nafion tubing or a water trap to avoid inaccuracies or failure of the system

3. Perfusion Index (PI) and Plethysmograph Variability (PVI)

PI reflects the amplitude of the pulse oximeter waveform, used as an indicator of perfusion. PVI measures the changes in PI over time within the respiratory cycle; it uses the plethysmograph waveform as a tool to assess fluid resuscitation. This is in the process of being validated in veterinary species to optimize goal-directed fluid therapy.

C. Thermoregulation

1. Temperature probes

Esophageal temperature probes work nicely to give continuous, accurate monitoring of core body temperature. Once the ET tube is securely in place, the tongue of the patient is drawn rostrally and the temperature probe is guided into the esophagus. There should be little to no resistance until the gastroesophageal sphincter is encountered; the anesthetist need not advance the probe beyond the distal third of the esophagus and so the temperature probe should reside rostral to the gastroesophageal sphincter. Further advancement may increase the potential for regurgitation.

   Rectal temperature probes work well as an alternative, if the anesthetist is unable to use an esophageal temperature probe; however, continuous monitoring is not as easily accomplished due to fecal accumulation and difficult access during a surgical procedure.

2. Devices for patient warming

Sedated and anesthetized patients lack the ability to move away from things such as warming devices. This makes the ideal warming device one that circulates heated air, water, or other heating distributed across a large surface area such as a blanket (Box 2.11). It is also

---

Box 2.11 Safe patient warming devices

- *Circulating warm water blanket*: this device typically goes underneath the patient and uses a water reservoir pump with the blanket. Disadvantages include unequal distribution of heat and limited temperature range. Additionally, the blankets are subject to frequent leaks and are relatively expensive to replace.
- *Fluid warmers* are used to warm the patient's fluid line prior to entry into the IV catheter. This device is relatively inexpensive and reusable. However, it is also bulky and not effective alone to correct hypothermia.
- *Forced air warmers (FAW, e.g., Bair Hugger®)*: common in practice, these devices are effective at prewarming and rewarming patients. The placement of this device has tremendous flexibility (around, under, or above the patient). It is advisable to turn this device off until the patient/sterile field is draped into surgery. It is best to use this with intended FAW blankets or it could cause thermal burns.
- *Heated breathing circuits (e.g., Darvall)*: these circuits are used to warm inhaled gases being delivered to the patient; while they are not effective alone, they can prevent worsened heat loss. It is important these circuits are not wrapped around a patient as this can lead to thermal burns.
- *Low-flow anesthesia (rates of 5–10 mL/kg on a rebreathing circuit, with a minimum of 500 mL/min when using nonprecision veterinary anesthesia machines)*: this is a technique, rather than a device, to prevent worsened hypothermia. Low oxygen flow rates during maintenance of general anesthesia will minimize heat loss through evaporation. This also decreases the amount of oxygen and inhalant anesthetic used, and decreases the amount of waste gas generated. One must also be aware that to facilitate rapid changes in anesthetic depth, it is necessary to turn the flow rate up.
- *Restrictive polymer device (e.g., Hot Dog®)*: This device is a conductive pad with temperature sensors throughout the blanket. Like the FAW, the placement of this device has tremendous flexibility (around, under, or above the patient). The reusability of the blankets reduces cost of upkeep. However, when equipment needs to be replaced, it is expensive, and blankets require a specific cleaner which is not peroxide based. If cautery is used, the device needs to be at medium setting.

---

advantageous for a device to have a constant temperature unless adjusted by a technician or veterinarian. Although patient warming devices are effective to rewarm patients, simple things like plastic covering and socks, bubble wrap, or cling wrap on extremities are inexpensive and easily used to maintain temperature (although they will seldom raise temperature).

Devices including heating pads, warm water bottles, or reusable discs are not recommended as the heat generated may result in thermal burns.

D. *Blood gas analysis*

Blood gas (or acid–base) analysis allows the anesthetist to evaluate the pH of the patient and partial pressure of important respiratory gases (oxygen and carbon dioxide). Blood gas analysis allows identification of V/Q mismatch or shunting (see Chapter 3). Depending on the machine used to perform this analysis, additional information such as electrolytes, glucose, hematocrit, and lactate is also obtained (Table 2.11).

Table 2.11 Normal arterial blood gas values for canine and feline patients.

	Dogs	Cats[a]
pH	7.36–7.46	7.32–7.42
$PaCO_2$ (mmHg)	38–48	32–42
PaO_2[b] (mmHg)	80–110	80–115
HCO_3 (mEq/L)	19–27	16–24
BE (mEq/L)	(–4)–4	(–6)–2

[a]Normal cats may have CO_2 and pH values lower than those provided here.
[b]PaO_2 depends on fraction of oxygen delivered (FiO_2).

1. Collecting a blood sample

To obtain a blood sample for evaluation of oxygenation, arterial sampling is necessary. For most other parameters, a venous sample is adequate. If an arterial sample is not possible, use a blood sample from the lingual vasculature; arterial and venous anastomosis is present. This is not entirely representative but gives more useful information than a venous sample in regard to oxygenation. The syringe is heparinized to avoid clot formation, which damages the analyzer and gives inaccurate results. Make sure air bubbles are removed from the sample, and it is capped to avoid exposure to air. Run the sample according to the analyzer manufacturer directions. If electrolytes are analyzed, use of a lithium heparin syringe is advised.

For more information on interpretating abnormal blood gases, please see Chapter 3.

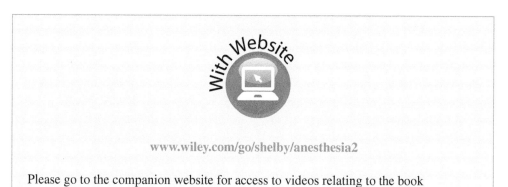

www.wiley.com/go/shelby/anesthesia2

Please go to the companion website for access to videos relating to the book

References

1. Dorsch J, Dorsch S. *Understanding Anesthesia Equipment*, 2nd edn. Baltimore, MD: Williams & Wilkins; 1975.
2. Eger E, Epstein R. Hazards of anesthetic equipment. Anesthesiology. 1964;25:490–504.
3. Eichhorn V, Trepte C, Richter HP et al. Respiratory systolic variation test in acutely impaired cardiac function for predicting volume responsiveness in pigs. Br J Anaesth. 2011;106(5):659–64.

Chapter 3

Adverse events/anesthetic complications

Carolyn M. McKune and Angela Borchers

Chapter 3

Even in patients deemed healthy, anesthesia is not always uneventful. In fact, when broken down by ASA status (see Chapter 1), even patients considered ASA 1–2 have a risk of death of 0.05% (canine) and 0.11% (feline). This equates to roughly 1 in 2000 dogs and 1 in every 875 cats, who are healthy enough to assign a low ASA score, actually dying within 48 hours of anesthesia. When evaluating patients with higher risk (ASA 3–5), that number jumps significantly to between 1.33% (canine) and 1.4% (feline), or approximately 1 in every 75 dogs and cats which die within 48 hours of anesthesia [1]. Given these odds, which are far worse than human anesthetic risk odds, it stands to reason that even in the healthy patient, complications occur. It is not always death which is the result of anesthetic complications; up to 6% of cases which experienced an adverse event required management in the intensive care unit (ICU) in one study [2].

This section describes complications encountered during anesthesia and recovery, their potential consequences, causes and treatments. Complications are mitigated when they are anticipated and appropriately addressed. To minimize adverse outcomes during anesthesia, it is recommended that a thorough preanesthetic workup is performed and a trained, experienced member of the veterinary team is dedicated to continuously monitoring anesthesia and recovery (see Chapter 1). It is important to have dedicated monitoring (even in the healthy patient) to help with early recognition of complications; indeed, in one study, up to 63% of cases had anesthetic safety events mitigated by the intervention of a knowledgeable anesthetist [3].

Some of the most common complications experienced during routine procedures include breakthrough pain, bradycardia, hypotension, hypoventilation, and hypothermia due to anesthesia's physiologically deregulating effects. It is imperative to monitor for these problems during any anesthetic event. Other aspects of the patient and the procedure will determine which additional complications the anesthetist prepares for.

I. Cardiovascular complications

Arrhythmias frequently present in the anesthetized patient. Often anesthetic and analgesic drugs, as well as preexisting cardiovascular disease, perpetuate arrhythmias. The use of an electrocardiogram (ECG) to monitor the heart's electrical activity is important in confirming

Table 3.1   Systematic evaluation of electrocardiogram.

Method
1. What is the heart rate, and are the atria and ventricles beating at the same rate?
2. Are the atrial and ventricular rhythms regular?
3. What is the relation between the P wave (if present) and the QRS complex?
4. How are the P, QRS and T waves configured?

arrhythmias, which occur in up to 5.8% of cases [2]. A Doppler is a helpful tool as well. A systematic approach to ECG evaluation helps to determine which arrhythmia the anesthetist faces (Table 3.1).

A. Sinus bradycardia

Sinus bradycardia is one of the most common anesthetic complications experienced, and likely is a result of high vagal tone [4], coupled with the (thankfully) ubiquitous use of opioids (Figure 3.1). This arrhythmia has a normal sinus rhythm (P wave for every QRS, QRS for every P) but the heart rate (HR) is slower than the patient's normal resting HR. Typically, in dogs, this is less than 60 beats per minute (bpm) and 100–120 bpm in cats; however, the patient's normal resting HR is considered when determining bradycardia. The prevalence of bradycardia significantly increases in certain disease conditions, with up to 21.6% of cats presenting for urethral obstruction also having concurrent bradycardia (presumably due to hyperkalemia) [5]. In dogs, up to 36.3% of retrospectively reviewed anesthesia cases reported bradycardia as a complication [6].

1. *Consequences*: Sinus bradycardia is not always detrimental. However, bradycardia causes a reduction in cardiac output (CO), resulting in decreased blood pressure (BP) and organ perfusion. Additionally, if left untreated, it may develop into more adverse arrhythmias.
2. *Causes*: Sinus bradycardia is secondary to drugs used during anesthesia, including opioids, alpha-2 agonists, and beta-blockers. Other causes include high vagal tone and hypothermia.
3. *Treatment*: Not all sinus bradycardias require treatment. The anesthetist determines if the bradycardia is affecting CO and perfusion. If CO and perfusion are compromised, immediate treatment is required. Anticholinergics (atropine or glycopyrrolate) are administered IV or IM depending on urgency. Depending on the nature of the case, having an anticholineregic drawn and ready is appropriate. For example, in dogs undergoing hemilaminectomies, up to 24.6% required pharmacologic intervention for heart rate correction [7]. Atropine is faster

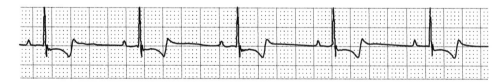

Figure 3.1   Sinus bradycardia in a dog. 25 mm/s, from an automated monitor.

Chapter 3

acting but has a shorter duration than glycopyrrolate; however, glycopyrrolate produces fewer tachyarrhythmias. While not recommended for routine use as a premedication [8], anticholinergics are given preemptively for patients who are suspected to have high vagal tone (brachycephalic patients, gastrointestinal [GI] disease, etc.) and when sinus brady-cardia is induced by opioids or beta-blockers. Opioids are reversed if necessary. Caution is exercised in the administration of anticholinergics to treat sinus bradycardia caused by alpha-2 agonists. Reversal of the alpha-2 agonist is recommended to alleviate possible vasoconstriction (bearing in mind this will also reverse any analgesia and minimum alveolar concentration [MAC]-sparing effects). If the HR does not increase following reversal, an anticholinergic is administered. Patients who are hypothermic (less than 92 °F) are unlikely to respond to anticholinergics. Aggressive warming of the patient is warranted.

B. Atrial ventricular (AV) block

Atrial ventricular block results from a delay or disruption in the conductance of depolarization between the sinus atrial (SA) node and the atrial ventricular (AV) node. First-degree AV block is characterized by a prolonged P-R interval; however, all atrial impulses are conducted to the ventricle. Second-degree AV block is characterized by intermittent conduction from the SA node to the AV node, resulting in "dropped beats" or absent QRS complexes following P waves (Figure 3.2). Second-degree AV block is further classified into Mobitz type I and Mobitz type II based on assessment of the P-R interval. A progressively prolonged P-R interval is characteristic of Mobitz type I, whereas an unchanged P-R interval but failure of normal conduction is characteristic of Mobitz type II. Third-degree AV block is a complete disassociation between the SA and AV node. The SA node has a consistent yet independent rate from the ventricle, which often conducts an escape rhythm (see Figure 3.2).

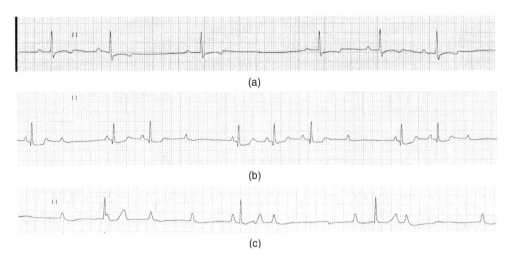

(a)

(b)

(c)

Figure 3.2   (a) First-degree AV block, 50 mm/s, 10 mm/mV. (b) Second-degree AV block, 50 mm/s, 10 mm/mV. (c) Third degree AV block, 50 mm/s, 10 mm/mV in canine patient. *Source:* Courtesy of Jorge L. Vila.

1. *Consequences*: Under anesthesia, any conduction disturbance results in a decrease in CO, because the compensatory mechanisms present when a patient is conscious are diminished (if not absent). However, the degree to which the cardiovascular system is impacted varies based on the form of AV block, with the most serious impacts resulting from high-grade second-degree and third-degree AV block.
2. *Causes*: Anesthetic drugs, including opioids, alpha-2 agonists, calcium channel blockers, and beta-blockers, may result in first- and second-degree AV block. Electrolyte abnormalities (such as hyperkalemia) and hypothermia result in bradycardia, as does increased vagal tone (for example, in patients with GI disease [9]). Second-degree AV block also occurs in extremely athletic patients, following low doses of anticholinergic administration [10], and secondary to arrhythmias like atrial flutter or fibrillation. Third-degree AV block in small animals occurs for a variety of reasons, including infectious diseases such as Chagas disease or Lyme disease, or neoplastic disease. In humans, there appears to be a genetic basis [11].
3. *Treatment*: The first line of treatment in cases of first- and second-degree blocks is the administration of anticholinergics. Third-degree AV block is diagnosed based on failure to respond to an atropine challenge and ECG analysis. Administering anticholinergics to patients with third-degree AV block is unlikely to produce a reliable increase in HR (although it is often attempted). In cases of third-degree AV block where anesthesia is indicated, placement of a pacemaker is necessary. Placement of an introducer and temporary pacemaker or external pacing provides control of the HR during short elective procedures or for placement of a permanent pacemaker. A constant-rate infusion (CRI) of isoproterenol will increase the HR in cases where a temporary pacemaker is not an option (see Drug Formulary).

C. Bundle branch blocks

Bundle branch block (BBB) results from abnormal conduction between the bundle of His and the Purkinje fibers of the ventricles. BBB affects the right, left or both branches of the conduction pathway. This rhythm is often mistaken for a pathologic ventricular arrhythmia although its origin is above the ventricle, as evidenced by P waves preceding each wide QRS complex (particularly a wide or "slurred" S wave; Figure 3.3). Auscultation of a right BBB may have a split second heart sound.

1. *Consequences*: Most dogs with BBB are minimally affected and do not require treatment. Under anesthesia, however, it is prudent to monitor BP to ensure hemodynamics are unchanged.
2. *Causes*: Myocardial fibrosis or ischemic damage may result in BBB. BBB may also manifest after procedures such as pulmonic balloon valvuloplasty.
3. *Treatment*: This rhythm itself needs no treatment. However, it is ideal to have a cardiovascular workup including an ECG prior to anesthesia to identify any underlying cardiovascular disease, predisposing to BBB. If the patient is hypotensive during anesthesia, positive inotropes and MAC-sparing drugs (e.g., opioid CRI) coupled with MAC reduction are useful to maintain BP. Fluid therapy is adjusted accordingly depending on underlying heart disease.

Chapter 3

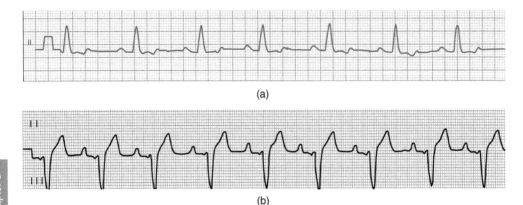

(a)

(b)

Figure 3.3 (a) LBBB, 50 mm/s, 10 mm/mV. (b) RBBB, 50 mm/s, 10 mm/mV. *Source:* Courtesy of Jorge L. Vila.

D. Atrial flutter and fibrillation

These arrhythmias are remarkably fast supraventricular tachycardias (Figure 3.4a). Atrial rates of greater than 350 bpm and 500 bpm occur with atrial flutter and fibrillation, respectively. These arrhythmias result from disorganized reentrant pathways which are then filtered by the AV node. Atrial flutter has a characteristic "saw tooth" baseline appearance of F waves. Atrial fibrillation has no distinguishable P waves, is irregularly irregular, and has a "wavy" baseline (Figure 3.4b).

1. *Consequences*: Atrial flutter and fibrillation have some adverse outcomes, including decreased CO, stroke volume (SV), and perfusion, and sudden death [12].

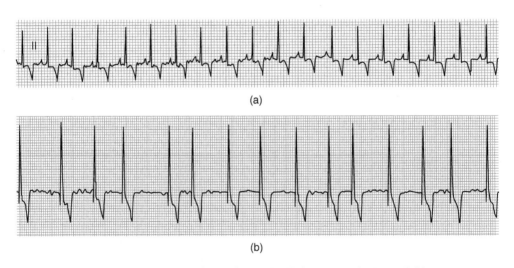

(a)

(b)

Figure 3.4 (a) SVT, 25 mm/s, 10 mm/mV. (b) Atrial fibrillation, 25 mm/s, 10 mm/mV. *Source:* Courtesy of Jorge L. Vila.

2. *Causes*: The cause of atrial fibrillation and flutter in a patient may be unknown, but ruling out congestive heart failure (CHF), dilated cardiomyopathy (DCM), and digoxin toxicity is warranted with a thorough cardiac workup.
3. *Treatment*: If there is an underlying cause for the arrhythmia, it is prudent to address and resolve this prior to anesthesia. If the arrhythmia manifests itself under anesthesia, the HR and hemodynamic consequences will help to determine the need for intervention. If rate control is necessary, esmolol is a selective ultra-short-acting beta-1-blocker metabolized by plasma esterases and thus has a short half-life. A bolus dose of 0.05–0.1 mg/kg is administered followed by a CRI of 6–24 mg/kg/h, if necessary. Cardioconversion using a defibrillator is useful when atrial fibrillation is unresponsive to pharmacologic intervention, and quality of life is impacted.

E. Ventricular arrhythmias

The ventricles are capable of generating impulses to pace the heart, although this rate is much slower (40–60 bpm) than the rhythm generated by the SA node, as it does not use the normal conduction pathway but rather conducts from cell to cell. Simple ventricular premature complexes (VPCs) result in a wide, bizarre appearance to the QRS, with no P waves (Figure 3.5b).

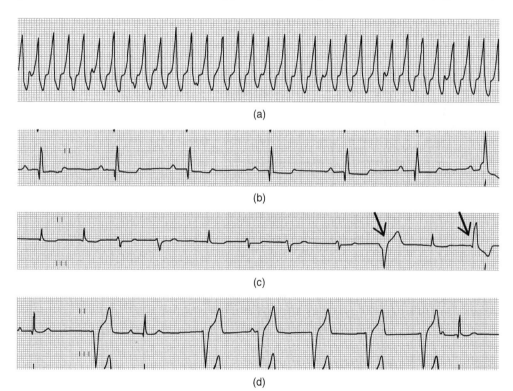

(a)

(b)

(c)

(d)

Figure 3.5   (a) VT, 50 mm/s, 10 mm/mV. (b) Uniform VPCs, 50 mm/s, 10 mm/mV. (c) Multiform VPCs (large arrow), 50 mm/s, 5 mm/mV. (d) AIVR, 50 mm/s, 5 mm/mV. *Source:* Courtesy of Jorge L. Vila.

VPCs are classified as uniform (similar in appearance) or multiform (varying in appearance). A ventricular rhythm with a rate above 160–180 bpm in dogs or 220 bpm in cats is classified as ventricular tachycardia (VT; Figure 3.5a). Accelerated idioventricular rhythm (AIVR) is a ventricular rhythm with a rate between a normal sinus rate and VT (usually 100–140 bpm). Distinguishing between VT and AIVR is important because VT may respond to lidocaine, whereas AIVR will not. Sustained VT lasts longer than 30 seconds, whereas nonsustained VT is less than 30 seconds, and thus may not require treatment.

1. *Consequences*: Runs of VPCs and sustained VT result in a decrease in ventricular filling time, leading to a decrease in SV and CO. This compromises perfusion, leading to tissue hypoxia, lactic acidosis, myocardial hypoxia, and additional cardiac arrhythmias. Sudden death may also result from sustained VT. Multiform VPCs and fast sustained VT may deteriorate into ventricular fibrillation (VF), a life-threatening emergency.
2. *Causes*: Hypoxemia, electrolyte abnormalities (hypokalemia, hypomagnesemia, hypocalcemia), acid–base imbalances, pain, and sympathetic stimulation are leading causes of VPCs and VT under anesthesia. Primary cardiac disease, such as myocarditis, endocarditis, and cardiomyopathy, may result in ventricular arrhythmias as well. Ventricular arrhythmias might also occur in patients with certain systemic diseases, such as splenic masses or gastric dilation-volvulus (GDV).
3. *Treatment*: The first step for most complications is to identify and correct any contributing cause. For example, VT or runs of VPCs from hypoxemia usually resolve if the patient receives supplemental oxygenation. AIVR or the occasional uniform VPC rarely requires treatment. VPCs only require treatment if they meet the certain criteria (Table 3.2). Indeed, treatment of VPCs without the above criteria is often unsuccessful, because lidocaine (our first line of treatment for ventricular tachyarrhythmias other than ventricular flutter or fibrillation) relies on the presence of abnormal Na^+ channels to work effectively. Recommended treatments of ventricular rhythms are listed in Table 3.3.

F. Cardiac arrest rhythms: asystole, pulseless electrical activity (PEA), and ventricular fibrillation (VF)

Cardiac arrest rhythms are terminal arrhythmias. Asystole, classically known as a "flat line," indicates there is no electrical activity occurring in the heart. PEA occurs when an ECG tracing is present – and may even look somewhat normal – but on palpation, there is no pulse present. In VF, there is no electrical organization to the heart, creating a chaotic ECG (Figure 3.6). Coarse VF may deteriorate into fine VF; however, coarse fibrillation responds

Table 3.2 Criteria for determining treatment of ventricular premature complexes (VPCs).

Multiform in appearance
Heart rate is greater than 160 bpm
Runs of VPCs occur (more than 30 in a minute)
R on T phenomenon occurs
There is compromise to the rest of the hemodynamic system (such as low blood pressure when VPCs occurs)

Table 3.3   Treatment of ventricular rhythms.

AIVR	VT, multiform or runs of VPCs		VF or unresponsive/ sustained VT
	Dogs	**Cats**	
No treatment may be necessary	Lidocaine 1–2 mg/kg IV followed by 3–6 mg/kg/h CRI	Lidocaine 0.25–0.5 mg/kg IV slowly; repeat up to twice more as needed	Defibrillation: External 2–4 J/kg Internal 0.2–0.4 J/kg Amiodarone 5 mg/kg IV/IO
Glycopyrrolate 0.01 mg/kg IV	Procainamide 5–10 mg/ kg IV followed by 1.5–3 mg/kg/h CRI	Esmolol 0.2–0.5 mg/kg IV, CRI 1.5–12 mg/kg/h	
Dobutamine 0.3– 0.6 mg/kg/r IV		Propranolol 0.02 mg/kg slow IV; dose is repeated up to four times	

AIVR, accelerated idioventricular rhythm; CRI, constant-rate infusion; IO, intraosseous; IV, intravenous; VF, ventricular fibrillation; VPC, ventricular premature complex; VT, ventricular tachycardia.

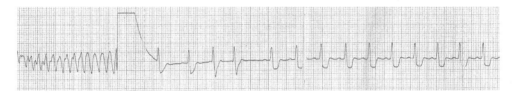

Figure 3.6   VF converted to ventricular rhythm following external defibrillation, 25 mm/s. *Source:* Courtesy of Jorge L. Vila.

better to electrical defibrillation. Therefore, rapid recognition and treatment are crucial to a successful intervention.

1. *Consequences*: There is no coordinated mechanical function of the heart, and thus no circulation or perfusion to any organ, with all three rhythms.
2. *Causes*: Asystole and PEA have numerous causes, and occur without warning even in healthy patients under anesthesia. Heart disease (such as DCM), acid–base and electrolyte abnormalities, as well as sepsis, are leading causes of VF.
3. *Treatment*: When perfusion to the body ceases, the brain no longer receives oxygen. Thus, immediate recognition and treatment (i.e., CPR) are critical components not only for a successful return to spontaneous circulation, but to discharging the patient. RECOVER guidelines support beginning CPR in all patients who have cardiac arrested (or are suspected to have cardiac arrested), without pausing to palate for a pulse [13] (see Appendix B), although it is the authors' recommendation to utilize 5 seconds or less to assess supporting monitoring (EtCO$_2$, Doppler, SpO$_2$ for wave form) if the patient is under anesthesia, as a rapid confirmation. Additionally, life-saving treatment for VF is electrical

defibrillation [14]. However, few veterinarians have a defibrillator readily available and charged. Therefore, it is most practical if CPR is initiated immediately with high-quality cardiac compressions, while the defibrillator is positioned and charged. It is important to understand that the action of the defibrillator is to either stop electrical fibrillation of the heart (i.e., "flatline", so hopefully normal electrical conduction returns) or to generate a normal sinus rhythm. It is the current recommendation in humans receiving defibrillation to deliver one large shock rather than incrementally increasing the dose delivered; this is because it is important to minimize the time between interruptions of chest compressions [15]. Dose for external defibrillation is 2–4 J/kg or 0.2–0.4 J/kg internally. An immediate return to chest compressions is imperative to oxygenate the myocardium and increase success of resuscitation.

G. Isorhythmic dissociation

This conduction disturbance in the cat is often observed under anesthesia [16]. Fortunately, it is rarely associated with any disease. The arrhythmia is characterized by a P and QRS which are unassociated, so one will observe the P wave "wandering" back and forth through the preceding or following QRS. The rate of the atria and ventricle are the same.

1. *Consequences*: There are no pathologic consequences of this arrhythmia.
2. *Causes*: While this arrhythmia commonly manifests under anesthesia, it occurs in the awake feline as well. A definitive cause is unknown, although cats being aliens is suspected.
3. *Treatment*: This arrhythmia is benign and requires no treatment. There is some suggestion that increasing sinus rate by the use of anticholinergics may correct this.

II. Blood pressure

A. Hypertension

Hypertension is defined as systolic arterial pressure (SAP) over 160 mmHg [17]; no consensus guidelines of mean arterial pressure associated with hypertension are available. Hypertension is rarely seen under anesthesia due to the vasodilatory effect of most anesthetic drugs, only occurring in about 1.7% of cases [2]. It is important to identify if the patient has preexisting hypertension, in order to work up the underlying cause, and because this helps to direct what target pressure under anesthesia should be.

1. *Consequences*: Prolonged hypertension damages many vital organs, such as the kidney and brain. High BP does not necessarily ensure improved perfusion. Hypertension as a result of increased systemic vascular resistance (SVR) may cause states of decreased perfusion and tissue hypoxia.
2. *Causes*: Systemic diseases including renal disease, diabetes mellitus, intracranial diseases with a secondary Cushing reflex (see Chapter 5), hyperthyroidism, hyperadrenocorticism (i.e., Cushing disease), and pheochromocytomas all result in hypertension. Hypertension occurring under anesthesia in a previously normotensive patient requires two primary rule-outs: a light plane of anesthesia or a physiologic response, most often to noxious stimuli. Noxious stimuli and light anesthesia occur in a significant number of patients [2].

Table 3.4 Treatment options for hypertension.

1. Increase gas inhalant
2. Administer low dose of vasodilator such as 0.005–0.01 mg/kg intravenous acepromazine
3. Nitroprusside constant-rate infuson 0.06–0.3 mg/kg/h

Note: One should use nitroprusside with extreme caution and only if necessary. See Chapter 7 "Nitroprusside," p.346.

3. *Treatment*: Invasive blood pressure (IBP) monitoring is recommended (see Chapter 2) to ensure accuracy of therapeutic interventions, for patients with hypertension identified pre-operatively. Management of, or at the very least awareness of, diseases known to increase BP in a patient prior to anesthesia is crucial to understanding the management of hypertension during anesthesia. If hypertension persists from an underlying disease, and becomes severe, intervention may be necessary (Table 3.4). If one is unsure whether a preexisting condition exists, it is helpful to watch for trends in BP. Patients who are hypertensive from a preexisting disease are often consistently hypertensive. Using good technique to assess anesthetic depth (see Chapter 1) will allow the anesthetist to adjust the anesthetic plane accordingly. If the anesthetic depth is adequate, no preexisting disease exists, and the BP is increased, noxious stimuli are addressed. Analgesia in the dog is provided with the use of either a bolus or CRI of opioids, local anesthetics, or an NMDA antagonist; or, if the patient is already receiving a CRI, the dosage is increased or something extra is added. See "noxious stimuli" on p. 86 for information on the cat. Chapter 7 details regional analgesic techniques that are also beneficial for prevention of nociception.

B. Hypotension

Hypotension is one of the most common complications experienced during anesthesia [18], occurring in anywhere between 10.5% and 37.9% of cases [2,6]. This number climbs significantly depending on the comorbidities a patient may have; for example, in a study evaluating phacoemulsification performed in diabetic or nondiabetic dogs, diabetic patients were far more likely to experience moderate to severe hypotension than their nondiabetic counterparts [19]. Dogs undergoing hepatic surgery with or without cholecystectomies experienced hypotension in anywhere from 66% to 74% of cases [20]; cats undergoing biliary tract surgery fared worse than their canine counterparts, with a case series describing five cats which experienced unresponsive and persistent hypotension without blood loss, and postoperative renal failure [21]. Dogs undergoing hemilaminectomy for severe, acute thoracolumbar disc herniation experienced hypotension in 59% of cases [22].

In a survey of diplomates of the American or European College of Veterinary Anesthesia and Analgesia (DACVAA or DECVAA, respectively), consensus was that hypotension is defined as a MAP of 62 +/– 4 mmHg, or in cases were MAP is not evaluated (i.e., when using only a Doppler and sphygmomanometer), a SAP less than 87 +/– 8 mmHg. This same group of DACVAAs or DECVAAs agreed that intervention was best performed when MAPs were less than 61 +/– 4 mmHg or 85 +/– 13 mmHg in surgical cases [23].

Perfusion of the body is dependent on oxygen content of the blood (see "Hypoxemia," p. 66) and CO. CO is seldom measured in routine anesthesia cases; gold standards for CO measurement (i.e., dilutional techniques) require invasive equipment (i.e., pulmonary arterial catheter). Instead, knowing that CO is defined by HR, contractility, preload, and afterload, veterinarians often choose to measure a more readily available means of hemodynamic evaluation, BP, which gives information about afterload. It is important, however, that the anesthetist keep the "big picture" in mind; during anesthesia, we are ultimately striving for perfusion of organs, and BP evaluation is only one (albeit very important) part of the puzzle (Figure 3.7).

1. *Consequences*: Hypotension results in decreased perfusion to vital organs (heart, brain, kidneys, skeletal muscle, etc.). This may lead to tissue hypoxemia, anaerobic metabolism, lactic acidosis, and organ damage. The kidneys are highly susceptible to this kind of damage [21], especially given the confounding nature of additional drugs administered around the perioperative period for patient comfort (e.g., nonsteroidal antiinflammatory drugs, NSAIDs).

2. *Causes*: Hypotension is primarily caused by a decrease in SVR ("vasodilation") and decreased contractility ("cardiovascular depression") from anesthetic agents such as propofol and inhalant anesthetics. Hypotension is also the result of a decrease in CO secondary to bradycardia or hypovolemia (e.g., dehydration or blood loss) resulting in a decreased preload and thus stroke volume. Attempts are made to correct these abnormalities prior to anesthesia.

3. *Treatment*: The anesthetist must always anticipate hypotension due to the routine use of anesthetic agents and gas inhalants. Treatment of hypotension is based on the underlying cause and is approached systematically (Table 3.5). If the patient is dehydrated or anemic, interventions are made prior to anesthesia (preferably) with the administration of fluids or blood products. In the cat, thoughtful use of fluids is recommended, as up to 15.5% of apparently healthy cats actually have underlying cardiovascular disease [24]. Evaluation of HR is important. CO is dependent on HR; as a result, hypotension manifests because of reduced CO secondary to bradycardia. When administering drugs known to result in bradycardia (i.e., fentanyl) to patients in a laboratory setting where CO was monitored, even in cases of normotension, CO decreased with a decrease in HR [25]. Positive inotropes such as dopamine and dobutamine are commonly used as CRIs to increase contractility. As the dose of dopamine increases, so will SVR (however, this is not the case with dobutamine). Positive inotropes are initiated prior to the use of vasopressors because of their ability to increase contractility with minimal vasoconstriction at low to moderate

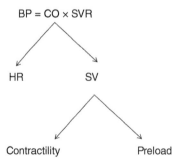

Figure 3.7   Blood pressure equation.

Table 3.5 Treatment options for hypotension in the otherwise healthy patient.

1. Minimize effect of inhalants.
   (a) Check anesthetic depth of the patient. If the gas inhalant can be reduced, do so.
   (b) Add MAC-sparing drug support such as CRIs of opioids, lidocaine or ketamine where appropriate, to reduce MAC.
2. Administration of fluids or blood products.[a]
   (a) Isotonic crystalloids are given as a bolus of 5–20 mL/kg IV.
   (b) Hypertonic saline at 3–5 mL/kg IV with concurrent isotonic crystalloids.
   (c) Colloids at 2–5 mL/kg IV. Not to exceed 20 mL/kg/day in dogs; 10 mL/kg/day in cats. This should be used only as a last resort, as mounting evidence suggests possible increase in mortality and acute kidney injury secondary to the use of colloids [69].
3. Treat bradycardia if present.
   (a) Reverse alpha-2 agonists.
   (b) Atropine 0.02 mg/kg (can double if no response) IV or glycopyrrolate 0.01 mg/kg IV.
4. Inotropic/vasopressor support (see Drug Formulary).
   (a) Dopamine or dobutamine CRI.
   (b) Bolus or CRI of phenylephrine, vasopressin, epinephrine or ephedrine.
   (c) Norepinephrine CRI.
5. Discontinue MV.
6. Abort procedure until patient is better stabilized.

[a]See "Hemorrhage/blood loss" for information regarding administration of blood products, 64.
CRI, constant-rate infusion; IV, intravenous; MAC, minimum alveolar concentration; MV, mechanical ventilation.

doses. Each animal has a variable response to dopamine or dobutamine, meaning that the dosage of drug is tailored to each patient [26]. It is important to note that in some patients, an increase in contractility is absolutely indicated (such as the dog with DCM) while in others it is absolutely contraindicated (cats with hypertrophic cardiomyopathy [HCM] who already have a remarkable increase in myocardial workload). In cases where positive inotropes are ineffective, only marginally effective or contraindicated, vasopressors are used to support BP. Common vasopressors include phenylephrine, vasopressin, norepinephrine, and epinephrine. The risk of using vasopressors is tightening vascular tone too profoundly, resulting in decreased perfusion to vital tissues. The anesthetist may not know a decrease in perfusion is occurring because the BP values will be normal. Therefore, if vasopressive drugs are utilized, it is imperative to monitor lactate levels. If lactate values exceed 2.0 mMol/L, these drugs are reduced or discontinued, as they are likely reducing perfusion to vital organs, although they are creating desirable numbers. Mechanical ventilation (MV) negatively impacts BP by worsening hemodynamics. MV fills the thorax with positive pressure, which collapses weak-walled vessels (e.g., the vena cava), reducing the returning blood to the heart (thus reducing preload). While MV effectively addresses hypoventilation and may improve delivery of oxygen to the lungs under anesthesia, this oxygen is saturated with inhalant, which results in inadvertent "overdosing" of a patient and worsening contractility. Finally, MV will reduce CO_2, which peripherally (although *not* centrally) will stimulate catecholamine release. This lack of catecholamine stimulation will worsen hemodynamics. In cases where the anesthetist has taken all the above steps and hemodynamics are still compromised, the surgeon is counseled to terminate the procedure as quickly as possible so anesthesia is discontinued expeditiously.

Table 3.6   Maximum blood loss estimations.

2 × 2 sponge/gauze	5 mL
4 × 4 sponge/gauze	10 mL
Laparotomy sponge	100 mL
Suction jar	See equation 3.1

Note: These are estimations with sponges completely soaked. Weighing soiled sponges and subtracting weight of unsoiled is more accurate at estimating blood loss.

C. Blood loss/hemorrhage

During a surgical event, hemorrhage is difficult to estimate accurately. It is important to have a preoperative assessment of packed cell volume (PCV), total proteins (TP), hemoglobin (Hb), and hydration. Volume replacement is imperative even for low-level losses, because CO relies on effective circulating volume (ECV). Volume replacement is initially achieved with crystalloid fluid therapy. However, as blood loss increases and hemodynamics begin to suffer, a transfusion is warranted. The total blood volume estimation based on a normovolemic patient for a dog is 80–90 mL/kg or 8% of total body weight and 50–60 mL/kg or 6% of total body weight in the cat. The PCV of the patient may not reflect the total blood loss the patient has experienced, due to splenic contraction [27]. Also, a decrease in total proteins may result from dilution secondary to fluid therapy, so sometimes an educated assessment of the patient is necessary. Blood loss estimation is accomplished by evaluation of soaked gauze squares, lap sponges, and suction collection jars. Estimations are made by adding the number of soaked sponges following assumptions in Table 3.6 or, more accurately, by weighing the sponges and subtracting the weight of unsoiled sponges (1 g = 1 mL of blood).

Equation 3.1 Blood loss estimation from suction jar.

$$\frac{\text{PCV of suction jar}}{\text{Pre-op PCV of patient}} \times \text{Volume of suction jar} = \text{estimated mL of blood in suction jar} \qquad (3.1)$$

1. *Consequences*: Intraoperative blood loss leads to reduced preload, decreased CO, decreased perfusion, and hypotension. Excessive blood loss may result in lactic acidosis and cardiovascular collapse.
2. *Causes*: Intraoperative hemorrhage results from unidentified source of bleeding, iatrogenic causes of hemorrhage, low platelet counts, coagulopathies, or altered physiology affecting coagulation.
3. *Treatment*: If blood loss exceeds 20% of total blood volume or PCV falls below 20%, a transfusion is indicated. Ideally, a cross-match and blood type is performed to select a compatible blood transfusion; follow the protocol for your own institution in this regard. Whole blood (WB) is ideal; however, packed red blood cells (pRBC) with fresh frozen plasma (FFP) are alternatives. The goal is to maintain adequate blood volume to provide adequate oxygen delivery to tissues. WB replaces deficit at a volume of 1:1. When delivering blood products in a nonemergent situation, start with a slow rate of 1–3 mL/kg/h for

the first 15 minutes and evaluate the patient for a transfusion reaction. Signs of an immediate transfusion reaction include hypotension, tachycardia, hives, and increased temperature. It is important to note these signs may be masked in the anesthetized patient. If no reaction is appreciated, the transfusion rate is adjusted to the patient's need. If a transfusion reaction is evident, discontinue the transfusion and give diphenhydramine at 1 mg/kg IM (note: some clinicians may include this preemptively, prior to transfusion; please use best clinical judgment). Blood products containing citrate as an anticoagulant are not administered with fluids that contain calcium (such as LRS), sodium bicarbonate or positive inotropes. If more than one transfusion is necessary, it is prudent for ionized calcium levels to be evaluated as hypocalcemia may result. Ionized calcium values of 0.75 mM/L require treatment as a "rule of thumb" (see Table 3.13).

III. Respiratory complications

A. Hyperventilation (hypocapnia)

Hyperventilation, or hypocapnia, is defined by $EtCO_2$ or $PaCO_2$ levels below normal range (less than 35 mmHg). If the anesthetist believes the patient is truly hypocapnic, an arterial blood gas sample is collected to evaluate $PaCO_2$.

1. *Consequences*: Brief episodes of hyperventilation or periods of low CO_2 are not detrimental. Prolonged hypocapnia results in respiratory alkalosis and decreased cerebral perfusion; this results in localized ischemic damage to areas of the brain. The brain will also begin to reset its own baseline CO_2 level when exposed to prolonged periods of hypoventilation [28].
2. *Causes*: The most common cause of hyperventilation under anesthesia is aggressive MV. Other causes include neurologic disease, trauma, pain, noxious stimuli or compensatory respiratory alkalosis. Hypoxemic patients may compensate by increasing RR, thus sacrificing CO_2 to improve oxygenation.
3. *Treatment*: Treatment is focused on the underlying cause for hyperventilation; collection of an arterial blood gas guides therapy and helps with assessment of treatment. Adjustment of ventilation is required if hyperventilation is iatrongenic. If the patient is hyperventilating due to noxious stimuli during a surgical procedure, drugs to provide analgesia are indicated. When hyperventilation is secondary to a metabolic acidosis, the primary acid–base abnormality is corrected. Treatment for the hypoxemic patient is based on the cause of hypoxemia (see "Hypoxemia," p. 66). If the primary cause is not determined and treated, the patient can relapse or decompensate in recovery.

B. Hypoventilation (hypercapnia)

Hypoventilation is one of the most common complications experienced during anesthesia, occurring in anywhere from 13.5% to 63.9% of cases [2,6]. Hypoventilation (hypercapnia) is present when the $PaCO_2$ is greater than 45 mmHg. Alveolar ventilation is defined in Equation 3.2.

Equation 3.2 Alveolar ventilation equation. V_A is alveolar ventilation, V_t is tidal volume, V_d is dead space, and f is frequency (RR).

$$V_A = (V_t - V_d) \times f \tag{3.2}$$

Under general anesthesia, when the patient is intubated, V_d is fixed. Therefore, V_A is dependent on V_T and RR. In cases of hypoventilation, adjustments are made to V_T and RR.

1. *Consequences*: Mild increases in CO_2 levels are of little consequence in the healthy patient. As CO_2 increases, respiratory acidosis becomes evident, although the long-term impact of this is likely of little consequence when the recovered patient resumes normal ventilation. As CO_2 levels exceed 95 mmHg, CO_2 may induce anesthesia, suggesting this level of CO_2 is certainly unacceptable. In patients with neurologic disease, hypoventilation results in increased intracranial pressure (ICP); if there is space-occupying disease (e.g., a brain tumor) or intracranial hemorrhage, a brain herniation may result. CO_2 is carefully controlled in these patients. For patients with potential for a sudden increase in ICP, hyperventilation to maintain $PaCO_2$ levels near 32–35 mmHg may be beneficial until the ICP issue is directly treated (see Chapter 5).

2. *Causes*: Typically hypoventilation results from dose-dependent respiratory depressants (inhalant anesthetics) and worsens with a deep plane of anesthesia. Although rare, malignant hyperthermia (MH) will present as an increasing temperature and $EtCO_2$, and is a life-threatening condition. Neurologic disease may affect the chemoreceptors' sensitivity to CO_2 and the respiratory muscles' mechanical function, causing hypercapnia. Tight bandages restricting inspiratory efforts may also cause an increase in CO_2. A rise in CO_2 is evident in cases of pneumothorax (with a concurrent decline in oxygenation). A rise in $PaCO_2$ without a rise in $EtCO_2$ suggests CO_2 is unable to diffuse out of blood efficiently; pulmonary thromboembolism will lead to such a discrepancy (see "Pulmonary thromboembolism," p. 69).

3. *Treatment*: Identification of the cause of hypoventilation is key for treatment. RR, capnography, minute volume, and V_T are parameters used to monitor ventilation. Reducing excessive dead space (e.g., small or no "Y" piece for small patients) is helpful in minimizing hypoventilation. Check the patient's anesthetic plane and decrease the depth of anesthesia if possible. Supporting ventilation in the anesthetized patient is initiated by manual or MV (see Chapter 2). Reverse drugs that may cause respiratory depression (e.g., opioids), if hypoventilation is severe, especially during the recovery period. If there is a restrictive bandage, remove it until the patient is recovered and it can be loosely reapplied. If MH is the cause, treatment with dantrolene is indicated (see Drug Formulary). Cases of pulmonary thromboembolism (PTE) require extensive interventions (see "Pulmonary thromboembolism," p. 69).

C. Hypoxemia/inappropriate P:F ratio

Desaturation of a patient results in hypoxemia, which occurs in 2.8–16.4% of patients [2,6]. Hypoxemia is officially defined as a PaO_2 less than 60 mmHg. PaO_2 is evaluated from an arterial blood sample, analyzed with blood gas analysis. In animals with normal lung function, PaO_2 is approximately 4–5 times the fraction of inspired oxygen (FiO_2). For example, in a patient breathing room air (FiO$_2$ = 21% O$_2$), PaO$_2$ should equal approximately 100 mmHg. If a patient is anesthetized and breathing 100% oxygen, PaO$_2$ equals approximately 500 mmHg. The ratio of PaO$_2$ to FiO$_2$ is referred to as the P:F ratio; normal P:F ratio is 5:1. A change in this ratio to less than 5:1 is important because of its impacts during the animal's recovery, when the patient returns to room air (21% O$_2$). For example, if a patient has severely compromised lung function with a PaO$_2$ of 100 mmHg when breathing 100% oxygen, that patient's P:F ratio is 1:1. This example patient, while not currently hypoxemic (because the PaO$_2$ is not less than 60 mmHg), has a severely inappropriate P:F ratio. When that patient moves into recovery, 100% oxygen is discontinued and 21% room air is breathed while the P:F ratio is unchanged, PaO$_2$ will fall to 21 mmHg – a severe and life-threatening hypoxemia. If blood gas analysis is unavailable, a pulse oximeter provides valuable information on oxygenation for patients breathing room air.

As one can see from Figure 3.8, a pulse oximeter is of limited use in patients with normal lung function on 100% oxygen (i.e., under anesthesia); the anesthetized patient must have severely compromised lung function before the pulse oximeter will read less than 98–100%. Even the patient in the previous example will have a PaO$_2$ of 100 mmHg and thus a pulse oximeter reading of 98–100% while on 100% oxygen.

1. *Consequences*: Inadequate oxygenation leads to tissue hypoxemia, lactic acidosis, and ultimately organ failure. Arrhythmias such as VPCs and VT followed by VF become evident if perfusion to the heart is compromised; organs like the brain and kidney are sensitive to reduced perfusion, and often this compromise is not detected until the post-operative period.

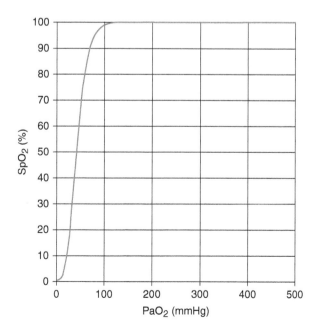

Figure 3.8   Oxygen hemoglobin desaturation curve.

2. *Causes*: The causes of hypoxemia fall into five categories.
   - Decreased FiO_2 (unlikely in anesthetized patients breathing an FiO_2 of 100%)
   - Diffusion impairment (such as chronic fibrosis of the lungs or severe pulmonary edema)
   - Right to left shunt (such as a reverse PDA)
   - Hypoventilation (a common cause in patients breathing room air, but uncommon cause for hypoxemia in anesthetized patients with an FiO_2 of 100%)
   - V/Q mismatch (the most common cause of hypoxemia under anesthesia)

   Patients with diaphragmatic hernias, pneumothorax, foreign body airway obstructions, asthma, pneumonia, pleural effusion, large abdominal masses, ascites or free fluid in the abdomen, among others, are at high risk for hypoxemia. Certain procedures, such as feline bronchoscopy, have a remarkable incidence of desaturation associated with them [29].

3. *Treatment*: If the patient is hypoxemic or has increased respiratory effort prior to induction, preoxygenation will prolong the time before a patient desaturates [30] (Table 3.7). In particular, preoxygenation with a facemask as opposed to simple flow-by greatly improves oxygenation of the patient [31] (Table 3.8). Most patients are tolerant of a facemask, after effective premedication. In the anesthetized patient, if the PaO_2 is less than expected (even if above 60 mmHg), the abnormality resulting in the low PaO_2 is addressed. For example, in cases of low FiO_2 (for example, a patient receiving nitrous oxide), FiO_2 is increased. If the patient is recovering from anesthesia, supplemental oxygen options include placement in an oxygen cage or nasal oxygen cannulas for increased FiO_2. If diffusion impairment occurs because of a treatable cause, treatment is instituted. For example, evidence of pulmonary edema warrants the use of furosemide. While the primary indication for MV is hypoventilation, there are several maneuvers with MV that will improve oxygenation. First, it is imperative that the patient receives an adequate V_T for each breath. Increasing the I:E ratio allows a long duration of inspiration for oxygen exchange to occur; however, I:E ratio should not exceed 1:2, as that will not allow enough time for expiration to efficiently occur. A "sigh" breath is a recruitment maneuver intended to prevent collapse of marginally inflated alveoli. To deliver a sigh breath, one breath of every 4–5 breaths is delivered at a high positive inspiratory pressure (PIP), of 25–30 cmH_2O. The use of positive end expiratory pressure (PEEP) will not improve oxygen content, but it may

Table 3.7   Treatment of hypoxemia.

1. Preoxygenate with 100% oxygen for minimum of 5 minutes up to point of intubation
2. Initiate assisted ventilation immediately
3. Ensure adequate tidal volume (increase I:E ratio) and respiratory rate
4. Administer sigh breath (PIP 25–30 cmH_2O) every 4–5 breaths
5. Add PEEP valve
6. Administer albuterol
7. When the above fail: maximize perfusion (positive inotrope for cardiac output, appropriate fluid or blood product therapy)

PEEP, positive end-expiratory pressure; PIP, positive inspiratory pressure.

Table 3.8 Supplemental oxygen methods.

Method of O_2 supplementation	O_2 Flow Rate	Maximum FiO_2 (%)
Flow-By	2–3 L/min	20–40%
Oxygen mask	2–5 L/min	40%
Oxygen cage	Varies by cage size	40–60%
Nasal cannula	50–150 mL/kg/min	30–70%
Endotracheal Intubation	200–300 mL/kg/min on NRB system, 20–30 mL/kg/min RB system	100%

prevent worsening P:F ratios by preventing marginal alveoli from collapsing. PEEP valves come in different sizes, typically 5, 7.5 and 10 cmH_2O. Large PIP and PEEP valves will decrease CO by decreasing preload secondary to increased and sustained positive pressure in the chest. Benefits are compared to risks when deciding to use these tactics to reduce the V/Q mismatch. The use of an inhaled bronchodilator (i.e., albuterol) may also improve oxygen exchange in the lungs; contraindications include the presence of tachycardia, which may worsen secondary to the use of a bronchodilator. In cases where in spite of all attempts to improve oxygenation, there is no improvement in PaO_2, the anesthetist's efforts move to improving perfusion by focusing on CO and maintaining normal hemodynamics while the procedure is rapidly concluded.

D. Pulmonary thromboembolism

A PTE is a clot, forming an obstruction in the lung's vasculature, thus severely reducing or eliminating perfusion to the section of lung tissue that would normally be perfused. This is the most severe form of V/Q mismatch in that there is little to no perfusion to an area of adequate ventilation. This is identified under anesthesia by a sudden and drastic drop in $EtCO_2$, and possible desaturation of the patient (drop in SpO_2). Blood gas analysis demonstrates a large gradient between $PaCO_2$ (which is often markedly elevated) and $EtCO_2$ (which is often quite low). A decrease in PaO_2 will also be present if compared with a pre-thromboembolism blood gas.

1. *Consequences*: The anesthetist will struggle with hypoxemia and possibly bradycardia (if emboli lodge in the coronary vasculature). Respiratory arrest is a possible consequence of a PTE. A thrombotic patient likely has more systemic problems than the anesthetist may appreciate, in that it is unlikely the lung is the only organ affected. For example, if a thrombus reached the brain, neurologic signs may not be evident until recovery. Ultimately, recovery is complicated as the patient may require MV for support while the thromboembolic disease and subsequent hypoxemia are addressed.
2. *Causes*: Patients who are hypercoagulable, such as those with Cushing disease, or have heartworm disease are predisposed. There is some evidence that laparoscopic procedures may result in air emboli to the lungs [32].

3. *Treatment*: Unfortunately, treatment options are limited under anesthesia. Supportive ventilation and diligent monitoring of blood gases are instituted. Treatment of other comorbidities is warranted. Anticholinergics cause bronchodilation [33] as well as increasing HR if a patient becomes bradycardic. Very few therapies, however, will eliminate an embolism once it is formed and thus recovery maneuvers are supportive rather than curative.

E. Pneumothorax

A pneumothorax occurs when air enters the pleural space and physically reduces lung volume, due to a loss of negative pressure. In the dog, there is no functional communication between sides of the thorax via the mediastinum, meaning pneumothorax on one side does not appear to affect the other [34]; it appears this is true for the cat as well, although they are their own unique creatures. Under anesthesia, a spontaneous pneumothorax presents as increased resistance during inspiration, decreased SpO_2, increase in RR, and initial decrease in $EtCO_2$. If the patient is on a ventilator, the V_T will decrease significantly while the PIP will drastically increase. A blood gas analysis will demonstrate an inappropriate P:F ratio (see "Hypoxemia," p. 66) or hypoxic PaO_2, a V/Q mismatch and an increase in $PaCO_2$.

1. *Consequences*: A pneumothorax causes hypoxemia and hypoventilation by limiting lung expansion, reducing compliance, and increasing resistance to ventilation. A severe pneumothorax may result in respiratory distress or arrest.
2. *Causes*: Iatrogenic causes of pneumothorax include any thoracoscopic or thoracotomy procedures; these intentional pneumothoraxes must be managed the same way postoperatively as a spontaneous pneumothorax. Trauma and ruptured bullae are leading causes of spontaneous pneumothorax. Additionally, pneumothorax is caused by extreme overinflation of the lung such as occurs when the adjustable pressure limiting ("pop off") valve is closed/occluded or when overly aggressive ventilation is used. The anesthetist must exercise caution when ventilating a patient with potential trauma to the thoracic cavity, such as a patient hit by car, as damaged lung tissue is fragile and susceptible to rupture.
3. *Treatment*: If a pneumothorax is present prior to surgery, the chest is tapped and/or a chest tube placed to allow for continuous drainage of air from the chest prior to induction of anesthesia (Tables 3.9 and 3.10). If a pneumothorax will be intentionally created (i.e., during a thoracoscopy), use of a PEEP valve (which maintains a constant end expiratory pressure in the lungs) during the procedure will prevent the lung from collapsing down to residual volume (RV) and thus reduce the risk of alveolar trauma for reopening completely collapsed alveoli; the use of positive pressure may improve oxygenation intraoperatively as well [35]. Treatment of a spontaneous pneumothorax involves immediate decompression of the air within the thorax. This is achieved by a chest tap or placement of a chest tube. Manual or MV with positive pressure is required to preserve adequate ventilation, as the animal will no longer have negative pressure to expand the lung, thus making its own attempts to breathe inadequate. Goals of ventilation include maintaining CO_2 levels within normal (35–45 mmHg) and providing adequate oxygenation (PaO_2 >60 mmHg). When ventilating these patients, use of longer inspiratory times and low PIP is helpful. Blood gas analysis is part of routine monitoring and patient assessment well into the recovery period.

Table 3.9 Placement of traditional chest tube.

Materials: Chest tube, clippers, aseptic preparation, sterile gloves, suture (Nylon), hemostats, Christmas tree adaptor, orthopedic wire, three-way stopcock, scalpel blade, bulldog clamp or "C" clamp

Technique: *Follow manufacturer's instructions for chest tube placement, as it can be specific to brand.*

1. Clip large area over chest with intercostal spaces 7–9 in center; aseptically prepare. Wearing sterile gloves, palpate rib space 7–9; select one of these rib spaces.
2. Stretch skin cranially over the site; make stab incision with the scalpel blade through the skin at the intercostal space selected on the cranial aspect of the rib.
3. Using hemostats, dissect down to the pleural lining.
4. Hold the chest tube perpendicular to the chest wall. Hold chest tube with one hand at the selected intercostal space; with other hand pop end of chest tube into the pleural space.
5. Rest chest tube parallel with the chest and advance into thoracic cavity.
6. Aspirate to ensure chest tube is in thoracic cavity. Remove any air or fluid from chest (quantify amounts) until negative pressure is achieved.
7. Relax skin to "normal" position over chest tube.
8. Secure in place with a mattress knot or Chinese finger trap. A bulldog or "C" clamp is placed on the tube to prevent air from entering the chest should the stopcock become dislodged.
9. A Christmas tree adaptor is commonly placed on the end of the chest tube with a three-way stopcock to maintain a seal. The stopcock and Christmas tree are soundly secured to the tube with orthopedic wire.

Note: Negative pressure is not always achieved. If the chest is "open" (meaning there is a wound leading from the outside into the chest), negative pressure is not achieved. These patients require surgical closure and are placed on a vacuum system.

Table 3.10 Chest tap.

Materials: Over-the-needle catheter (16–18 G) or butterfly catheter, three-way stopcock, fluid extension set, large syringe, sterile gloves, clippers, aseptic prep

Technique:

1. Clip area over intercostal spaces 7–9 (towards the dorsum for air, more ventral for fluid). Aseptically prepare the site.
2. While wearing sterile gloves, insert the catheter between the intercostal spaces of choice, on the cranial aspect of the rib. A "pop" is felt when entering the pleural space. If using an over-the-needle catheter, advance catheter into chest and remove stylet.
3. Attach one end of the fluid extension line to end of catheter, and attach a three-way stopcock to the other end of the extension set.
4. Place syringe on end of stopcock. Turn stopcock off to room air (but open between patient and the syringe); withdraw fluid or air until negative pressure is obtain with syringe. It is important to not place extreme negative pressure on the syringe or damage to the lung tissue could result. Once the syringe is full of air or fluid, turn the stopcock off to the patient and empty syringe. This process is repeated until negative pressure is obtained.
5. When negative pressure is achieved, the stopcock is turned off to the patient. Remember to record the total volume of air or fluid removed.

F. Postanesthetic aspiration pneumonia

Studies looking at the prevalence of postanesthetic aspiration pneumonia shed light on our need for preemptive planning, to prevent this possibly disastrous event. Authors report that this particular complication occurs in anywhere between 0.17% and 4.5% of patients [7, 36, 37].

1. *Consequences*: Aspiration pneumonia, especially of GI contents where pH has not been neutralized, can result in extensive hospitalization and necessitate oxygen supplementation, as well as causing death secondary to acute respiratory distress syndrome.
2. *Causes*: In a large multicenter study, two anesthesia-related events were significantly associated with the development of aspiration pneumonia: regurgitation (see p. 83) and the use of hydromorphone as a premed [36]. Presumably, this is because hydromorphone is such a ubiquitous premedication; however, the alternative way to consider this information is that if one uses hydromorphone regularly, including something to reduce the acidity of the stomach contents – such as alternative fasting plans, H2 blockers or proton pump inhibitors – may be wise. Certain procedures, such as laparotomies, upper airway surgery, neurosurgeries, thoracotomies, and endoscopy, were associated with increased incidence of aspiration pneumonia, while other procedures (for example, neuters and dental procedures), were not [36]. Of note, 96% of canine patients with two or more of the following diseases went on to develop aspiration pneumonia: a history of preexisting respiratory or neurologic disease, or megaesophagus [36]. It is often speculated that brachycephalic patients, due to elevated negative intrathoracic pressures necessary to overcome their inherent upper airway obstruction, are predisposed to gastroesophageal reflux, and therefore possible aspiration pneumonia. Large-scale studies do not support this conclusion, although smaller studies do [36–38].
3. *Treatment*: Should aspiration pneumonia occur, treatment is largely supportive in nature, including supplemental oxygen therapy for patients who are hypoxemic, possible need for mechanical ventilation, broad-spectrum antibiotic therapy as indicated for secondary infections, and other intensive care unit support as indicated. Therefore, prevention is a superior strategy when possible. While no one drug is capable of preventing regurgitation and subsequent aspiration pneumonia, it is best to avoid elective anesthesia for animals which have not been properly fasted. The 2020 anesthesia and monitoring recommendations from the American Animal Hospital Association (AAHA) give comprehensive fasting guidelines, for those with interest in this [39]. In the authors' opinion, it is preferable to provide gastrointestinal protection, such as an H2 blocker, to patients predisposed to aspiration pneumonia.

G. Respiratory distress or arrest

Respiratory distress or arrest occurs for a variety of reasons but ultimately leads to cessation of breathing, either because the patient is unable to breathe or is incapable of taking adequate breaths. Under anesthesia, respiratory characteristics such as effort and rate are very important to monitor. Other key respiratory parameters include SpO_2, PaO_2, and capnography. Because the patient is vigilantly monitored, it is unlikely this complication would occur during anesthesia; the anesthetist usually notes hypoventilation and either manually or mechanically assists the patient. However, respiratory arrest is one of the three major causes of postoperative morbidity and mortality [1], indicating the need for careful monitoring in the postoperative period.

1. *Consequences*: Respiratory distress or arrest may result in fatality of the animal.
2. *Causes*: Respiratory fatigue, pneumothorax, and increased intraabdominal pressure from diseases such as GDV, pregnancy, large mass or foreign body, and diaphragmatic hernia may all result in respiratory distress or arrest. Additionally, an animal that is inadequately recovered from anesthesia in the postoperative period and is not appropriately monitored/supported may have respiratory distress or arrest that is unnoticed.
3. *Treatment*: Recognizing the cause of respiratory distress or failure is important for treatment decisions. MV is indicated in a patient which may have compromised respiratory effort under anesthesia or postoperatively. If a pneumothorax is suspected, tapping the chest is indicated (see Table 3.10). Continuous monitoring of the patient's respiratory effort, blood gas, and SpO$_2$ is important throughout the recovery period. Supplemental oxygen may be necessary and the patient must be observed for at least 3 hours postoperatively [40].

IV. Acid–base disturbances

Acid–base disturbances are common complications under anesthesia, especially in the critical patient, and may provide insight on prognosis [41]. Knowing the patient's clinical history allows the anesthetist to differentiate between a primary problem and compensation. The ability to measure blood pH is essential to detecting an acid–base disorder. This is done as part of a routine blood gas analysis and obtained with point-of-care monitors or benchtop lab equipment.

There are two approaches to diagnosing an acid–base disturbance: a traditional approach based on the Henderson–Hasselbalch equation and the Stewart approach. The traditional approach is described. For those interested in the Stewart approach and other new models evaluating acid–base disturbance, additional resources are available [42].

To evaluate changes in pH, other components of a blood gas, including PaCO$_2$, bicarbonate (HCO$_3$), and base excess (BE), are necessary. The first step is to evaluate pH – is it normal (7.35–7.45), acidotic (less than 7.35) or basic (above 7.45)? PaCO$_2$ and HCO$_3$ changes will indicate whether pH changes are caused by a respiratory or metabolic disorder. The primary disorder follows the change in pH (Table 3.11). For example, in a patient with acidosis, PaCO$_2$ is elevated (respiratory acidosis) or HCO$_3$ is decreased (metabolic acidosis). In a patient with alkalosis, PaCO$_2$ is decreased (respiratory alkalosis) or HCO$_3$ is increased (metabolic alkalosis). The compensatory mechanism attempts to "mitigate" this problem. In disturbances with mixed/multiple issues, the pH is often normal with values of PaCO$_2$ and HCO$_3$ in opposite directions. One "rule of thumb" is the body will never *over* correct. In other words, it is not possible to have a pH that is acidotic or alkaline because the body has overcompensated for a disease.

Arterial whole blood or heparinized samples (depending on the analyzer) are used for accurate acid–base analysis. Room air has its own level of PaCO$_2$ (that is, zero) and PaO$_2$, and therefore is removed from the syringe; the sample is then analyzed immediately for accurate results. If an arterial sample is not available, a blood sample from the tongue (considered a mixed arterial and venous sample) is the next most accurate sample for acid–base analysis.

Table 3.11   Simple acid–base disorders and compensatory mechanism.

Primary disorder	Change in pH	Primary cause	Compensatory mechanism
Respiratory acidosis	Decreased	Increased $PaCO_2$	Increased HCO_3
Respiratory alkalosis	Increased	Decreased $PaCO_2$	Decreased HCO_3
Metabolic acidosis	Decreased	Decreased HCO_3	Decreased $PaCO_2$
Metabolic alkalosis	Increased	Increased HCO_3	Increased $PaCO_2$

A. Metabolic acidosis

Metabolic acidosis is characterized by a pH less than 7.35 with a low HCO_3, negative BE, and decreased $PaCO_2$ (Table 3.12).

1. *Consequences*: Acidosis regardless of origin causes a decrease in myocardial contractility, a decrease in CO, and vasodilation. It also leads to arrhythmias, including VF. During anesthesia, acidosis makes the patient less responsive to catecholamines. The conscious patient with metabolic acidosis will hyperventilate, which leads to respiratory exhaustion. However, under anesthesia, this compensatory mechanism is diminished.
2. *Causes*: When using a traditional approach to blood gas analysis, anion gap is evaluated to determine, from a list of rule-outs, the cause of metabolic acidosis. One particularly concerning rule-out is lactic acidosis caused by hypoperfusion, resulting in cells under-going anaerobic metabolism and producing lactate. Indeed, in a recent study, mortality was 59.8% in dogs and 49% in cats with lactic acidosis [41]. Acquiring a lactate value helps to eliminate lactic acidosis as a rule-out. Other causes include liver or renal failure, diabetic ketoacidosis, GI losses of HCO_3 and a variety of toxicities.
   * Calculation of anion gap: the anion gap is the difference between measured cations and measured anions; the size of this difference assists in determining the cause of metabolic acidosis. A normal anion gap is usually less than or equal to 10 mEq/L. A low anion gap is unlikely. A high anion gap results from increase in unmeasured anions, such as lactate or ketones.

$$\text{Anion gap}\left(\text{mEq/L}\right) = \left(Na^+ + K^+\right) - \left(Cl^- + HCO_3^-\right)$$

Table 3.12   Acid–base disorder examples.

Acid–base disorder	pH	$PaCO_2$ (mmHg)	HCO_3 (mmol/L)	Base excess (mmol/L)
Metabolic acidosis	7.28	21.8	10.2	−17
Metabolic alkalosis	7.55	52.6	27.8	9
Respiratory acidosis	7.23	58.6	25.1	−5
Respiratory alkalosis	7.49	20.3	16.5	5
Mixed/complex	7.38	19.9	30.4	Highly variable

An alternative to anion gap is the use of Stewart's equation, a mathematically complex formula using serum biochemistry values; the reader is referred elsewhere for further information.

3. *Treatment*: Treatment depends on identifying the primary problem causing metabolic acidosis. However, under anesthesia, the anesthetist's goals include maximizing perfusion with fluids or blood products, positive inotropes to increase CO, and supporting the patient's ventilation (usually hyperventilation). For most cases, hemodynamic and ventilation support prevents the metabolic acidosis from becoming extreme. For life-threatening cases of metabolic acidosis while under anesthesia (pH less than 7.1), supplementation of sodium bicarbonate is used to increase pH for temporary preservation of life while continued efforts are made to identify and correct primary cause of the acid–base abnormality (see p. 74). If sodium bicarbonate is supplemented, additional CO_2 is produced; augmentation of ventilation to adjust for this is necessary.

B. Metabolic alkalosis

Metabolic alkalosis is characterized by an increase in pH (above 7.45), in HCO_3, positive BE and compensating increased $PaCO_2$ (see Table 3.12).

1. *Consequences*: Alkalosis (whether metabolic or respiratory in origin) results in impaired cerebral and coronary blood flow that ultimately leads to seizures, obtundation, and/or death. Cardiovascular consequences include vasoconstriction and possible ventricular arrhythmias. Conscious patients compensate with hypoventilation (increase in $PaCO_2$). Severe metabolic alkalosis leads to calcium binding to albumin, causing hypocalcemia and precipitating muscle weakness and decreased contractility. Other common electrolyte abnormalities seen with alkalosis include hypochloremia and hypokalemia.
2. *Causes*: Leading causes of metabolic alkalosis include patients with significant renal insufficiencies that affect the reabsorption of bicarbonate, excessive vomiting causing a loss of hydrogen and chloride ions (as occurs with a proximal obstruction of the duodenum), and hypovolemia. Oversupplementation of sodium bicarbonate also leads to metabolic alkalosis.
3. *Treatment*: Adequate volume resuscitation with possible supplementation of chloride and potassium is most important when treating or stabilizing this patient.

C. Respiratory acidosis

Respiratory acidosis is characterized by a low pH with a high $PaCO_2$ (see Table 3.12).

1. *Consequences*: This is the most frequent cause of acidosis under anesthesia. It is usually of little long-term consequence but cardiac arrest and hypoxemia may result if it is severe and left untreated. Acidosis regardless of origin causes a decrease in myocardial contractility, a decrease in CO and hypotension, as well as possible arrhythmias, including VF. During anesthesia, acidosis causes decreased responsiveness to catecholamines.
2. *Causes*: The leading cause of respiratory acidosis under anesthesia is hypoventilation due to a deep anesthetic plane or drug overdose. Other causes include airway obstruction, pleural effusion, MH, and chest wall disruption.

3. *Treatment*: Respiratory acidosis is most commonly the result of hypoventilation from excessive anesthetic depth. Depth of anesthesia is adjusted initially. Assisted ventilation is started once the anesthetic plane is addressed effectively. Assisted ventilation is achieved either by manually supplementing breaths or placing the patient on a ventilator. If the patient is currently on a ventilator, increasing the RR or V_T will usually decrease $PaCO_2$.

D. Respiratory alkalosis

Respiratory alkalosis is characterized by a low $PaCO_2$ and resulting increase in pH, typically above 7.45 (see Table 3.12).

1. *Consequences*: Severe alkalosis (pH greater than 7.6) regardless of metabolic or respiratory origin results in similar consequences, including decreased cerebral blood flow, seizures, and possible ventricular arrhythmias. Electrolyte abnormalities may also include hypocalcemia and hypokalemia.
2. *Causes*: The most common cause of respiratory alkalosis is iatrogenic hyperventilation. Other causes may include central nervous system injuries, pregnancy, hyperthermia, and pain.
3. *Treatment*: Identifying the primary causes of respiratory alkalosis and treating that cause is most effective. Under anesthesia, the most effective treatment involves controlling ventilation so $PaCO_2$ may increase, correcting pH. Typically, decreasing the V_T or RR will allow $PaCO_2$ to increase, correcting the acid–base abnormality. It is important to continue to try to identify and correct the underlying cause to avoid relapse at recovery.

V. Electrolyte disturbances

Electrolyte disturbances have negative ramifications if left unmonitored or without treatment. As with all patient complications, correction of these imbalances occurs prior to anesthetizing the patient when possible. Normal values are influenced by the electrolyte analyzer. The normal ranges listed are general guidelines to follow; however, the anesthetist must be familiar with the reference ranges specific to their own laboratory.

A. Calcium

Calcium plays an important role in muscle contraction, with the anesthetist's primary muscle of concern being myocardial (contractility). Changes in albumin levels (which occur with fluid therapy) do not impact ionized calcium and therefore under anesthesia, ionized calcium levels are used for therapeutic decisions (Table 3.13).

Hypercalcemia

Hypercalcemia is defined as an ionized calcium value greater than 6 mg/dL or 1.5 mmol/L in the dog and 5.7 mg/dL or 1.4 mmol/L in cats.

1. *Consequences*: The acuteness of hypercalcemia will determine if a patient has any consequences from it. For example, a patient that gradually becomes hypercalcemic from

Table 3.13 Treatment of hypercalcemia and hypocalcemia, once underlying disease is addressed.

Hypercalcemia	Hypocalcemia [70]
1. Fluid bolus/anesthetic maintenance of noncalcium-containing fluids: 0.9% NaCl or Plasma-Lyte	Treatment is a recommended dose of 5–15 mg/kg of elemental calcium slowly over 10–30 mins, or as a constant-rate infusion, 2.5–3.5 mg/kg/h of elemental calcium is targeted. There are two different formulations of calcium available: *Calcium gluconate* 10% (9.3 mg of elemental calcium/mL): 0.54–1.6 mL/kg of calcium gluconate over 10–30 mins, or 0.27–1.5 mL/kg/h *Calcium chloride* 10% (27.3 mg of elemental calcium/mL): 0.18–0.55 mL/kg of calcium chloride over 10–30 mins, or 0.092–0.128 mL/kg/h

Notes: When supplementing calcium, continuous monitoring of the ECG is important. Oversupplementation will cause bradycardia and possibly cardiac arrest.

neoplasia may exhibit few if any adverse problems under anesthesia. However, it is possible for hypercalcemia, especially if it is acute in nature, to cause muscle twitches or weakness and myocardial irritation. Myocardial effects include increased myocardial contractility and bradyarrhythmias (including AV block, asystole, and possible cardiac arrest).

2. *Causes*: Immature animals (especially large-breed dogs) may have higher calcium values. One study examined the most common pathologic causes of hypercalcemia. In dogs, this included malignancy-associated (12.9%), parathyroid-dependent (4.6%) and hypoadrenocorticism-associated (1.7%) hypercalcemia [43]. In feline patients, this included malignancy-associated hypercalcemia (22.7%), kidney injury (13.4%) and idiopathic hypercalcemia (12.6%) [43]. Under anesthesia, oversupplementation (for example, as a CRI during anesthesia to counter the hypocalcemic effects of EDTA or citrate in blood products) may also cause hypercalcemia.

3. *Treatment*: When treating electrolyte abnormalities, it is important to determine the potential cause or primary disease and correct it prior to anesthesia, if possible. A thorough evaluation of cardiac function is warranted. Diuresis with fluids that do not contain calcium (such as 0.9% NaCl) is ideal. Acid–base status is monitored as this alters calcium levels.

Hypocalcemia

Hypocalcemia is defined in dogs as ionized calcium less than 5 mg/dL or 1.25 mmol/L and less than 4.5 mg/dL or 1.1 mmol/L in cats. As a "rule of thumb," ionized calcium values below 0.75 mM/L require treatment [44].

1. *Consequences*: Hypocalcemia contributes to decreased myocardial contractility, resulting in low cardiac output. Hypocalcemia also results in tetany ("milk fever"). Muscle tremors and seizures may be seen in conscious patients. Under anesthesia, hypotension, tachycardia, respiratory depression or arrest may be seen. Narrow QRS complexes, decreased PR intervals, flattened T waves, and prolonged QT interval may be evident on the ECG.

2. *Causes*: In dogs, there are several common causes of hypocalcemia, including critical illness (17.4%), kidney injury (10.4%), and toxicity (7.5%). Moderate to severe hypocalcemia in the canine patient is significantly more likely with hypoparathyroidism, kidney injury, eclampsia or critical illness. Kidney injury (21.6%), urethral obstruction (15.1%), and critical illness (14.7%) were the most frequent pathologic causes of hypocalcemia in cats. Kidney injury, soft tissue trauma or urethral obstruction were significantly more likely in the feline population which presented with moderate to severe hypocalcemia [43]. Lactation may also result in hypocalcemia. The anesthetist frequently faces hypocalcemia following a massive blood transfusion with citrate as the anticoagulant.

3. *Treatment*: Determining the primary cause of the electrolyte imbalance is important. Treatment of life-threateningly low calcium is accomplished by slow supplementation with calcium gluconate or calcium chloride (see Table 3.13). When supplementing calcium, it is imperative the ECG is closely monitored for signs of hypercalcemia and ionized calcium is checked at frequent intervals to avoid oversupplementation.

B. Potassium

Potassium is an important electrolyte that influences the normal resting cell membrane potential. Normal range for potassium is 3.5–5.5 mEq/L.

Hyperkalemia

Hyperkalemia is defined as a serum potassium level above 5.5 mEq/L. Hyperkalemia is life-threatening above 7.5 mEq/L.

1. *Consequences*: As serum potassium levels rise (especially acutely), severe and possibly life-threatening bradycardia occurs [5]; up to 18.9% of cats died postoperatively in one study. At potassium levels greater than 5.5 mEq/L, T waves become peaked and narrow. At 6.5 mEq/L, the PR interval becomes prolonged followed by wide QRS complexes. At 7 mEq/L, the P waves become depressed or absent and there is a potential for atrial standstill. Above 8.5 mEq/L, cardiac arrest may occur. See Figure 3.9 for ECG changes in the patient with hyperkalemia.

2. *Causes*: Urinary obstruction or bladder rupture, hypoadrenocortism, uncontrolled diabetes mellitus (secondary to insulin deficiency), renal failure, and reperfusion injury following thromboembolism potentially result in hyperkalemia. Iatrogenic causes may include administration of expired pRBCs or oversupplementation of potassium. There is also a report of two greyhounds who developed spontaneous, life-threatening hyperkalemia under anesthesia without a preexisting reason [45].

3. *Treatment*: Cardiac bradyarrhythmias are life-threatening and require immediate treatment. Table 3.14 outlines guidelines for treatment of hyperkalemia.

Hypokalemia

Hypokalemia is characterized by serum potassium levels less than 3.5 mEq/L.

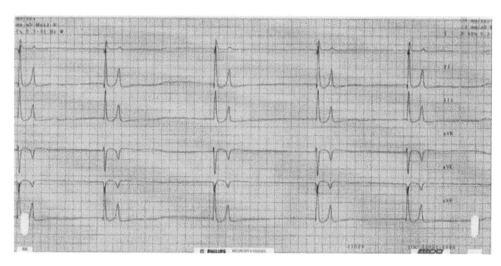

Figure 3.9   ECG in a patient with acute hyperkalemia, 50 mm/s, 10 mm/mV. *Source:* Courtesy of Jorge L. Vila.

Table 3.14   Treatment of hyperkalemia.

1. 0.9% NaCl is the crystalloid fluid of choice for anesthetic maintenance or bolus.
2. Administer regular insulin at 0.1–0.2 IU/kg with/without a CRI of 0.1 IU/kg/h IV. It is prudent to administer a 50% dextrose bolus at 0.25 g/kg slow over 3–5 mins diluted at least 1:4 with 0.9% NaCl, followed by 2.5–5% dextrose added to 0.9% NaCl run at anesthetic fluid maintenance rate.
3. Calcium gluconate 0.54–1.6 mL/kg over 10–30 mins may be cardioprotective.
4. Sodium bicarbonate at 0.5–1.0 mEq/kg IV over 15–30 mins will force potassium intracellularly.
5. Beta agonist such as dopamine or dobutamine will decrease K+ via the ATPase pump.

Notes: While treating hyper- or hypokalemia, continuously monitor the ECG and serum potassium levels. If administering insulin, dextrose, calcium supplements or sodium bicarbonate, blood gas, blood glucose, and electrolyte values must be monitored closely.
CRI, constant-rate infusion; IU, international unit; IV, intravenous.

1. *Consequences*: Muscle weakness, respiratory depression, and cardiac arrest may occur secondary to hypokalemia [46].
2. *Causes*: A decrease in potassium intake, vomiting, diarrhea, certain drugs (such as administration of loop diuretics, beta agonists or insulin overdose), chronic renal disease or post obstructive diuresis without appropriate fluid supplementation, and diabetic keto-acidosis all potentially result in hypokalemia.
3. *Treatment*: Supplementation of potassium is necessary; however, one needs to be very careful when supplementing potassium under anesthesia. As with all complications, it is best to correct any potassium deficits prior to anesthesia. The authors suggest supplementing potassium if serum potassium is below 2.5 mEq/L. A general rule for supplementation is no faster than 0.5 mEq/kg/h IV; often times, during anesthesia, potassium supplementation

is much less. Adding supplemental potassium to a bag of fluids to bring the total potassium concentration of the fluids to 20–40 mEq/L and administering at the surgical fluid rate is a conservative means of preventing an iatrogenic hyperkalemia, as long as one is careful not to bolus these fluids (separate, potassium free fluids are available to bolus, if needed). ECG and electrolyte values are continuously monitored for signs of hyperkalemia.

C. Sodium

Sodium is an important electrolyte in maintaining plasma osmolality and cellular hydration. Free water moves to areas of higher sodium concentrations. As serum sodium levels increase outside the cell, water leaves cells and the cells risk becoming dehydrated. As serum sodium decreases below the concentration in cells, free water moves into these cells, resulting in cellular edema. The kidney tightly regulates sodium concentrations, with very little fluctuation throughout the day.

Hypernatremia

Sodium concentrations above 165 mEq/L indicate hypernatremia.

1. *Consequences*: As with other electrolyte imbalances, how quickly a change in electrolyte status occurs influences the severity of consequences. Altered neurologic function, muscle tremors, seizures, and death can result from hypernatremia.
2. *Causes*: Hypernatremia occurs due to severe dehydration (possibly due to lack of available water or exposure to high temperatures), vomiting, diarrhea, and renal failure. Iatrogenic causes include administration of solutions containing sodium, such as hypertonic saline or sodium bicarbonate. Diseases such as diabetes insipidus and neurologic alterations may also cause increases in serum sodium.
3. *Treatment*: Treatment includes diagnosing the underlying cause of hypernatremia and evaluating the patient's hydration status. The brain compensates for hypernatremia by accumulating its own osmolytes to prevent dehydration. Rapidly decreasing sodium concentrations do not allow the brain enough time to compensate, which leads to neuronal swelling and rupture. Care is taken to only decrease serum sodium levels 0.5–1 mEq/kg/h to avoid cerebral edema. If anesthesia absolutely must occur prior to sodium regulation, the anesthetist should administer a fluid solution that is the same mEq/L concentration of sodium as the patient's own serum sodium. This is achieved by taking a solution like 0.9% NaCl and adding hypertonic saline to that fluid to raise sodium concentration. This fluid is then used as the patient's maintenance fluid, and correction of the sodium imbalance begins in the postoperative period. Serum sodium levels are diligently monitored throughout anesthesia.

Hyponatremia

Hyponatremia is defined as serum sodium level below 130 mEq/L, and is considered severe below 120 mEq/L.

1. *Consequences*: Hyponatremia causes changes in mentation status, seizures, coma, and possibly death due to cerebral edema and increasing ICP. Rapidly correcting hyponatremia results in myelinolysis, making it advisable to slowly correct this abnormality before anesthesia, although there is some leeway for very acute cases.
2. *Causes*: Causes of hyponatremia include fluid retention secondary to disease states (such as CHF), ascites or other body cavity effusions (i.e., uroabdomen or chylothorax), loss of sodium through the GI system or renal system, psychogenic polydipsia, and hypoadrenocorticism, as well as iatrogenic causes including excessive use of diuretics or hypotonic fluid administration.
3. *Treatment*: Treatment involves correction with sodium supplementation no faster than 0.5 mEq/kg/h. If the patient is concurrently hypovolemic, rehydration with fluid therapy is also necessary. If anesthesia must occur, hypotension is likely and requires treatment (see "Hypotension," p. 61).

VI. Glycemic control

Serum blood glucose (BG) is regulated by a variety of hormones, including insulin (which lowers BG) and glucagon, epinephrine, cortisol and growth hormones (which increase BG). Measuring BG concentrations is easily done with small, portable point-of-care monitors; however, one limitation of such monitors is their inaccuracy at very high or very low glucose concentrations. Familiarity with the analyzer's guidelines regarding sampling provides more accurate results.

A. Hyperglycemia

Hyperglycemia is defined as serum glucose greater than 180–200 mg/dL.

1. *Consequences*: Given the choice between hyper- or hypoglycemia in a patient, the anesthetist would prefer hyperglycemia. However, there is continued controversy about glycemic control under anesthesia in humans, with some studies demonstrating an improvement in morbidity for critically ill patients whose serum glucose is tightly regulated. This has lead to evidence-based literature reviews which concluded that a target BG range of 150–180 mg/dL may improve outcome in perioperative patients [47]. Up to 44% of diabetic canines will experience an episode of hyperglycemia over 250 mg/dL during a procedure (in this case, phacoemulsification) [19]. However, the same review cautions vigilance for hypoglycemia and having the means to correct it in the event of aggressive glucose management. Additionally, patients which have a history of hyperglycemia (diabetics) that have had restricted access to water may be dehydrated or hypovolemic, worsening hypotension, which is more prevalent in diabetics versus nondiabetic dogs [19]. Extreme hyperglycemia (greater than 600 mg/dL) may cause a prolonged recovery, seizures or coma.
2. *Causes*: Some diseases may perpetuate hyperglycemia or extreme fluctuations in glucose. The classic veterinary disease resulting in hyperglycemia is diabetes mellitus. Pancreatitis or acromegaly (felines) concurrently with diabetes may make BG more difficult to manage.

Chapter 3

Stress causes increases in glucose, especially in the feline. Hyperglycemia also occurs in patients with adrenal abnormalities, such as hyperadrenocortism (Cushing disease) or pheochromocytomas, or from adrenal changes secondary to supplementation with gluco-corticoids. Iatrogenic hyperglycemia results from oversupplementation with dextrose.

3. *Treatment*: Regular insulin is ideal during anesthesia and is dosed at 0.25–0.5 IU/kg IV or at a CRI of 0.05–0.1 IU/kg/h. Glucose is closely monitored every 30–45 minutes to prevent hypoglycemia. Because of frequent blood draws to assess glucose, a sampling line is typically placed in these patients.

B. Hypoglycemia

Hypoglycemia is a serum glucose less than 40–60 mg/dL.

1. *Consequences*: Glucose is a necessary energy source for cellular reactions and is critically important in the brain. Seizures may occur in the conscious, hypoglycemic patient; however, the neurologic damage that occurs is often masked in the anesthetized animal, as seizures will not be externally visible until recovery. Generalized weakness is evident during recovery. Hypoglycemia prolongs recovery, especially in small, exotic animals and young patients.

2. *Causes*: The most common cause of hypoglycemia in adult patients which are not obtunded/ otherwise appear normal is an insulinoma, as these patients have become "tolerant" of their hypoglycemia. Other causes of hypoglycemia include liver insufficiencies (secondary to PSS), hypoadrenocorticism (Addison disease), and sepsis. Iatrogenic causes include overdoses of insulin and extended fasting, especially in young animals.

3. *Treatment*: It is important to know if a patient has an insulinoma before they are treated for hypoglycemia. If an insulinoma is present, aggressively supplementing dextrose will cause the insulinoma to release more insulin and further worsen hypoglycemia. Therefore, in the insulinoma patient, dextrose supplementation is only used if the patient is severely hypoglycemic (less than 40–50 mg/dL) and then usually as a CRI of a 2.5–5% dextrose solution in the fluids, with target BG levels of 50–60 mgl/dL. In patients with other reasons for severe hypoglycemia, especially iatrogenic reasons, a bolus of dextrose at 0.5 g/kg diluted (due to the highly osmotic nature of dextrose) at least 1:3 with saline, and admin-istered IV slowly over 5 minutes, is warranted, as are fluids with dextrose supplementation to follow this bolus. In cases of mild to moderate hypoglycemia, the anesthetic fluids are supplemented with 2.5–5% dextrose and given at desired anesthetic fluid rate (usually 5–10 mL/kg/h).

VII. Other complications

A. Anaphylaxis/anaphylactoid reaction

Anaphylaxis is a type I (acute reaction mediated by immunoglobin E [IgE] attaching to mast cells resulting in degranulation) hypersensitivity. An anaphylactoid reaction is a reaction that, although clinically similar, is not mediated by IgE. Most reactions under anesthesia are anaphylactoid caused by mast cells and basophils releasing histamine in response to drugs and chemicals. Both reactions are treated in the same way.

1. *Consequences*: The degranulation of mast cells results in serious, adverse events including urticaria (hives), bronchospasm (although most patients are already intubated and so this is only evident at recovery), laryngeal and/or pulmonary edema, vasodilation, and tachycardia.
2. *Causes*: Drugs that prompt reactions include opioids (i.e., morphine), contrast media, antibiotics, and neuromuscular blocking agents. However, there are reports of certain induction agents, including alfaxalone and propofol, causing anaphylactic reactions, although not necessarily anaphylactic shock [48,49]. Blood products also have the potential to cause a reaction, especially when used in an untyped and uncross-matched patient.
3. *Treatment*: Discontinue any drug suspected to result in the reaction. If the response has not become severe, diphenhydramine (0.5–2.0 mg/kg IV) may reduce symptoms (although it does not "reverse" degranulation, as its action is to blockade H1 receptors, and prevent further engagement of these receptors by the mast cell tumors). Epinephrine (0.01 mg/kg IV) is warranted if symptoms progress to anaphylactic shock, or are initially very pronounced. The addition of a H2 blocker, such as famotidine (1.0 mg/kg IV), is warranted to prevent the GI side-effects of mast cell release. Other supportive measures (fluid therapy, inotropes, furosemide, etc.) are administered as needed.

B. Gastrointestinal dysfunction secondary to anesthesia

Gastrointestinal dysfunction takes many forms under anesthesia, including regurgitation (see "Respiratory complications," p. 65), gastroesophageal reflux (GER), nausea, vomiting or diarrhea, and functional ileus [50]. Regurgitation is the passive flow of stomach contents or gastric secretions into the esophagus, and occurs in up to 4.9% of certain procedures [7]. Regurgitation is clinically recognized by yellowish or brown fluid in the mouth or nares of the patient, and is concerning in that it can lead to aspiration pneumonia (see "Postanesthetic aspiration pneumonia," p. 72). Unfortunately, some dogs will silently regurgitate or have GER, meaning the anesthetist may not be aware of the regurgitation until the dog returns to the hospital at a future date with an esophageal stricture [51]. This may occur more commonly than visible evidence of regurgitation, and in one study the incidence was as high as 17.3% of patients [50].

Postoperative nausea and vomiting is a well-documented scenario secondary to anesthesia for human patients [52]. Nausea is hard to detect in the animal patient, as it is by definition a *feeling*. However, we do have literature to suggest that vomiting occurs in up to 5.5% or patients, and diarrhea in up to 10.5% of patients [50].

Patients who have a history of vomiting, regurgitation, gastric obstruction such as a foreign body, or increased intraabdominal pressure due to a mass or GDV are monitored closely for GI disturbance. A "test suction" is done in patients where silent regurgitation is suspected. When positioning a patient for a procedure, care is taken to avoid positioning the head below the stomach if possible, especially in patients known to have regurgitated during previous anesthetic procedures.

1. *Consequences*: The pH of the stomach is extremely acidic. Over time, gastric contents in contact with the esophagus's lining result in endothelial damage and possibly lead to

strictures. If the GI contents are aspirated into the lungs, aspiration pneumonia can result (see "Postanesthetic aspiration pneumonia," p. 72). Aspiration pneumonia of gastric contents greatly increases morbidity and mortality.

2. *Causes*: Some predisposing factors for gastrointestinal dysfunction secondary to anesthesia include intraabdominal surgery, changes in body position, and the length of anesthesia influencing the potential for GER [50]. In fact, many incidences of GER occurred immediately after anesthesia induction [53]. In the case of postoperative vomiting, factors including changes in the ventilation mode during surgery, length of anesthesia, and rescue synthetic colloid support due to hypotension were positively associated [50].

   There is some debate over the effect of preoperative fasting and the incidence of GER, with some authors suggesting prolonged fasting may worsen the incidence of reflux [53]. The AAHA has issued feeding guidelines as part of its 2020 recommendations for anesthesia and monitoring [39].

   It is often speculated that brachycephalic patients, due to elevated negative intrathoracic pressures necessary to overcome their inherent upper airway obstruction, are predisposed to gastroesophageal reflux; large-scale studies do not support this conclusion, although smaller studies do [36–38].

3. *Treatment*: Prevention is the best cure in the case of gastrointestinal dysfunction under anesthesia. While no one drug is capable of preventing gastrointestinal dysfunction, it is best to avoid anesthesia for animals which have not been properly fasted. The 2020 anesthesia and monitoring recommendations from the AAHA give comprehensive fasting guidelines, for those with interest in this [39]. In the authors' opinion, it is preferable to provide gastrointestinal protection to patients predisposed to gastrointestinal dysfunction, as it is unlikely to harm the patient. This is in fact the authors' own practice, to provide H2 blockers to all patients undergoing general anesthesia.

If regurgitation is noticed, the esophagus is immediately suctioned and lavaged with normal saline or tap water. Lavage of the esophagus is continued until the fluid removed is clear. It is important to always properly inflate the ET tube's cuff immediately following induction of anesthesia, as this decreases the chance of aspiration. Prior to extubation, the patient must be able to lift its head and swallow; the cuff is left partially inflated for removal of the tube. Instillation of sodium bicarbonate (after suction and lavage of the esophagus) increases the esophageal pH [54], which may reduce the incidence of esophageal stricture.

C. Hyperthermia

Thermal dysregulation occurs into up to 5% of patients [2]. Hyperthermia is defined as a body temperature above 103–104 °F (39.4–40 °C) in dogs and cats.

1. *Consequences*: Increased body temperature causes an increase in metabolic rate and oxygen consumption, which increases workload of important organs like the heart, skeletal muscles, and brain. Severe hyperthermia (temperatures >107 °F or 41.7 °C) may disrupt the body's normal enzymatic function and damage organs, including the brain (resulting in obtundation and seizures) and heart (ventricular arrhythmias), as well as leading to other organ failure and possibly death.

2. *Causes*: The most common cause of intraoperative hyperthermia in the healthy patient is iatrogenic oversupplementation of heat, usually through the use of circulating water blankets or forced air warming units. Hypermetabolic patients may present with hyperthermia. Malignant hyperthermia (MH) is a rare condition in which a defective ryanodine receptor allows for uncontrolled skeletal muscle activity, resulting in high temperatures, high EtCO$_2$, increased HR, RR and muscle tone. While primarily occurring in pigs, this disease has been reported in dogs [55] in response to anesthetic drugs. With the advent of drugs such as tramadaol, it is also important to note that serotonin syndrome, a syndrome reported in humans secondary to the use of drugs preventing serotonin reuptake, also results in hyperthermia. This syndrome is reported in a single feline case [56] but may become more prevalent, especially if multiple drugs that inhibit serotonin reuptake are combined.

   Postoperative hyperthermia is a phenomenon unique to the cat secondary to the combination of the use of opioids and intraoperative hypothermia [57]. Some feline patients reached temperatures greater than 107 °F (41.6 °C) postoperatively, a situation that warrants aggressive intervention. While opioids such as hydromorphone, when used in the cat, resulted in postoperative hyperthermia in up to 40% of the cases [58], all opioids have at least some documented incidence of postoperative hyperthermia [59]. Work by Posner's group identified the relationship between the degree of intraoperative hypothermia and postoperative hyperthermia in cats receiving opioids [57]. This highlights the importance of thermoregulation and monitoring in the feline.

3. *Treatment*: If the healthy patient has become hyperthermic under anesthesia, the anesthetist removes the source of heat. If using a forced air warming device, ambient air (68 °F) is circulated (i.e., the forced air warming unit is used to cool the patient). For extremely high temperatures (>107 °F or 41.6 °C), more drastic measures are taken. Oxygen supplementation is important in the face of hyperthermia due to the increased oxygen consumption at the tissue level. High flows (>300 mL/kg/min) will help cool the patient, as well as provide supplementation. Acepromazine at 0.01–0.03 mg/kg IV will cause vasodilation that will also assist with cooling. Cool icepacks are applied, particularly around the head to help keep the brain cool. Alcohol is applied to the foot pads as well. If severe hyperthermia is experienced under anesthesia along with an increase in EtCO$_2$ or PaCO$_2$, the anesthetist must rule out MH. The patient is disconnected from the current breathing circuit and placed only on oxygen, via a fresh circuit if available (injectable agents are used to maintain anesthesia if a procedure cannot be discontinued), in addition to the previously mentioned maneuvers. Controlling any arrhythmias and possible hyperkalemia are necessary steps as well. Definitive treatment includes the use of dantrolene at 1–5 mg/kg IV slowly, although this is infrequently available at most veterinary clinics, due to cost and short shelf-life. If a patient is suspected to have MH, dantrolene is obtainable from most human hospitals in advance of the procedure.

D. Hypothermia

Hypothermia is one of the most common complications of anesthesia, with thermal dysregulation occurring in up to 5% of overall cases [2, 6], and hypothermia reported in up to 63.8% of dogs undergoing certain procedures, such as thoracolumbar hemilaminectomy [7]. In dogs and cats, normothermia is 99.5 °F and 102 °F (37.5 °C and 38.9 °C), respectively. In the conscious human, body temperature rarely fluctuates more than 0.4 °F [60]; however, general anesthesia induces swings of 4–7 °F [61]. Mild hypothermia is somewhat beneficial to anesthetized patients in that myocardial and cerebral metabolic oxygen consumption is decreased, and inhalant requirement is reduced by approximately 5% for each 1.8 °F decline [62]. Hypothermia is possibly "neuroprotective" by limiting brain damage following cardiac arrest. As temperatures drift below 95 °F (35 °C), hypothermia requires intervention, unless deliberate hypothermia is utilized for anesthesia.

1. *Consequences*: Consequences of hypothermia depend on the degree of body heat loss. Generally, hypothermia causes decreased metabolism of drugs, mild metabolic acidosis, delayed wound healing, and coagulopathies. Mild to moderate hypothermia results in vasoconstriction and decreased tissue perfusion. As hypothermia progresses, patients become bradycardic and unresponsive to anticholinergics, causing a decrease in cardiac output resulting in hypotension, further worsening tissue perfusion. Cardiac arrhythmias such as AV block, VPCs and VF are evident as temperature drops further. Below 85 °F (29.4 °C), the anesthetist will commonly see these arrhythmias, which are often unresponsive to defibrillation, should cardiac arrest occur. Hypothermia results in prolonged anesthetic recoveries and shivering. Although shivering may seem insignificant, it increases a patient's metabolic rate and oxygen consumption by 200–600% [63]; this cost is profound to a patient with organ compromise.

2. *Causes*: Hypothermia most commonly results from lack of prevention. Small patients, neonates, debilitated, or emaciated patients are predisposed to hypothermia. In cases of cardiopulmonary bypass, hypothermia is deliberately induced; this is a complex procedure and is only taken on by an experienced anesthesia team.

3. *Treatment*: Treatment is aimed at maintaining the current body temperature and preventing it from worsening. If sedating the patient prior to induction, the patient is kept warm to avoid unnecessary losses in body temperature. Common equipment used to maintain patients' body temperature includes circulating water blankets, forced air warming blankets, electric warming units, plastic surgical drapes, and warmed intravenous fluids. Additional methods of warming the patient during a surgical procedure include warm abdominal lavage, decreasing oxygen flow rates to minimum requirement (rebreathing system 10–20 mL/kg/min, nonrebreathing system 200 mL/kg/min), preparation of surgical site with warm saline and antiseptic scrub (no alcohol), and minimizing anesthesia time. Aggressive warming and prevention is necessary in patients predisposed to hypothermia, although disappointingly, the literature shows little advantage to prewarming [64, 65].

E. Noxious stimuli ("breakthrough pain" or "arousal")

True pain is a conscious perception, and is defined as "an unpleasant sensory and emotional experience associated with actual or potential tissue damage, or resembling that associated with damage" [66]. Therefore, under anesthesia, upregulation of pain pathways is termed "noxious stimuli" to differentiate it from the cognizant perception that is pain. Nociception is the body's physiologic response to pain (Figure 3.10).

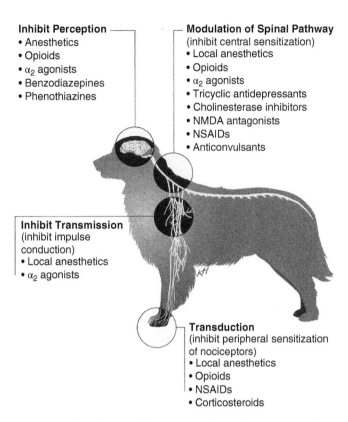

Inhibit Perception
- Anesthetics
- Opioids
- α_2 agonists
- Benzodiazepines
- Phenothiazines

Modulation of Spinal Pathway
(inhibit central sensitization)
- Local anesthetics
- Opioids
- α_2 agonists
- Tricyclic antidepressants
- Cholinesterase inhibitors
- NMDA antagonists
- NSAIDs
- Anticonvulsants

Inhibit Transmission
(inhibit impulse conduction)
- Local anesthetics
- α_2 agonists

Transduction
(inhibit peripheral sensitization of nociceptors)
- Local anesthetics
- Opioids
- NSAIDs
- Corticosteroids

Figure 3.10   Nociception pain pathways with analgesic drugs that target specific areas of the pathway. *Source:* Courtesy of Teton NewMedia.

However, the scientific literature may still refer to this as "breakthrough pain" or "arousal" and overall, this was the most commonly reported adverse event during the anesthetic period in one study, with an incidence of up to 14.9% [2].

1. *Consequences*: Upregulation of noxious pathways, even under anesthesia, results in modulation of the pain processing centers, which sets the stage for chronic pain, should treatment remain inadequate. Long-term consequences of mismanaged pain (i.e., postoperatively) are the subject of much debate, but ultimately the presence of pain undeniably reduces quality of life.

2. *Causes*: Primary causes of pain under anesthesia are a result of inadequate analgesia during a surgical procedure; that is, it is not enough to simply turn up the vaporizer without providing additional analgesic interventions.

3. *Treatment*: The target for treatment of pain is a preemptive and multimodal approach in the anesthetic plan. A multimodal approach is one that combines a variety of analgesic drugs, which target different receptors – for example, an opioid targeting opioid receptors, ketamine for NMDA antagonism, and lidocaine to target abnormal sodium channels. Premedication typically involves including an analgesic and sedative. Ideally, if the patient has an anticipated surgery scheduled such as an orthopedic correction or fracture repair,

appropriate analgesia is instituted prior to the preanesthetic phase. In this day and age, it is highly inappropriate for a patient to "earn" its analgesia; it is up to the anesthetist to anticipate pain and preemptively attempt to address it.

It is difficult under anesthesia to differentiate noxious stimulation from a patient who is inadequately anesthetized. End-tidal agent analysis assists with this; if the end-tidal agent values are at or above surgical MAC for the agent and patient, and the patient has hypertension, increased HR, or RR, noxious stimuli are suspected and responsiveness to analgesic drug administration (opioids, ketamine, etc.) is assessed. In the absence of an end-tidal agent analysis, the determination is much more speculative; however, responsiveness to analgesic drug administration (which, in dogs, will often reduce the need for inhalant) is also used. If the animal is responsive to a bolus of the analgesic agent, a CRI is an option to deliver a background of analgesic drug.

Noxious stimuli are much more difficult to address in a cat under anesthesia. Very few drugs reduce their inhalant requirements. Indeed, administration of some opioids may actually *increase* their MAC values. Yet, when these same cats were assessed conscious, the opioids administered clearly reduced the amount of pain experienced [67]. Therefore, it is advisable in the cat to assume an invasive procedure will be painful and to preemptively provide analgesia for such a procedure. See Appendix C for calculations and suggestions for CRI drug combinations.

It is important to address pain following the procedure in the anesthetic recovery phase. Conscious pain is evaluated with the assistance of pain-scoring techniques (see Appendix A).

F. Recovery complications

Target goals of recovery are that a patient is warm, comfortable and pain free; the environment that patient recovers in should be conducive to these target goals. This phase warrants continued observation, in that in large-scale studies examining the incidence of anesthetic-related mortality, anywhere between 47% and 60% of that mortality occurred in the first 3 hours postoperatively [1]. A patient should remain in hospital for at least this 3-hour period, postoperatively, and be closely monitored during this time. It is also prudent to leave the intravenous catheter in place during this phase [39]. Certain breeds warrant a special mention here: brachycephalic patients which have undergone a brachycephalic airway surgery have a remarkable incidence of postoperative complications, up to 23.4% [37]. It is prudent and advisable that these patients have intravenous access and access to oxygen supplementation.

One of the most common complications during recovery is excitation, which is present in up to 4.6% of patients [2].

Excitation during recovery

1. *Consequences*: Often referred to as either "dysphoria" (which may be the culmination of things like uncontrolled pain) or "emergence delirium" (uncontrolled struggling of a patient which is not yet fully conscious), this excitement is often abrupt and requires rapid intervention to prevent a patient from harming itself or others.

2. *Causes*: Dysphoria results from either a patient's vital need (uncontrolled pain, hypoxemia) not being addressed, or in the case of emergence delirium, a patient who is not fully conscious, and therefore uncoordinated in a possibly uninhibited state.
3. *Treatment*: An analgesic drug is appropriate in the case where one is unsure about pain levels. In the case where a patient is experiencing an altered state, the addition of a sedative may allow signs to subside. Because the sedative and analgesic drugs may work in a synergist fashion, as is the case with opioids and alpha-2 agonists [68], it is often advantageous to administer these drugs concurrently. Other urgent needs, such as hypoxemia, should be addressed specifically, such as through the use of supplemental oxygenation via facemask, nasal cannulas, oxygen cage, reintubation, etc.

Delayed recovery

1. *Consequences*: A delay in recovery requires additional staff to nurse the patient, and supportive measures, such as manual ventilation and thermal support, while a course of action is determined.
2. *Causes*: When recovery is delayed, it is imperative to determine whether it is because the patient cannot return to normal function (excessive anesthetic depth, hypothermia, administration of certain drugs, metabolic abnormalities [hypoglycemia, hypokalemia], etc.) or does not want to return to normal function (i.e., pain).
3. *Treatment*: Treatment is targeted at the underlying cause. If no underlying cause is found, and recovery is profoundly prolonged (i.e., greater than 1 hour), reversal of those drugs which are reversible may be considered. See Drug formulary for reversal drugs and dosages. If reversal is chosen, ensure the patient has adequate analgesia prior to reversing any drugs which may provide analgesia (alpha-2 agonists, opioids).

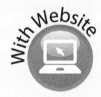

www.wiley.com/go/shelby/anesthesia2

Please go to the companion website for access to videos relating to the book

References

1. Brodbelt D, Blissitt K, Hammond R et al. The risk of death: the confidential enquiry into perioperative small animal fatalities. Vet Anaesth Analg. 2008;35(5):365–73.
2. McMillan M, Darcy H. Adverse event surveillance in small animal anaesthesia: an intervention-based, voluntary reporting audit. Vet Anaesth Analg. 2016;43(2):128–35.

3. McMillan MW, Lehnus KS. Systems analysis of voluntary reported anaesthetic safety incidents occurring in a university teaching hospital. Vet Anaesth Analg. 2018;45(1):3–12.

4. Schuessler RB, Ishii Y, Khagi Y, Diabagate K, Boineau JP, Damiano RJ Jr. The effects of inflammation on heart rate and rhythm in a canine model of cardiac surgery. Heart Rhythm. 2012;9(3):432–9.

5. Garcia de Carellan Mateo A, Brodbelt D, Kulendra N, Alibhai H. Retrospective study of the perioperative management and complications of ureteral obstruction in 37 cats. Vet Anaesth Analg. 2015;42(6):570–9.

6. Redondo JI, Rubio M, Soler G, Serra I, Soler C, Gomez-Villamandos RJ. Normal values and incidence of cardiorespiratory complications in dogs during general anaesthesia. A review of 1281 cases. J Vet Med A Physiol Pathol Clin Med. 2007;54(9):470–7.

7. Bruniges N, Rioja E. Intraoperative anaesthetic complications in dogs undergoing general anaesthesia for thoracolumbar hemilaminectomy: a retrospective analysis. Vet Anaesth Analg. 2019;46(6):720–8.

8. Erhardt W, Bohn FK, Ehmann H. [Anticholinergic medication in the dog before and during anesthesia]. Berl Munch Tierarztl Wochenschr. 1990;103(2):42–9.

9. Sartor DM. Sympathoinhibitory signals from the gut and obesity-related hypertension. Clin Auton Res. 2013;23(1):33–9.

10. Cho SK, Hwang GS, Kim YK, Huh IY, Hahm KD, Han SM. Low-dose atropine amplifies cardiac vagal modulation and increases dynamic baroreflex function in humans. Auton Neurosci. 2005;118(1-2):108–15.

11. Benson DW. The genetic origin of atrioventricular conduction disturbance in humans. Novartis Found Symp. 2003;250:242–52; discussion 52–9, 76–9.

12. Chen L, Sotoodehnia N, Bûžková P et al. Atrial fibrillation and the risk of sudden cardiac death. JAMA Intern Med. 2013;173(1):29–35.

13. Fletcher DJ, Boller M. Updates in small animal cardiopulmonary resuscitation. Vet Clin North Am Small Anim Pract. 2013;43(4):971–87.

14. Scapigliati A, Ristagno G, Cavaliere F. The best timing for defibrillation in shockable cardiac arrest. Minerva Anestesiol. 2013;79(1):92–101.

15. Xanthos T, Karatzas T, Stroumpoulis K et al. Continuous chest compressions improve survival and neurologic outcome in a swine model of prolonged ventricular fibrillation. Am J Emerg Med. 2012;30(8):1389–94.

16. Little SE. *The Cat: Clinical Medicine and Management*. St Louis, MO: Elsevier Saunders; 2012.

17. Acierno MJ, Brown S, Coleman AE et al. ACVIM consensus statement: Guidelines for the identification, evaluation, and management of systemic hypertension in dogs and cats. J Vet Intern Med. 2018;32(6):1803–22.

18. Gordon A, Wagner A. Anesthesia-related hypotension in a small-animal practice. Vet Medi. 2006;101:22–6.

19. Oliver JA, Clark L, Corletto F, Gould DJ. A comparison of anesthetic complications between diabetic and nondiabetic dogs undergoing phacoemulsification cataract surgery: a retrospective study. Vet Ophthalmol. 2010;13(4):244–50.

20. Burns BR, Hofmeister EH, Brainard BM. Anesthetic complications in dogs undergoing hepatic surgery: cholecystectomy versus non-cholecystectomy. Vet Anaesth Analg. 2014;41(2):186–90.

21. Monticelli P, Stathopoulou TR, Lee K, Adami C. Life-threatening perianaesthetic complications in five cats undergoing biliary tract surgery: case series and literature review. J Feline Med Surg. 2017;19(6):717–22.

22. Dixon A, Fauber AE. Effect of anesthesia-associated hypotension on neurologic outcome in dogs undergoing hemilaminectomy because of acute, severe thoracolumbar intervertebral disk herniation: 56 cases (2007–2013). J Am Vet Med Assoc. 2017;250(4):417–23.

23. Ruffato M, Novello L, Clark L. What is the definition of intraoperative hypotension in dogs? Results from a survey of diplomates of the ACVAA and ECVAA. Vet Anaesth Analg. 2015;42(1):55–64.

Chapter 3

24. Paige CF, Abbott JA, Elvinger F, Pyle RL. Prevalence of cardiomyopathy in apparently healthy cats. J Am Vet Med Assoc. 2009;234(11):1398–403.

25. Ilkiw JE, Pascoe PJ, Haskins SC, Patz JD, Jaffe R. The cardiovascular sparing effect of fentanyl and atropine, administered to enflurane anesthetized dogs. Can J Vet Res. 1994;58(4):248–53.

26. Pascoe PJ, Ilkiw JE, Pypendop BH. Effects of increasing infusion rates of dopamine, dobutamine, epinephrine, and phenylephrine in healthy anesthetized cats. Am J Vet Res. 2006;67(9):1491–9.

27. Ojiri Y, Noguchi K, Chibana T, Sakanashi M. Effects of adrenergic stimulants on the splenic diameter, haemoglobin content and haematocrit in anaesthetized dogs: determination of the adrenoceptor subtype responsible for changes in the splenic diameter. Acta Physiol Scand. 1993;149(1):31–9.

28. Curley G, Kavanagh BP, Laffey JG. Hypocapnia and the injured brain: more harm than benefit. Crit Care Med. 2010;38(5):1348–59.

29. Tucker PK, MacFarlane P. Incidence of perianaesthetic complications experienced during feline bronchoscopy: a retrospective study. J Feline Med Surg. 2019;21(10):959–66.

30. McNally E, Robertson S, Pablo L. Comparison of time to desaturation between preoxygenated and nonpreoxygenated dogs following sedation with acepromazine maleate and morphine and induction of anesthesia with propofol. Am J Vet Res. 2009;70(11):1333–8.

31. Ambros B, Carrozzo MV, Jones T. Desaturation times between dogs preoxygenated via face mask or flow-by technique before induction of anesthesia. Vet Anaesth Analg. 2018;45(4):452–8.

32. Richter S, Matthes C, Ploenes T et al. Air in the insufflation tube may cause fatal embolizations in laparoscopic surgery: an animal study. Surg Endosc. 2013;27:1791–7.

33. Gal TJ, Suratt PM. Atropine and glycopyrrolate effects on lung mechanics in normal man. Anesth Analg. 1981;60(2):85–90.

34. von Recum AF. The mediastinum and hemothorax, pyothorax, and pneumothorax in the dog. J Am Vet Med Assoc. 1977;171(6):531–3.

35. Rubio J, Rodríguez A, Varela A et al. [Evaluation of 2 techniques for ventilation support during single-lung ventilation]. Rev Esp Anestesiol Reanim. 1992;39(1):14–18.

36. Ovbey DH, Wilson DV, Bednarski RM et al. Prevalence and risk factors for canine post-anesthetic aspiration pneumonia (1999–2009): a multicenter study. Vet Anaesth Analg. 2014;41(2):127–36.

37. Lindsay B, Cook D, Wetzel JM, Siess S, Moses P. Brachycephalic airway syndrome: management of post-operative respiratory complications in 248 dogs. Aust Vet J. 2020;98(5):173–80.

38. Shaver SL, Barbur LA, Jimenez DA et al. Evaluation of gastroesophageal reflux in anesthetized dogs with brachycephalic syndrome. J Am Anim Hosp Assoc. 2017;53(1):24–31.

39. Grubb T, Sager J, Gaynor JS et al. 2020 AAHA anesthesia and monitoring guidelines for dogs and cats. J Am Anim Hosp Assoc. 2020;56(2):59–82.

40. Brodbelt D. Perioperative mortality in small animal anaesthesia. Vet J. 2009;182(2):152–61.

41. Kohen CJ, Hopper K, Kass PH, Epstein SE. Retrospective evaluation of the prognostic utility of plasma lactate concentration, base deficit, pH, and anion gap in canine and feline emergency patients. J Vet Emerg Crit Care. 2018;28(1):54–61.

42. Corey HE. Stewart and beyond: new models of acid-base balance. Kidney Int. 2003;64(3):777–87.

43. Coady M, Fletcher DJ, Goggs R. Severity of ionized hypercalcemia and hypocalcemia is associated with etiology in dogs and cats. Front Vet Sci. 2019;6:276.

44. Tranquilli W, Thurmon J, Grimm K (eds) *Lumb and Jones' Veterinary Anesthesia and Analgesia*, 4th edn. Ames, IA: Blackwell Publishing Professional; 2007.

45. Jones SJ, Mama KR, Brock NK, Couto CG. Hyperkalemia during general anesthesia in two Greyhounds. J Am Vet Med Assoc. 2019;254(11):1329–34.

46. Kjeldsen K. Hypokalemia and sudden cardiac death. Exp Clin Cardiol. 2010;15(4):e96–9.

47. Jacobi J, Bircher N, Krinsley J et al. Guidelines for the use of an insulin infusion for the management of hyperglycemia in critically ill patients. Crit Care Med. 2012;40(12):3251–76.

48. Haworth M, McEwen M, Dixon B, Purcell SL. Anaphylaxis associated with intravenous administration of alphaxalone in a dog. Aust Vet J. 2019;97(6):197–201.

Chapter 3

49. Onuma M, Terada M, Ono S, Murakami A, Ishida T, Sano T. Incidence of anaphylactic reactions after propofol administration in dogs. J Vet Med Sci. 2017;79(8):1446–52.

50. Torrente C, Vigueras I, Manzanilla EG et al. Prevalence of and risk factors for intraoperative gastroesophageal reflux and postanesthetic vomiting and diarrhea in dogs undergoing general anesthesia. J Vet Emerg Crit Care. 2017;27(4):397–408.

51. Wilson DV, Walshaw R. Postanesthetic esophageal dysfunction in 13 dogs. J Am Anim Hosp Assoc. 2004;40(6):455–60.

52. Cao X, White PF, Ma H. An update on the management of postoperative nausea and vomiting. J Anesth. 2017;31(4):617–26.

53. Galatos AD, Raptopoulos D. Gastro-oesophageal reflux during anaesthesia in the dog: the effect of preoperative fasting and premedication. Vet Rec. 1995;137(19):479–83.

54. Wilson DV, Evans AT. The effect of topical treatment on esophageal pH during acid reflux in dogs. Vet Anaesth Analg. 2007;34(5):339–43.

55. Adami C, Axiak S, Raith K, Spadavecchia C. Unusual perianesthetic malignant hyperthermia in a dog. J Am Vet Med Assoc. 2012;240(4):450–3.

56. Indrawirawan Y, McAlees T. Tramadol toxicity in a cat: case report and literature review of serotonin syndrome. J Feline Med Surg. 2014;16(7):572–8.

57. Posner LP, Pavuk AA, Rokshar JL, Carter JE, Levine JF. Effects of opioids and anesthetic drugs on body temperature in cats. Vet Anaesth Analg. 2010;37(1):35–43.

58. Niedfeldt R, Robertson S. Postanesthetic hyperthermia in cats: a retrospective comparison between hydromorphone and buprenorphine. Vet Anaesth Analg. 2006;33(6):381–9.

59. Posner L, Gleed R, Erb H, Ludders J. Post-anesthetic hyperthermia in cats. Vet Anaesth Analg. 2007;34(1):40–7.

60. Lopez M, Sessler DI, Walter K, Emerick T, Ozaki M. Rate and gender dependence of the sweating, vasoconstriction, and shivering thresholds in humans. Anesthesiology. 1994;80(4):780–8.

61. Støen R, Sessler DI. The thermoregulatory threshold is inversely proportional to isoflurane concentration. Anesthesiology. 1990;72(5):822–7.

62. Vitez TS, White PF, Eger EI. Effects of hypothermia on halothane MAC and isoflurane MAC in the rat. Anesthesiology. 1974;41(1):80–1.

63. Horvath SM, Spurr GB, Hutt BK, Hamilton LH. Metabolic cost of shivering. J Appl Physiol. 1956;8(6):595–602.

64. Rigotti CF, Jolliffe CT, Leece EA. Effect of prewarming on the body temperature of small dogs undergoing inhalation anesthesia. J Am Vet Med Assoc. 2015;247(7):765–70.

65. Aarnes TK, Bednarski RM, Lerche P, Hubbell JA. Effect of pre-warming on perioperative hypothermia and anesthetic recovery in small breed dogs undergoing ovariohysterectomy. Can Vet J. 2017;58(2):175–9.

66. IASP. Part III: Pain Terms, A Current List with Definitions and Notes on Usage. www.iasp-pain.org/AM/Template.cfm?Section=Pain_Definitions&Template=/CM/HTMLDisplay.cfm&ContentID=1728#Pain

67. Brosnan R, Pypendop B, Siao K, Stanley S. Effects of remifentanil on measures of anesthetic immobility and analgesia in cats. Am J Vet Res. 2009;70(9):1065–71.

68. Valtolina C, Robben J, Uilenreef J et al. Clinical evaluation of the efficacy and safety of a constant rate infusion of dexmedetomidine for postoperative pain management in dogs. Vet Anaesth Analg. 2009;36(4):369–83.

Chapter 4

Anesthetic considerations for specific procedures

Amanda M. Shelby and Carolyn M. McKune

This chapter provides suggested protocols for specific procedures and is heavily influenced by the author's opinions; however, the most suitable protocol for any procedure is based on familiarity of the anesthetist with anesthetics and analgesics available and the patient's preanesthetic assessment. Therefore, the user is highly encouraged to try various protocols in healthy patients prior to attempting these protocols for the first time in compromised animals. Procedures are listed in categorical orders (see guide below). Also listed are possible common complications, and prevention methods, as they relate to anesthesia for patients undergoing the specified procedure.

Sedation versus anesthesia

In some cases, sedation is a suitable alternative to full general anesthesia. Procedural selection is important when making this choice. For example, minimally invasive, elective, soft tissue procedures make up the vast majority of acceptable surgeries under sedation. Examples include laceration repairs, minor mass removals, enucleations, and feline neuters. Surgeon experience will determine the additions to such a list, with more experienced and expeditious surgeons electing to expand these offerings.

Characteristics of the patient also influence this choice. Generally speaking, sedation is an option when there is minimal risk of hemorrhage, pain is anticipated to be low to moderate, patients are ASA Category 1 or 2 and duration is short (60 minutes or less). Tables 4.3 and 4.7 list some common sedation options for a few of these procedures.

I. Soft tissue surgeries

A. Abdominal exploratory (exploratory laparotomy)

Abdominal exploratory is performed for a variety of reasons. Patient presentation varies substantially. It is important to assess each patient thoroughly with a thorough physical examination (PE), complete blood count (CBC) and chemistry, and appropriate imaging. Additional laboratory and diagnostics are performed as indicated by the differential list. Anesthetic protocols are based on the patient's presentation, PE, blood work (BW), diagnostic test results, and suspected differentials. The following information details anesthetic considerations, complications, and suggested protocols for common abdominal exploratory procedures (Box 4.1).

1. Anesthetic protocol (Table 4.1)

Drug selection depends greatly on the patient's presentation. In ASA 1–2 patients requiring an exploratory, IM premedication is acceptable. In ASA 3–5 patients, IV catheters are often

---

Box 4.1 Anesthetic concerns/common complications for abdominal exploratory.

- *Arrhythmias*: Arrhythmias (e.g., ventricular premature contractions [VPCs], ventricular tachycardia) commonly occur in patients requiring an abdominal exploratory. They are due to hypoxemia, anemia, metabolic abnormalities, and/or abdominal pain. Often, as in the case of gastric dilation-volvulus (GDV) or splenectomy, these may not resolve immediately after the procedure, and continued monitoring of the patient throughout the postoperative period is warranted.
- *Electrolyte abnormalities and metabolic acid–base disturbances*: Vomiting or diarrhea secondary to gastrointestinal (GI) disease results in electrolyte imbalances and altered acid–base balance. Dehydration will also affect electrolyte imbalances. These are corrected prior to surgery when possible.
- *Hemorrhage*: The abdomen contains highly vascular organs such as the liver, kidneys, and spleen. Blood loss is quantified for an accurate estimation (see Chapter 3, "Blood loss/hemorrhage", p.64). Patients requiring a splenectomy often present with a hemoabdomen. Preoperative packed cell volume (PCV) is very important before inducing anesthesia. Efforts to increase PCV to >25% before induction are made with a transfusion of packed red blood cells (pRBC) or whole blood product. In an active bleed, there is often a challenging balance between optimizing PCV above 25% to anesthetize the patient and allowing for "low" volume resuscitation to avoid exacerbating the bleed. A second catheter is placed to provide a port for transfusion, should it become necessary.
- *Hypoproteinemia (loss of protein or bleeding in the gastrointestinal tract, sepsis, severe liver disease)*: This contributes to a reduction in effective circulating volume and subsequent hypotension. Additionally, many anesthetic drugs are protein bound. In the hypoproteinemic patient, this results in increased unbound drug, causing a more profound effect. Hypoproteinemia also influences oncotic pressure and third space shift of fluid.
- *Hypoventilation*: Abdominal distention impedes normal respiration; this is compounded by anesthesia reducing diaphragmatic tone, thus reducing the natural barrier preserving thoracic space. Hypoventilation results in respiratory acidosis via increased CO_2 and worsens overall acidosis (see Chapter 3, "Hypoventilation").
- *Hypovolemia*: Often experienced in patients with GI disease, GDV, and splenetic masses, hypovolemia leads to a decrease in effective circulating volume, which worsens hypotension occurring under anesthesia (see Chapter 3, "Hypotension"). Volume resuscitation prior to anesthesia is warranted.
- *Pain (conscious patient)/noxious stimuli (unconscious patient)*: Pain pathways in the GI tract are triggered by distention. Distention secondary to gas occurs with blockage of the GI tract and results in severe patient discomfort.
- *Regurgitation*: Regurgitation may occur passively secondary to disease or during the procedure from high intraabdominal pressure. Patients who experience regurgitation are more likely to experience aspiration pneumonia [1], esophagitis, and potentially esophageal strictures.
- *Sepsis*: GI perforations or necrosis of areas of the GI tract result in leakage of bacteria into the abdominal cavity, which induces an inflammatory reaction in the body and bacteria in the blood. This leads to septic shock, a state of profound vasodilation that is exacerbated under anesthesia.

Table 4.1 Suggested anesthesia protocol for an abdominal exploratory.

	Opioid premed (mg/kg)	Sedative premed (mg/kg)	Induction (mg/kg)	Maintenance	Intraoperative analgesia (mg/kg/h)	Postoperative analgesia (mg/kg)
ASA 1–2	(a) Methadone 0.3–0.5 IM, 0.2–0.3 IV OR (b) Hydromorphone 0.1 IM, 0.05 IV	(a) Acepromazine[a] 0.01–0.02 OR (b) Dexmedetomidine 0.003–0.005	(a) Propofol to effect +/– midazolam 0.2 and/or lidocaine[b] 1.0 IV to reduce total dose of propofol OR (b) Ketofol (ketamine and propofol, 2–mg/kg each combined in the same syringe) to effect +/–midazolam 0.1 mg/kg IV OR (c) Alfaxalone 2–4 to effect +/–midazolam 0.1–0.2 IV	Sevoflurane OR isoflurane	(a) Opioid CRI 　(i) Fentanyl 0.01–0.042 OR 　(ii) Hydromorphone CRI 0.03 (b) Lidocaine CRI 1.5–3 (dogs only)[b]	(a) Opioid CRIs: 　(i) Fentanyl 0.002–0.005 OR 　(ii) Hydromorphone 0.01 (b) Lidocaine CRI 1.5 OR (c) Intermittent bolus (select one): 　(i) Methadone 0.3 IV q 4–6 h OR 　(ii) Hydromorphone 0.05–0.1 IV q 4–6 h AND (d) Lidocaine patch over incision OR (e) Liposomal encapsulated bupivacaine 5.3 mg/kg diluted to required volume injected subcutaneously over incision

(Continued)

Table 4.1 (Continued)

	Opioid premed (mg/kg)	Sedative premed (mg/kg)	Induction (mg/kg)	Maintenance	Intraoperative analgesia (mg/kg/h)	Postoperative analgesia (mg/kg)

ASA 3–5	(a) Fentanyl bolus 0.002–0.005 IV	+/–
		(a) Midazolam 0.1–0.1 IV
		AND
		(b) Lidocaine[b] 1–2 IV (dogs only)
			(a) Alfaxalone 1–2 to effect +/– midazolam 0.1–0.2 IV
			OR
			(b) Propofol to effect +/– midazolam 0.1–0.2 IV to reduce propofol
			OR
			(c) Ketofol (ketamine and propofol, 2 *each* combined in the same syringe) to effect +/– midazolam 0.1 IV
				Sevoflurane
				OR
				isoflurane
				+
				CRIs for reduction of inhalant requirement
					(a) Opioid CRI
					  (i) Fentanyl 0.01–0.042
					OR
					  (ii) Hydromorphone CRI 0.03
					(b) (b) Lidocaine[b] CRI 1.5–3 (dogs only)
						(a) Opioid CRIs:
						  (i) Fentanyl 0.002–0.005
						OR
						  (ii) Hydro-morphone 0.01
						(b) Lidocaine 1.5
						AND
						(c) Lidocaine patch over incision
						OR
						(d) Liposomal encapsulated bupivacaine 5.3 mg/kg diluted to required volume injected subcutaneously over incision

[a]Avoid in cases of splenectomy.

[b]Lidocaine CRI is contraindicated in cats.

CRI, constant-rate infusion; IM, intramuscular; IV, intravenous.

placed without sedation, and fluids are given prior to anesthesia to correct electrolyte abnormalities and stabilize hemodynamic parameters. In general, reversible drugs are ideal in critical patients. Opioid and lidocaine constant-rate infusions (CRIs) are excellent analgesics in the canine patient and greatly reduce minimum alveolar concentration (MAC) of inhalants intraoperatively. Opioid CRIs are used in cats for analgesia but do not produce a profound reduction in MAC of inhalant compared to dogs [2]. CRIs help balance the anesthetic technique and assist in stabilization of hemodynamic parameters. Postoperatively, CRIs are often necessary for pain management. Liposomal encapsulated bupivacaine is an option for use during closure of the incision as an alternative to the lidocaine patch. Appropriate fluid therapy to correct anemia, electrolyte imbalances, and acid–base disturbances is continued and tailored to the individual patient (Boxes 4.2–4.8).

Box 4.2 Adrenalectomy.

An adrenalectomy is indicated in cases of functional (e.g., nonpituitary-dependent hyperadrenocorticism) adrenal tumors or pheochromocytoma. These tumors result in inappropriate hormone secretion and have very different presentations.

- *Comorbidities*: Patients with functional adrenal tumors face several concerning comorbidities, including hypertension, hypercoagulability, and posttumor removal hypoadrenocorticism (resulting in hypotension and electrolyte imbalances).
- *Hemodynamic changes*: Patients with pheochromocytoma face life-threatening conditions intraoperatively. These include severe and remarkable tachycardia, arrhythmias, and blood pressure that fluctuates wildly. The use of phenoxybenzamine prior to surgery significantly reduces mortality from removal of the pheochromocytoma [3]. Recent work suggests that labetalol may be beneficial in reducing blood pressure without impacting heart rate, in cases where a pheochromocytoma is diagnosed intraoperatively [4]. See Chapter 3 for discussion of tachyarrhythmias and hypertension.
- *Hemorrhage*: Invasiveness of the tumor into surrounding vasculature is associated with the degree of hemorrhage a patient may experience. Interestingly, a low esophageal temperature was statistically associated with the incidence of hemorrhage [5], so temperature monitoring may give the anesthetist another key for when hemorrhage may be occurring. Cross-matching and blood typing are imperative for these cases as the probability of a transfusion is high. A second catheter is placed to provide a port for transfusion, should it become necessary.
- *Hypotension*: This was the most common complication observed (51.2%) in canine adrenalectomies in a small-scale study done in 2019 [5].
- *Mortality*: In a small-scale study, mortality rate was as high as 14.6% for canine patients undergoing an adrenalectomy. Mortality rate improved with the use of intraoperative hydrocortisone [5].

Box 4.3 Cholecystectomy.

Gallbladder mucocele (GBM) is an extrahepatic biliary disease found in dogs, and infrequently in cats [6,7] for which a cholecystectomy may be indicated. The presentation for these cases ranges from stable dogs whose proactive owners would like surgical management for the GBM (which is associated with improved survival compared to medical management [8]), to dogs who are septic from a ruptured GBM and are remarkably ill. Overall, the prognosis is guarded for animals with a GBM, with up to 17.4% of them being euthanized or dying during hospitalization in one study [9], and a range of mortality between 7% and 45% noted in another [10]. Of note,

Pomeranians were at an increased risk of death in a large multicenter study, although Shetland Sheepdog, American Cocker Spaniel, Chihuahua, Border Terrier and Miniature Schnauzer are also considered predisposed to this disease [11].

Therefore, patient presentation and breed will make a huge difference in the choice of anesthetic protocols. Please see Table 4.1.

- *ASA score*: Dogs presenting for a cholecystectomy with a higher ASA score appear to have a higher risk of mortality, which is anticipated [12]; see Chapter 1 for discussion on ASA scoring. As alluded to for cholecystectomies, worsening clinical signs (and thus a higher ASA score) reinforce the need for anesthetic management geared toward the critically ill patient. See Table 4.1 ASA 3–5 patients for the most suitable plan in these cases.
- *Hypotension*: While hypotension was no more frequent for patients undergoing cholecystectomies versus other hepatic surgery, it was still frequently encountered. Hypotension was evident in 74% of cholecystectomies in one study, and required inotropic support in about half of the cases [13]. It is prudent to have inotropic support prepared and available for these cases as part of the preparatory setup. Of note, hypotension intraoperatively did not worsen postoperative prognosis for these patients [12].
- *Prolonged anesthetic event*: Dogs undergoing cholecystectomies had an increased anesthesia duration compared to dogs undergoing other hepatic surgeries [13], so it is appropriate to anticipate that routine anesthetic complications such as hypothermia, hypotension, and hypoventilation may be encountered. See Chapter 3 for more information on common anesthetic complications applicable to all procedures. While it was not statistically significant, time to extubation (30 versus 49 minutes) was longer for patients which underwent cholecystectomies, so postoperative recovery will likely require continued patient support for considerable time.
- *Vagal event*: Some anesthesiologists report that manipulation of the gallbladder may result in a vagal (bradycardic) event. There is no published information to support this. However, it stands to reason that bradycardia could contribute to the high prevalence of hypotension in these cases. Having atropine or glycopyrrolate available to correct bradycardia associated with hypotension is good patient management.

Box 4.4 Gastric dilation and volvulus (GDV).

- *Hypovolemia*: The first priority for a patient with a GDV is volume resuscitation. At least two large gauge IV catheters are placed, preferentially in the cranial half of the patient; initiate IV fluid shock boluses to prevent circulatory collapse.
- *Regurgitation*: The patient is stabilized prior to induction. It is important to secure an airway quickly. Inflate the endotracheal (ET) tube cuff immediately to minimize the chance of aspiration of stomach contents.
- *Monitoring*: Utilize invasive blood pressure (IBP) monitoring, as rapid changes in hemodynamic variables occur. Central venous pressure (CVP) may be helpful to tailor fluid therapy. Monitoring serial serum lactate levels helps determine if fluid therapy and blood pressure supportive medications (i.e., positive inotropes and vasopressors) improve perfusion. Older dogs and those with disseminated intravascular coagulation were at an increased risk for development of hypotension [14].
- *Stomach distention*: Passing a stomach tube or (in cases where this is not possible) trocharizing a patient to relieve distention of the stomach prior to anesthesia is warranted. Decompression prior to anesthesia improves systemic vascular resistance (SVR), stroke volume (SV), and cardiac output (CO). Often, the surgeon needs a stomach tube passed intraoperatively, so it is warranted for the anesthetist to obtain this piece of equipment and bring it into the OR suite, if the tube is not passed preoperatively.
- *Ventricular arrhythmias*: Arrhythmias are common and may or may not respond to lidocaine (see Chapter 3, "Ventricular arrhythmias") or other antiarrhythmics.
- *Ventilation*: Assist ventilation, as the distended stomach functionally compromises ventilation.

Box 4.5 GI obstruction (i.e., foreign body, mass, resection/anastomosis, intussusception)

- *Vomiting*: Avoid premedication with drugs that result in vomiting, such as morphine or hydromorphone. Inclusion of ondansetron or maropitant in the preanesthetic plan is advised. See below for further important information when including maropitant in the premedication.
- *Regurgitation and aspiration pneumonia*: It is important to note that while an animal may not vomit with maropitant, fluid may still be retained in the stomach. When induced, this patient may regurgitate this fluid and because the airway is unprotected, aspiration pneumonia may result. It is advised that if there is distention of the stomach with fluid visible on imaging, a nasogastric tube be placed and the stomach emptied prior to induction, as well as administering fast-acting H2 blockers (e.g., famotidine) prior to anesthesia induction.
- *Hypovolemia and electrolyte abnormalities*: Patients with GI obstruction may have a history of vomiting and diarrhea. This further potentiates hypovolemia. Volume resuscitation is performed prior to anesthetic induction. Careful attention is paid to electrolyte abnormalities (specifically sodium and chloride), as this may dictate fluid selection.

Box 4.6 Nephrectomy.

- *Drug administration*: Avoid ketamine, especially in the cat, as the cat metabolizes ketamine only to norketamine, an active metabolite reliant on renal excretion [15].
- Additionally, there is much debate in the literature as to pharmacologic support for the kidney, with mannitol [16,17], dopamine in the dog [18], and fenoldopam [19] all having possible utility. It is, however, universally agreed that supporting blood pressure (BP) through the use of inotropes and/or vasopressors as necessary is best medical practice.
- *Hemorrhage*: Massive hemorrhage is possible; the anesthetist confirms the patient is blood-typed and cross-matched prior to anesthesia, and the compatible products are available to the anesthetist during the procedure. A second catheter is placed to provide a port for transfusion, should it become necessary.
- *Hypertension*: Patients with renal disease frequently have hypertension concurrently; obtain a BP prior to anesthesia to determine the patient's "normal" BP range.
- *Urine production*: Urine output will decrease under anesthesia [20]. The option of monitoring urine output with a urinary catheter and collection system is at the discretion of the surgeon. Normal urine output is approximately 0.5–1 mL/kg/h in the anesthetized patient [20]. If one is monitoring urine output and the patient is not producing enough urine, osmotic diuretics such as mannitol and furosemide may be used.

Box 4.7 Portosystemic shunt (PSS) (see Chapter 5, Hepatic function disease).

- *Decreased oncotic pressure*: If albumin is less than 2.2 g/dL, give a colloid, such as plasma, at 2–5 mL/kg/h to provide oncotic support instead of or concurrent with crystalloids.
- *Hemorrhage*: Prior to the procedure, a patient is cross-matched or blood-typed in case of hemorrhage. A second catheter is placed to provide a port for transfusion, should it become necessary.
- *Hypocoagulation*: Compared with healthy canines, the activity of clotting factors is decreased in dogs with a PSS; this results in a prolonged partial thromboplastin time (PTT) [21]. This can predispose the patient to increased hemorrhage.
- *Hypoglycaemia*: Because glycogen storage is one of the liver's primary functions, animals with PSS (i.e., decreased liver function) often have hypoglycemia. Monitor glucose and supplement fluids with 2.5–5% dextrose as necessary (see Appendix D).

- *Portal hypertension*: Post shunt occlusion, portal hypertension is possible and may contribute to neurologic decompensation and seizures postoperatively.
- *Decreased metabolism*: The liver's physiologic obligation is metabolism. This is important under anesthesia, as the majority of anesthetic drugs are metabolized hepatically. In a dog with a PSS, reduced liver function results in lower metabolism of anesthetic drugs, leading to relative overdose. Using the low end of drug dosages will reduce this impact.
- *Pain management*: The use of epidural morphine as a perioperative pain management tool reduces the requirement for additional analgesia postoperatively [22].

Box 4.8 Splenectomy.

- *Drug dosages*: Often, splenic masses are quite large and have a significant weight before they are discovered and surgically addressed. It is prudent to dose the patient at their normal weight without the contribution of the mass.
- *Hemoabdomen*: In cases of a ruptured splenic mass, hemoabdomen patients are typed and cross-matched; blood products must be readily available. A presurgical packed cell volume/total solid (PCV/TS), as well as intraoperative PCV/TS will guide blood product and fluid administration (see Chapter 3, "Blood loss/hemorrhage"), bearing in mind that, of the two, a decrease in TS is the more representative determinant of blood loss. A second catheter is placed to provide a port for transfusion, should it become necessary.
- *Hypotension*: In case of frank hemorrhage necessitating immediate intervention, the anesthetist does not have the luxury of preemptively volume stabilizing the patient. In this case, the patient is stabilized as well as possible in the OR. Positive inotropes (i.e., dobutamine, dopamine) and CRIs to decrease MAC requirements are helpful to maintain normotension while the anesthetist works to restore effective circulating volume.
- *Ventricular arrhythmias*: It is common to experience VPCs or even ventricular tachycardia with splenic masses. See Chapter 3 "Ventricular Arrhythmias," for instituting therapy.

B. Amputations (digits, forelimb, hindlimb, tail)

Amputations are often indicated for certain disease processes (e.g., osteosarcoma) or as a salvage procedure (e.g., financial limitations preventing fracture repair or a failed repair). They do not require specialized expertise or equipment and are performed in a broad range of veterinary hospitals (Box 4.9).

1. Anesthetic protocols

Drug selection is based on the patient's preanesthetic assessment (see Chapter 1). Analgesia is maximized. This starts with inclusion of a full agonist opioid with a sedative when needed for premedication. This procedure has no specific contraindications to a particular induction agent. Inhalant anesthetics are routinely used for maintenance. Regional blocks are ideal and highly recommended (see Chapter 7) where appropriate. Alternatively, the use of intraoperative CRIs of opioids, ketamine, and/or lidocaine (in the case of lidocaine, dogs only) is recommended when regional blocks are not performed. When the nerve is dissected, local anesthetic is applied perineural when provided sterilely to the surgeon. Postoperatively, nonsteroidal

---

Box 4.9 Anesthetic concerns/common complications for amputations.

- *Hemorrhage:* The higher the site of limb removal, the more substantial the risk of blood loss. This is because major arteries branch off the trunk at these regions (e.g., femoral artery or brachial plexus). As arterial branching progresses, arteries become smaller. However, a small artery allowed to hemorrhage still results in significant loss. While the anesthetist may focus on hemorrhage as the major cause of blood loss, it is important to remember that when the limb is removed, all the volume perfusing that limb is removed as well; therefore, even in situations of excellent hemostasis, hypovolemia may result. A second catheter is placed to provide a port for transfusion, should it become necessary.
- *Pain:* During the first year after an amputation, people commonly report phantom limb pain (PLP), with up to 76% of patients experiencing this phenomenon [23]. Although the incidence of PLP decreased to only 10% of patients over time in the previous study, our patients are not capable of verbalizing this phenomenon. Therefore, it stands to reason that as humans and animals share a similar pain pathway, our patients will experience PLP. To minimize the risk of occurrence, it is important to provide a balanced anesthetic technique with appropriate analgesia (see later discussion).

---

antiinflammatory drugs (NSAIDs) are administered if not contraindicated. A soaker catheter, liposomal encapsulated bupivacaine during surgical closure, or lidocaine patches postoperatively help with desensitizing this region. Pain scoring should continue and a rescue analgesia plan prepared. Rescue analgesia should include intermittent boluses of opioids at appropriate intervals or implementation of an opioid CRI. See Table 4.2 for analgesic plans for specific amputations.

C. Superficial mass removal

A variety of masses of varying size and degree of infiltration may require surgical removal. While it is impossible to present a protocol appropriate for all mass removals, general

Table 4.2 Suggested analgesic plan for amputations.[a]

Procedure	Intraoperative analgesia	Postoperative analgesia

Front limb amputation	(a) CRIs of opioid, lidocaine[b] (dogs only) and ketamine	(a) Opioid administration
		  (i) CRI
		OR
		  (ii) Intermittent opioid bolus
		AND
		(b) Local anesthetic
		  (i) Liposomal encapsulated bupivacaine 5.3 mg/kg diluted to required volume
		OR
		  (ii) Soaker catheter with lidocaine[b] CRI or bupivacaine every 4–6 h
		OR
		  (iii) Lidocaine patch

(Continued)

Table 4.2 *(Continued)*

Procedure	Intraoperative analgesia	Postoperative analgesia
Hindlimb amputation	(a) Lumbosacral epidural 0.1–0.2 mL/kg total volume (i) Preservative-free morphine 0.1 mg/kg AND/OR (ii) Preservative-free bupivacaine 0.5 mg/kg AND/OR (b) CRIs of opioid, lidocaine[b] (dogs only) and ketamine	(a) Opioid administration (i) CRI OR (ii) Intermittent opioid bolus AND (b) Local anesthetic (i) Liposomal encapsulated bupivacaine 5.3 mg/kg diluted to required volume OR (ii) Soaker catheter with lidocaine[b] CRI or bupivacaine every 4–6 h OR (iii) Lidocaine patch
Tail amputation	(a) Sacrococcygeal epidural 0.05–0.1 mL/kg total volume (i) Preservative-free bupivacaine 0.5 mg/kg OR (b) Lumbosacral epidural 0.1 mL/kg total volume with needle bevel facing caudally (i) Preservative-free bupivacaine 0.5 mg/kg AND/OR (c) CRIs opioid, lidocaine[b] (dogs only) and ketamine	(a) Opioid administration (i) CRI OR (ii) Intermittent opioid bolus AND (b) Local anesthetic (i) Liposomal encapsulated bupivacaine 5.3 mg/kg diluted to required volume OR (ii) Lidocaine patch
Toe amputation	(a) Ring block (i) Bupivacaine 3 mg/kg OR (b) RUMM block (forelimb) (i) Bupivacaine 1–3 mg/kg AND (ii) Dexmedetomidine 1 mcg/kg if not contraindicated OR (c) Lumbosacral epidural (hindlimb) 0.1–0.2 mL/kg total volume (i) Preservative-free bupivacaine 0.5 mg/kg	(a) Opioid administration (i) CRI OR (ii) Intermittent opioid bolus AND (b) Local anesthetic (i) Liposomal encapsulated bupivacaine 5.3 mg/kg diluted to required volume

[a]See Chapter 7 for description of blocks, suggested drugs, and dosages.
[b]Lidocaine CRI is contraindicated in cats.
CRI, constant-rate infusion; RUMM, radial, ulnar, median and musculoskeletal nerve.

> **Box 4.10** General anesthetic concerns/common complications for superficial mass removals.
>
> - *Analgesia*: The diagnosis, size, location, and invasiveness of the mass determine the level of analgesic intervention necessary (see below on preventing spread of disease). If possible, administration of a local anesthetic as a topical cream or infiltrative block is incorporated into the mass removal plan, in an attempt to stop pain transmission (see Chapter 7). NSAIDs, if not contraindicated, and opioids are the cornerstone of pain management strategies for these types of procedures. Liposomal encapsulated bupivacaine is useful when infiltrated into the tissues after mass removal.
> - *Preventing spread of disease*: If it is unknown whether the tumor is benign or malignant, it is best to avoid using an infiltrative local anesthetic strategy, as there is a hypothetical risk of spreading cancer cells along the needle tract in animals, as has been reported for people [24].
> - *Sedation versus general anesthesia*: If a mass is fairly small and the surgeon is comfortable with this technique, the combination of heavy sedation and a local technique (if not contraindicated; see "Preventing spread of disease") is often a reasonable alternative to general anesthesia for patients with a truly minor mass removal.

concepts are listed (Box 4.10). It is essential to have an idea based on cytology or previous biopsy for the anesthetist to prepare accordingly (i.e., to know whether to include a local block or forego it in the case of invasive masses).

1. Anesthetic protocol

Drug selection is based on the patient's preanesthetic assessment. This will also assist the anesthetist with the choice of general anesthesia or heavy sedation. In a patient with a mellow temperament, heavy sedation is quite useful. In a highly strung patient, general anesthesia (and thus better control over the patient) is often warranted. If procedures are of a short duration, the anesthetist may elect for a "middle of the road" approach and use partial or total intramuscular anesthesia (PIMA or TIMA) or total intravenous anesthesia (TIVA); see Table 4.3. Premedication is ideal in any case to provide preemptive analgesia, facilitate catheter placement, and reduce the requirement for other drugs necessary for induction or

Table 4.3 Suggested protocols for superficial mass removals without inhalant anesthesia.[a]

	Sedative premed (mg/kg)	Analgesic (mg/kg)	Anesthetic (mg/kg)
Heavy sedation (ideal for punch biopsy, minor cutaneous mass)	Dexmedetomidine 0.005 (IV)–0.01 (IM)	(a) Hydromorphone 0.1 (IV)–0.2 (IM) OR (b) Methadone 0.3 (IV)–0.5 (IM) OR (c) Butorphanol 0.2 (IV)–0.4 (IM) (requires local block)	(a) Infiltrative local block (i) Bupivacaine 3 AND (ii) Dexmedetomidine 0.001 if not contraindicated AND (b) Top up with propofol 1 IV if necessary

(Continued)

Table 4.3 *(Continued)*

	Sedative premed (mg/kg)	Analgesic (mg/kg)	Anesthetic (mg/kg)
TIMA[b] (ideal for no more than moderate mass removals)	Dexmedetomidine 0.01–0.015 IM	(a) Hydromor- phone 0.2 IM OR (b) Methadone 0.5 IM OR (c) Butorphanol 0.4 IM (requires local block)	(a) Alfaxalone 2–3 IM OR (b) Ketamine 5–7.5 IM AND (c) Infiltrative local block (i) Bupivacaine 3 AND (ii) Dexmedetomi- dine 0.001 if not contraindicated
TIVA[c] (Ideal for no more than moderate mass removals)	Dexmedetomidine 0.005 (IV)–0.01 (IM)	(a) Hydromorphone 0.1 (IV)–0.2 (IM) OR (b) Methadone 0.3 (IV)–0.5 (IM) OR (c) Butorphanol 0.2 (IV)–0.4 (IM) (requires local block)	(a) Propofol (with- out preservative) 6–24 mg/kg/h IV after induction with propofol 2 IV AND (b) Infiltrative local block (i) Bupivacaine 3 And (ii) Dexmedetomi- dine 0.001 if not contraindicated

[a]These protocols are for use in patients with minimal systemic disease. Sedation and analgesic drugs are combined and administered at the same time.
[b]Please note that with TIMA one should support the patient with an oxygen mask, and be prepared to intubate.
[c]With TIVA, intubation, oxygen support, and monitoring (as with general anesthesia) are standard practice.
IM, intramuscular; IV, intravenous.

anesthetic maintenance. Should general anesthesia be deemed necessary, a variety of induction drugs are used; propofol may result in a smooth recovery for short procedures. Maintenance
on an inhalant anesthetic often follows (Boxes 4.11 and 4.12).

D. Head and neck procedures

Head and neck surgeries, as a group, present the anesthetist with similar concerns (Box 4.13). Head
and neck surgeries include ocular surgeries, auricular surgery, airway surgeries, mass removals
commonly involving the thyroid and parathyroid glands, and feeding tube placements. However,
dental procedures often warrant the same considerations.

*1. Brachycephalic airway syndrome (BAS) procedures (laryngeal sacculectomy,
stenotic nares correction, soft palate resection)*

Head and neck procedures in the brachycephalic patient bear special mention, as soft tissue
surgery in this conformation of dog results in greater complications than does orthopedic

Box 4.11 Mast cell tumor (MCT).

- *Mast cell degranulation*: MCTs are sensitive to manipulation [25]. When aggressively manipulated, they can release histamine, serotonin, and heparin. Avoiding aggressive manipulation of the tumor is therefore warranted. While it does not prevent mast cell degranulation, preemptively administering an H1 blocker (e.g., diphenhydramine 1–2 mg/kg IM) and H2 blockers (e.g., famotidine 1 mg/kg IV) will prevent histamine from binding its receptors. If histamine release occurs, it is characterized by vasodilation, hypotension, and tachycardia. Supportive treatment is indicated, and additional diphenhydramine is administered. If the reaction is severe, epinephrine at 0.01 mg/kg IV may be necessary. Fluid boluses may mitigate the effects of vasodilation in the short term.
- *Anesthetic protocol modifications*: Some opioids are more likely to cause histamine release than others. Avoid opioids such as morphine and meperidine as secondary histamine release may occur. Methadone or hydromorphone is ideal for premedication. Acepromazine is the choice sedative if not otherwise contraindicated due to its antihistamine properties. Most induction agents are appropriate. If the mass is large or invasive, appropriate analgesia is required. Lidocaine patches over the incision are ideal postoperatively, along with systemic analgesics. Infiltrative local anesthetics are generally avoided due to the potential of seeding the tumor elsewhere.

Box 4.12 Mastectomy.

- *Pain*: This procedure is relatively painful, especially when it is a radical mastectomy [26]. The incision is extensive and inclusion of a lidocaine patch over the site, especially in the cat, provides an excellent option for local analgesia with minimal systemic impact [27]. Additionally, the expected postoperative pain level warrants aggressive preemptive analgesia and a well-balanced analgesic plan. Inclusion of local anesthetic as part of tumescent anesthesia reduces inhalant requirement and improves intraoperative and immediate postoperative analgesia, and was safe for use in clinical conditions in that it did not produce any adverse signs or toxic lidocaine plasma concentrations in dogs or cats [28–30]. Techniques such as the transverse abdominis plane (TAP) block, with intercostal nerve blocks as necessary in the case of radical mastectomy, show promise in reducing immediate postoperative pain [31]; see Chapter 7 for more information on TAP and intercostal nerve blocks. Infiltrative incisional application of liposomal encapsulated bupivacaine during closing eliminates use of the lidocaine patch and provides excellent desensitization to the area, as does the infiltration of traditional bupivacaine if liposomal bupivacaine is not available [32].
- *Ventilation*: Bilateral mastectomy performed in a single surgery may result in a tight skin closure (most common in the cat). While the skin becomes more supple over time, in the immediate postoperative period the patient may have difficulty ventilating due to this tight closure. While the patient is still intubated, this is identified by a high $EtCO_2$ reading. Once the patient is extubated, a venous blood gas is necessary to confirm this. If moderate to severe hypoventilation occurs, the patient must be reanesthetized to allow tension relief of the surgery site. Therefore, it is ideal for the anesthetist to evaluate for this possibility before general anesthesia is discontinued, and bilateral radical mastectomy is generally discouraged.
- *Anesthetic protocol modifications*: Drug selection is based on the patient's preanesthetic assessment. Intraoperative analgesia targets different pain receptors by use of multiple agents, including an opioid (morphine, hydromorphone, fentanyl), ketamine, and lidocaine (*note*: lidocaine CRIs are contraindicated in cats). Alternatively, a morphine epidural can be performed. Additionally, NSAIDs are a useful adjunctive analgesic postoperatively (see Chapter 7).

Chapter 4

Box 4.13 Anesthesia concerns/common complications for head and neck procedures.

- *Loss of access*: One of the most significant anesthetic concerns with head and neck procedures is loss of access to the patient. The anesthetist traditionally uses eye signs and jaw tone to assess anesthetic depth (see Table 1.6); now they must rely on monitoring equipment to compensate for the loss of ocular and oral access. Capnography is often a critical piece of monitoring, as disconnection of the ET tube, resulting in both lightening of the patient's anesthetic plane and desaturation, is a possible undesirable consequence with loss of access to the head. It is also the habit of most anesthetists to place IV catheters in the cephalic vein (patient's forelimb). Prudence suggests hindlimb catheterization in these patients for accessibility.
- *Trigeminal-vagal response*: The trigeminal nerve has three major branches (ophthalmic, mandibular, maxillary), which ultimately supply feedback into the parasympathetic system via the vagal nerve. Therefore, stimulation of these nerves (e.g., a surgeon resting their hands on a patient's face) may result in a profound bradycardia, potentially proceeding to asystole.
- *Aspiration*: Fluids from lavage and hemorrhage of the surgical site can compromise the integrity of the airway, leading to an increased potential for aspiration. The cuff of the ET tube is appropriately inflated at the beginning of the procedure, as blood from the surgical repair may otherwise be aspirated. When the ET tube is removed, the anesthetist has the option of incompletely deflating the cuff in order to remove accumulated blood or clots. Oropharyngeal packs or tonsil sponges are at times placed in the back of the throat to help minimize aspiration when they do not interfere with the surgery. It is the anesthetist's responsibility to remind the team to successfully remove these packs before discontinuation of maintenance anesthesia and extubation.
- *Desaturation*: Desaturation occurs rapidly in a patient after induction, prior to intubation [33]. Because the patient may not have a rapid intubation, it is best medical practice to preoxygenate all patients prior to and during the induction process. Supplemental oxygen may be required into the recovery period.
- *Sedation*: Premedication is used to facilitate handling of the patient, provide preemptive analgesia, and reduce the amount of induction and maintenance drugs. However, it also worsens the chance of airway obstruction in certain patients (i.e., brachycephalic patients or those with an airway obstruction). Conservative dosing and drug selection, as well as continuous patient observation post premedication, are necessary to prevent adverse consequences such as respiratory arrest. Avoiding premedications that cause vomiting reduces incidence of aspiration in an often already compromised airway. Additionally, consideration of administration of antivomiting or nausea medications is important (see Chapter 3).

---

surgery, for example [34] (Box 4.14). However, this may be a critical procedure to having fewer complications in future surgeries. Postanesthetic complications in subsequent anesthetic events were decreased by 79% in dogs with previous surgical correction of BAS [35].

(a) Anesthetic protocol (Table 4.4): Drug selection is based on the patient's preanesthetic assessment. Premedication is encouraged. An opioid such as methadone (which is unlikely to result in vomiting) is ideal. If hydromorphone or morphine is used, maropitant is administered prior to reduce the incidence of vomiting. Sedatives are used as needed to reduce anxiety, although it is important to monitor patients following administration. Propofol and alfaxalone are ideal induction agents because of their titratability, and at least one study suggests that ketamine with a benzodiazepine is best avoided [34]. If the surgeon elects to pack the back of the laryngeal area with gauze to absorb hemorrhage from the surgical sites, the anesthetist counts the number

---

Box 4.14 Anesthetic considerations/complications for BOAS procedures.

- *Airway obstruction and dyspnea*: Patients requiring head and neck procedures are at risk for airway obstruction pre-, intra-, and postoperatively. Often, the presurgical patient has learned to compensate for his or her inappropriate airway. However, following premedication, patients are monitored closely. Postoperatively, edema from surgical manipulation and correction may worsen the obstruction the patient experiences. This will often not manifest itself until extubation. Close monitoring of patients who have undergone a procedure involving the head or neck is required into the recovery period.
- *Equipment selection*: In addition to everted laryngeal saccules, stenotic nares, and elongated soft palate, these dogs also often have a hypoplastic trachea. The anesthetist must select a set of ET tube sizes that are smaller than expected for the average patient of the same weight.
- *Extubation*: The surgeon may request an airway examination during the induction process, to determine which of the procedures are necessary. It is advisable to have top-up of any induction drugs in case the patient becomes light during this period of extubation. Postoperatively, brachycephalic patients tolerate the ET tube because of misaligned teeth and relief of having a patent airway. Additionally, prior to extubation, the author finds swabbing the inflamed tissue with mannitol applied to cotton tip applicators helps decrease inflammation to the tissues. Because of the risk of postextubation airway obstruction, the anesthetist should have clean tubes available of half a size smaller, a laryngoscope, and enough induction drug to facilitate reintubation. Having a tracheostomy kit readily available is wise, as is continued observation for 24 hours postoperatively. Up to 24.1% of brachycephalic dogs for BAS had postoperative complications, including 8.9% who required a tracheostomy [37].
- *Increased postanesthetic risk*: Brachycephalic patients were roughly twice as likely to have postanesthetic complications as nonbrachycephalic dogs [34]. In this study (identifying risk factors), there were several things associated with complications in relation to anesthesia, including longer duration of anesthesia as well as the use of ketamine and a benzodiazepine for anesthetic induction, as opposed to propofol [34]. Other studies confirm the gravity of anesthesia in the brachycephalic patient; in one small study, mortality for brachycephalic patients was as high as 2.4%, almost double the overall mortality rate in ASA 3–5 canine patients [36,37].

Chapter 4

of gauze pads and ensures they are removed prior to discontinuing anesthesia. These surgical sites are extremely sensitive; it is common for patients to gag or swallow if not at an appropriate surgical plane of anesthesia. Some clinicians elect to administer systemic steroids at the time of incision to reduce the potential of excessive swelling; confirm with your team and if systemic steroids are administered, avoid NSAIDs.

2. Arytenoid lateralization (laryngeal tie back)

Laryngeal paralysis often affects older, large-breed dogs, which present in respiratory distress and are commonly given oxygen and low doses of acepromazine to decrease excitement and prevent hyperthermia (Box 4.15). Often, these patients are stabilized sufficiently with these measures to undergo surgery during normal business hours. During induction, an airway examination is performed by the surgeon, to determine which of the laryngeal cartilages are affected; make sure that the clinician performing the procedure is present at time of induction. Patients are routinely extubated following suture of the affected cartilage to visually ensure sufficient patency of the airway is present.

Table 4.4 Suggested anesthesia protocol for brachycephalic airway corrections.[a]

Opioid premed (mg/kg)	Sedative premed (mg/kg)	Induction (mg/kg)	Maintenance	Intraoperative analgesia (mg/kg/h)	Postoperative analgesia[b] (mg/kg)
(a) Methadone 0.5 IM OR (b) Hydromorphone[c] 0.05 IV OR (c) Buprenorphine 0.03 IM	(a) Acepromazine 0.03 IM	(a) Propofol 2–4 OR (b) Alfaxalone 1–3 IV to effect AND (c) +/– Midazolam[a] 0.2	(a) Isoflurane or sevoflurane AND (b) Metoclopramide CRI If patient must be extubated for procedure: (c) Propofol CRI 6–24 mg/kg/h IV OR (d) Alfaxalone CRI 4–8 mg/kg/h IV	(a) Intermittent bolus: (i) Methadone 0.3 IV OR (ii) Hydromorphone 0.05–0.1 IV OR (iii) Fentanyl 0.005 IV as needed OR (b) Opioid CRI (i) Fentanyl 0.01–0.042	(a) Intermittent bolus: (i) Methadone 0.3 (IV)–0.5 (IM) q 4–6 h OR (ii) Hydromorphone 0.05 (IM)–0.1 (IV) q 4 h OR (b) Buprenorphine 0.015 IV q 6–8 h

[a]The surgeon may want to evaluate airway/soft palate during induction; if so, avoid opioid, sedative premedication and benzodiazepines, if possible. It is best practice to administer GI protection, such as 1 mg/kg famotidine, after catheter placement but prior to induction. Preoxygenate patient.

[b]Because steroids may be necessary to reduce swelling, avoid NSAIDs.

[c]Administer maropitant 1 mg/kg IV prior to hydromorphone to avoid vomiting.

CRI, constant-rate infusion; IM, intramuscular; IV, intravenous.

Box 4.15 Anesthetic concerns for laryngeal tie back surgery.

- *Airway inflammation or edema*: Surgical manipulation of the airway may result in swelling or edema. NSAIDs are avoided, so dexamethasone can be administered if necessary.
- *Aspiration pneumonia*: Although the true cause of acquired idiopathic laryngeal paralysis is unknown, there is some evidence that it results from a neurologic dysfunction that also affects the esophagus [38]. Indeed, many of these dogs develop aspiration pneumonia after the tie back procedure [39]. Avoid drugs that cause regurgitation or vomiting (i.e., hydromorphone, morphine, alpha-2 agonists) postoperatively [40]. Sadly, evidence does not support a reduction in the incidence of aspiration pneumonia from simple interventions such as a metoclopramide CRI [41]. If oxygen saturation is inappropriate after extubation, thoracic films are warranted, as is supplemental oxygen.
- *Hyperthermia*: At presentation, many of these patients present stressed and hyperthermic. In addition to administration of acepromazine, cool fans and oxygen supplementation are often necessary.
- *Iatrogenic complications*: The surgeon may accidentally suture the cartilage to the ET tube; to ensure this has not happened, it is necessary to extubate the patient and assess the integrity of the sutures. Damage to the recurrent laryngeal nerve either during surgical dissection or subsequently from inflammation may lead to difficulty in swallowing, one of the signs the anesthetist uses to determine when to extubate the patient. In general, the ability to hold the head up also signifies appropriate muscle tone and readiness for extubation.

(a) Anesthetic protocol modifications (Table 4.5): Acepromazine produces mild sedation beneficial to patients in respiratory distress. Opioids that cause vomiting are avoided; methadone is the ideal opioid for these patients. Propofol or alfaxalone are the induction agents of choice, especially when the surgeon requires an airway examination during induction to check laryngeal function. The induction agent is administered slowly so the patient continues spontaneous ventilation for the surgeon to perform a laryngeal examination.

Premedication selection is based on the patient's preanesthetic assessment; it is not uncommon in the otherwise healthy and stable patient to forego premedication in order to obtain the most representative laryngeal exam. The induction agent is chosen based on each patient's profile, but often an induction agent's titratability makes it the agent of choice. Maintenance on a gas inhalant is used. If the procedure requires the patient to be extubated, intermittent bolus of induction agent or TIVA with propofol or alfaxalone is utilized.

3. Parathyroidectomy/thyroidectomy

This surgery involves dissection near and around many vital structures, including the major vessels, trachea, esophagus, and recurrent laryngeal nerve (Box 4.16).

(a) Anesthetic modifications protocol: No drugs are specifically contraindicated for this procedure in the canine patient; however, in cats undergoing thyroidectomy for hyperthyroidism, it is prudent to use a cardiac-friendly protocol, preferably based on cardiac ultrasound. Additionally, one may select fluids that do not contain calcium (although the calcium content in lactated Ringer's solution [LRS] is unlikely to change overall serum calcium levels). Ionized calcium levels are monitored postoperatively in parathyroidectomies. Patients are observed closely postoperatively for any signs of respiratory distress due to nerve damage as well as subsequent aspiration pneumonia.

Chapter 4

110

Table 4.5 Suggested anesthesia protocol for arytenoid lateralization (laryngeal tie back).[a]

Opioid premed (mg/kg)	Sedative premed (mg/kg)	Induction (mg/kg)	Maintenance	Intraoperative analgesia (mg/kg)	Postoperative analgesia (mg/kg)[c]
None per clinician request[b] OR (a) Methadone 0.5 IM OR (b) Hydromorphone[d] 0.05 IV	None per clinician request[b] OR (a) Acepromazine 0.02 IM	(a) Propofol 4–6 to effect OR (b) Alfaxalone 2–4 IV to effect	(a) Isoflurane or sevoflurane AND (b) Metoclopramide CRI If patient requires extubation for procedure: (c) Propofol CRI 6–24 mg/kg/h IV OR (d) Alfaxalone CRI 4–8 mg/kg/h IV	(a) Intermittent bolus: (i) Methadone 0.3 IV OR (ii) Hydromorphone 0.05–0.1 OR (iii) Fentanyl 0.005 IV as needed OR (b) Opioid CRI (i) Fentanyl 0.01–0.042 mg/kg/h	(a) Methadone 0.2 (IV)–0.5 (IM) OR (ii) Hydromorphone 0.05 (IM)–0.1 (IV) q 4 h

[a]Preoxygenate and preemptively provide GI protection.

[b]The clinician evaluating the larynx for laryngeal function may request no premedication. In this case, the "pre"-medication is given after induction. Make sure clinician evaluating larynx is present at induction.

[c]NSAIDs may be included if the clinician elects not to administer steroids to the patient.

[d]Administer maropitant 1 mg/kg IV before hydromorphone to avoid vomiting.

CRI, constant-rate infusion; IM, intramuscular; IV, intravenous.

Box 4.16 Anesthetic concerns regarding parathyroidectomy/thyroidectomy.

- *Cardiomyopathy*: In cases of thyroidectomy indicated for hyperthyroidism in cats, it is common (depending on the duration of the disease) to see changes to the myocardium, most often hyperthyroidism-induced concentric hypertrophy. An echocardiogram is warranted to help the anesthetist understand the extent of this comorbidity and adjust the anesthetic plan accordingly. Thyroidectomies of the cat result in minimal perioperative complications if a cardiac-friendly protocol is used [42].
- *Hemorrhage, swelling, hematoma*: Up to 7.7% of dogs undergoing a unilateral thyroidectomy had hemorrhage in one study [43]. This makes it reasonable to place direct blood pressure monitoring in these patients for anesthesia, as well as a second catheter to transfuse through, in the event a transfusion is warranted. If marked swelling or hematoma occurs in the area around the incision after closure, tracheal compression may occur.
- *Hormonal dysfunction*: The parathyroid gland secretes parathyroid hormone (PTH), which is responsible for the balance of calcium, phosphate, and vitamin D, among other things. After removal, it is necessary to monitor and address fluctuations of calcium, phosphate, and vitamin D. Hypercalcemia is common preoperatively, but is often of minimal impact to the anesthetist, although dilution with fluids that do not contain calcium preoperatively is good practice. The thyroid gland secretes thyroid hormone; see below.
- *Laryngeal nerve paralysis*: Laryngeal nerve paralysis from damage to the recurrent laryngeal nerve (secondary to inflammation or surgical trauma) results in laryngeal dysfunction. Because this nerve supplies the majority of motor function to the larynx, the patient often has difficulty swallowing and maintaining an open airway upon extubation. The extent of this damage is based on whether the nerve is damaged unilaterally or bilaterally. Aspiration pneumonia is also a concern postoperatively, so it may be beneficial to include GI protection in the perioperative period [43].
- *Thyroid storm*: Surgical manipulation or preoperative stress may trigger a thyroid storm in animals with a thyroid mass that is producing thyroid hormone; this manifests itself as an acute onset of tachycardia, hypertension and hyperthermia in response to the release of thyroid hormone. Treatment involves limiting increases in temperature with cool IV fluids and air circulating units. Beta-blockers (i.e., esmolol) are often needed to control tachycardia and subsequent hypertension.

---

4. Total ear canal ablation and bulla osteotomy (TECABO) and ventral bulla osteotomies (VBO)

A TECABO and a VBO are extremely noxious, stimulating procedures that are performed unilaterally or bilaterally. Patients often have chronic pain due to recurring infection and inflammation, in addition to the acute pain of their procedure (Box 4.17).

Box 4.17 Concerns regarding TECABOs.

- *Hemorrhage*: Because several major arteries course through this area, severe hemorrhage is possible, but uncommon when the procedure is performed by an experienced surgeon.
- *Horner's syndrome*: The incidence of postoperative Horner's syndrome is high [44]. Damage during surgical dissection or inflammation in the surrounding tissue to cranial nerve VII results in a prolapsed third eyelid and possible loss of palpebral reflex, as well as facial droop on the affected side. Patients should have their eyes well lubricated postoperatively.
- *Postoperative respiratory complications*: Up to 47% of cats who underwent a single-stage bilateral VBO developed severe respiratory complications and/or death related to surgery [45,46], so performing a bilateral single-stage VBO is discouraged. If this procedure is chosen, the anesthetist should prepare for postoperative reintubation by having appropriate drugs and equipment available, as well as having emergency drug doses calculated.

Chapter 4

(a) Anesthetic protocol modifications: Intraoperative noxious stimuli and postoperative pain are of primary concern for these animals. Anesthesia protocols must focus heavily on providing the best preemptive, intraoperative, and postoperative analgesia possible. See Table 4.6 as well as Chapter 7 for local blocks.

5. Deep ear flush/myringotomy

Deep ear flushes are performed in patients with chronic ear infections, to clear debris and purulent material from the ear. Often, these patients have painful ears and may or may not have an intact tympanic membrane. In cases where middle or inner ear infection is suspected, a myringotomy (incision into the tympanic membrane) is used to reduce pressure and pain (Box 4.18).

(a) Anesthetic protocol: Anesthetic protocol is based on the patient's preanesthetic assessment. Often these are short procedures (less than 20 minutes). Short-acting or reversible drugs are preferred (i.e., fentanyl and dexmedetomidine), bearing in mind that reversal of the sedative effects of the drug will reverse their analgesic benefits as well. The inclusion of alpha-2 agonists, if not contraindicated, and an opioid is suitable for premedication if warranted. Short-duration induction agents such as alfaxalone or propofol are ideal due to the short nature of the procedure, but do not offer additional analgesia. If not contraindicated, a low coinduction dose of ketamine can be considered to assist with chronic pain. Intermittent boluses or a CRI of opioids may be required to avoid stimulation during the procedure. Patients are intubated, and the ET tube cuff is properly inflated. Caution is suggested with inclusion of NSAIDs for these patients, as they may already be receiving steroids as part of their ear disease management. However, sending home postoperative analgesia is warranted.

6. Dentals with extractions

Routine dental cleanings have very few complications when one takes the proper precautions securing the patient's airway. Preanesthetic assessment with a complete PE, full BW, and indicated diagnostics is very important to ensure a suitable anesthetic plan. Many patients requiring extensive dental work are older with concurrent systemic issues, often times cardiac disease. At least one study indicates that if the anesthesia is performed by trained personnel who create a plan prioritizing cardiac disease, and the patient is carefully monitored, there is no increased risk in this population compared to those who do not have heart disease [47] (Box 4.19).

(a) Anesthesia protocol: Drug selection is based on the patient's preanesthetic assessment. As alluded to previously, many dental cases have other diseases in addition to requiring extensive dental work. These patients may require alterations in the anesthetic protocol to accommodate their concurrent diseases (see Chapter 5). Premedication involves an opioid appropriate for the extent of dental work intended (e.g., if several extractions are involved, a full agonist opioid is indicated) and a sedative if required. Induction and maintenance of anesthesia are accomplished by an agent appropriate for the patient. Dental nerve blocks are indicated for any patient with extractions (see Chapter 7). An opioid CRI may be required to reduce MAC and provide

Table 4.6 Suggested anesthesia protocol for a TECABO.

Opioid premed (mg/kg)	Sedative premed (mg/kg)	Induction (mg/kg)	Maintenance	Intraoperative analgesia (mg/kg/h)	Postoperative analgesia (mg/kg)
Full agonist opioid: (a) Hydromorphone 0.1 (IV)–0.2 (IM) OR (b) Methadone 0.3 (IV)–0.5 (IM)	(a) Dexmedetomidine 0.003 (IV)–0.005 (IM) OR (b) Acepromazine 0.01 (IV)–0.03 (IM)	(a) Ketamine 5 + midazolam 0.25 OR (b) Ketofol (ketamine and propofol, 2 mg/kg each combined in the same syringe) to effect +/–Midazolam 0.1 IV OR (c) Alfaxalone 2–4 to effect + Ketamine 0.5 +/–midazolam 0.1–0.2 IV	Isoflurane or sevoflurane	(a) Opioid CRI (i) Fentanyl CRI 0.01–0.042 OR (ii) Hydromorphone CRI 0.03 AND (b) Lidocaine CRI 1.5–3 (dogs only)[a] AND (c) Ketamine CRI 0.6	(a) Soaker catheter: (i) Lidocaine 1–2, followed by a CRI of 1.5 mg/kg/h OR (ii) Bupivacaine 2 followed by an intermittent dose of 1 q 4–6 h AND (b) Intermittent opioid bolus (select one): (i) Hydromorphone 0.1 q 4 h IV OR (ii) Methadone 0.2–0.3 q 4 h IV AND (c) NSAID

[a] Lidocaine CRI is contraindicated in cats.

CRI, constant-rate infusion; IM, intramuscular; IV, intravenous.

Box 4.18 Anesthesia considerations/common complications for deep ear flush.

- *Acute on chronic pain*: Patients that present for a deep ear flush often have chronic ear infections, which are a source of chronic pain. When the flush is performed in these patients, it adds an element of acute pain. This results in an "acute on chronic" noxious or painful event, which adversely affects quality of life. Every attempt to optimize analgesia is done for these animals.
- *Unintentional or unanticipated myringotomy*: The complications from a myringotomy are usually minimal, but may include vestibular disease present at recovery. Additionally, a myringotomy will create communication between the ear canal and trachea, possibly increasing chances for aspiration of fluid from ear flush. Make sure that the ET tube cuff is appropriately inflated.

Box 4.19 Anesthesia considerations/common complications for dental procedures.

- *Aspiration of fluid*: Copious amounts of fluid are present in the mouth during dental procedures, including fluid to keep the drill from overheating and blood from working in such a vascular area. To reduce the possibility of the patient aspirating these fluids, ensure the ET tube cuff is well inflated. Place sponge or gauze 4 × 4 with string secured to the ET tube (dental floss works well) in the back of the mouth to prevent aspiration; however, one must take extreme care to ensure the oropharyngeal pack is removed at the end of the procedure. It is recommended to record on the anesthesia record if a pack is placed and when it is removed. Simple positioning helps as well; elevating the neck with towels and trying to keep the nose down facilitates drainage of fluid from the mouth. In dogs, the anesthetist may choose to remove the ET tube with the cuff partially inflated if there is concern about fluid compromising the airway.
- *Noxious stimuli/pain*: Dental extractions are painful because of the innervation to the tooth as well as the sensitivity of the oral mucosa. Whenever possible, incorporation of a local block (see Chapter 7) is warranted, as this will prevent pain transmission.

---

additional analgesia in patients with extremely painful mouths. Patients are not extubated until they are capable of swallowing and lifting their head; again, confirm the dental pack is removed. Remember to include appropriate analgesia in the postoperative period, including NSAIDs, if not contraindicated.

7. Ocular procedures

These procedures are categorized into procedures involving the globe (i.e., enucleation, lens luxation, phacoemulsification) and those involving tissues surrounding the globe (i.e., cherry eye, entropion repair, mass removals) (Box 4.20).

(a) Anesthesia protocol: Full mu agonist opioids cause miosis in dogs and mydriasis in cats. Atropine, administered topically or systemically, will result in mydriasis and is often combined into the premedication protocol for the dog to avoid opioid-induced miosis. Alternatively, phenylephrine is used topically to dilate the pupil; systemic effects may be noticeable following topical application (i.e., profound hypertension secondary to vasoconstriction). Drugs causing vomiting (hydromorphone, morphine, dexmedetomidine) are avoided in patients where IOP is a concern. Ketamine increases IOP via muscle contracture around the globe, so it is only used

Box 4.20 Anesthesia concerns/common complications for ocular procedures.

- *Noxious stimuli/pain*: Because vision and thus the eye are key to survival, the eye is heavily innervated and therefore procedures involving the eye are very painful. Fortunately, local anesthetic delivered either topically or as a local block (see Chapter 7), when appropriately applied, prevents pain transmission. Indeed, when topical proparacaine is given as two drops, 1 minute apart, the cornea is anesthetized for up to 55 minutes in dogs [48]; the duration is much shorter in cats [49]. Combined with adequate premedication (i.e., a full mu agonist) and analgesic medication postoperatively (NSAIDs if not contraindicated), effective pain management is feasible.
- *Concurrent disease*: While not all patients with ocular disease have concurrent disease, a high prevalence of dogs presenting for phacoemulsification secondary to cataract disease are diabetic. Appropriate anesthetic management of the diabetic patient (see Chapter 5, "Diabetes mellitus") is necessary. Recent work also suggests between 11–20% of diabetic dogs undergoing phacoemulsification may experience hyperkalemia, so routine monitoring of intraoperative electrolytes is warranted in these patients [50].
- *Concurrent medications*: In addition to routine screening for concurrent medications as is done for any patient undergoing anesthesia, these patients may be receiving medication from the ophthalmologist to promote pupillary dilation (especially important in patients with a lens luxation or cataract) or to reduce intraocular pressure (IOP). These drugs (such as phenylephrine) manifest their presence during anesthesia, so it is good practice for the anesthetist to confirm what medications the patient is receiving, both from the owner and from the ophthalmologist.
- *Increased IOP*: Glaucoma compromises vision and therefore is an emergency which may require surgical intervention if medical therapy fails. The anesthetist's goal is not to worsen glaucoma through their actions. Drugs that worsen glaucoma are avoided (including atropine and ketamine). Anything that will cause vomiting (as vomiting increases IOP) is avoided. Coughing significantly increases IOP. The patient is intubated *only* at an adequate plane of anesthesia. Glaucoma is a very painful disease, and appropriate analgesia (opioids such as methadone) is incorporated into the analgesic plan.
- *Ocular positioning*: For certain procedures, such as phacoemulsification, a centrally located eye is necessary. In these cases, where a surgeon prefers not to use a stay suture for placement, a neuromuscular blocking agent (NMBA) is incorporated into the protocol. Prior to use of a NMBA, a nerve stimulator is placed on the patient, usually over the common peroneal nerve (Figure 4.1). A train of four (TOF) is observed, visually comparing the first twitch to the fourth twitch. While it is possible to provide neuromuscular blockade to only the eye, for safety reasons, the anesthetist must assume the NMBA will paralyze the respiratory muscles as well. Therefore, before administration of a NMBA, mechanical ventilation is begun (see Chapter 2, "Mechanical ventilation"). Once the NMBA is administered (see Chapter 7), the twitches will diminish from fourth to first before disappearing altogether. Ultimately, the appropriate effect of NMBA, regardless of how many twitches are present, is the ocular position for the ophthalmologist. Because the eye is very sensitive to the effect of neuromuscular blockade, even when four twitches are present post drug administration, the eye may still remain central. Readministration of the NMBA is at the discretion of the ophthalmologist.

  The next challenge is reversal of the blockade near the end of the procedure. The anesthetist's greatest concern with the use of NMBA is continued paralysis in recovery, which may go unnoticed. This iatrogenic respiratory arrest will proceed rapidly to cardiac arrest. Therefore, it is incumbent upon the anesthetist to ensure the patient is adequately ventilating before leaving the OR, regardless of when the procedure was completed (i.e., if timing is not optimized, the anesthetist may spend another hour in the OR after the procedure is completed, ensuring the patient is fit for recovery).

- No *specific drugs* are contraindicated for ocular procedures involving the tissues surrounding the eye. The protocol is selected based on the patient's preanesthetic assessment.

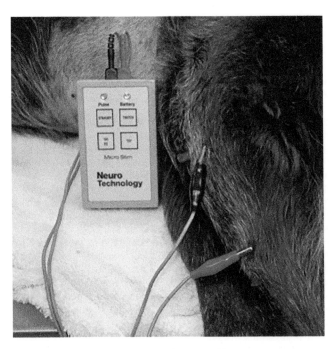

Figure 4.1   Patient with a nerve stimulator over the peroneal nerve (line). *Source:* Courtesy of Patricia Queiroz-Williams.

in a patient that has effective muscle relaxation from premedication or general anesthesia. There is debate about increases in IOP from the use of propofol [51,52] or alfaxalone [53,54]. In studies demonstrating an increase in IOP, the increase was 3–5 mmHg compared with dogs induced with thiopental, which is a small although statistically significant increase; these increases were transient for both drugs. However, these studies were also performed in clinically normal dogs (as opposed to dogs with glaucoma). Unfortunately, as thiopental is no longer commercially available in some parts of the world, propofol or alfaxalone are still preferable to etomidate in cases where pupillary diameter is of concern [55]. It is the author's recommendation to use thiopental, when available, as the induction agent of choice (unless contraindicated) in patients with glaucoma requiring anesthesia, or propofol or alfaxalone (after significant muscle relaxation) when thiopental is not available. Concurrent diseases may influence anesthetic protocol (see Chapter 5). In addition to applicable local blocks, intraoperative analgesia with lidocaine or opioid CRIs as well as intermittent opioid boluses is warranted. Eye ointment/ lubricant is not placed in the eye undergoing surgery, unless specifically requested by the ophthalmologist (usually after completion of procedure). If the ophthalmologist requires the eye to remain central, an NMBA is included (see Table 7.8).

E. Perianal surgeries (anal sacculectomy, perianal fistula, vulvoplasty)

These surgeries involve the area around the anus and vulva. This area is very sensitive to surgical stimulation. The surgical approach does not involve an open abdominal cavity, which makes temperature regulation much easier for the anesthetist (Box 4.21).

Box 4.21 Anesthesia concerns/complications for perianal surgeries.

- *Anal tone*: The surgical approach can disrupt innervation to the anus, resulting in postoperative fecal incontinence. For this reason and depending on the approach, some surgeons request that an epidural with local anesthetic is *not* performed, so an assessment of anal tone following recovery is possible. It is appropriate to discuss this with the surgeon preoperatively.
- *Noxious stimuli/pain*: Due to the level of innervation of this region, surgical stimulation results in a fair amount of noxious stimuli intraoperatively and pain postoperatively. An epidural with 0.1 mg/kg preservative0free morphine will provide suitable, long-lasting analgesia. If the surgeon is confident that they do not need to assess anal tone immediately following surgery, epidural administration of local anesthetic (such as 0.5 mg/kg bupivacaine), which desensitizes this region, improves the quality of the patient's anesthetic event significantly. When administering an epidural for analgesia in the perianal region, the bevel of the needle is directed caudally, allowing for drug delivery to the target dermatomes. An NSAID is warranted postoperatively, if not contraindicated.
- *Patient positioning*: For visualization, these patients are often placed on padding to elevate the hindquarters with the head/thorax directed downward. This results in hypoventilation because of the pressure of abdominal contents on the thorax, as well as difficulty in some monitoring placement (such as arterial line). $EtCO_2$ analysis is essential for these patients, and mechanical ventilation (MV) is often necessary. An indirect means for pressure monitoring is used instead of an arterial line or an arterial line is placed in an alternative location (i.e., front limb). As this is below the level of the heart, blood pressure may be artificially increased. Regurgitation also occurs; the patient's esophagus is suctioned postoperatively even if there is no evidence of regurgitation (to address "silent" regurgitation). If there is evidence of regurgitation upon suctioning, the esophagus is appropriately suctioned and lavaged (see "Regurgitation"). Preoperative GI protection, such as famotidine, is included.

1. Anesthetic protocol

Premedication and induction drugs are based on the patient's preanesthetic assessment. Full agonist opioid (methadone, morphine, hydromorphone or fentanyl) with or without a sedative when required is ideal for premedication. Specific to the procedure, there are no contraindications for specific induction agents. Intraoperative analgesia is best accomplished with coccygeal-sacral or low-volume (0.1 mL/kg) caudal-facing epidural, typically including a local anesthetic. Liposomal encapsulated bupivacaine may be used during closure of the incision. A sealing, protective ointment over the incision postoperatively helps soothe the wound as well as assisting in keeping fecal matter from contacting the incision. Often, these patients had a purse string suture placed preoperatively to close the anus; the anesthetist ensures this suture is removed before discontinuing anesthesia.

F. Reproductive procedures

Castrations and ovariohysterectomies are common procedures in a veterinary setting, with a low incidence of mortality [56]. A huge number of variations occur for anesthesia protocols for these cases, with studies reporting as many as 94 unique premedication/induction drug combinations for canine and feline ovariohysterectomies [57]!

While general anesthesia is used for most reproductive procedures, appropriate pain management has gained significant attention for these cases, and rightly so [58]. Pain is addressed for any animal undergoing a surgical procedure; however, it is important to recognize that an ovariohysterectomy (OVH) is an open abdominal procedure. It is imperative to provide routine surgeries such as OVH and castrations with appropriate pain management (Box 4.22).

1. Anesthesia protocol: cat castration

Castration of the cat is a quick procedure that rarely requires intubation. If the cat is a young healthy patient, a cat total injectable combination is administered. While several varieties of this cocktail exist, it usually involves the combination of an opioid (e.g., butorphanol or buprenorphine), sedative (e.g., dexmedetomidine), and dissociative (i.e., ketamine, although alfaxalone is an alternative). While most drug doses are calculated based on the patient's ideal body weight, cat total injectable combinations are commonly administered as a volume per cat. Table 4.7 shows some common cat total injectable combinations. An intratesticular block is encouraged (see Chapter 7). Postoperatively, a feline-appropriate NSAID (robenacoxib or meloxicam) is given SQ when not contraindicated.

Of note, there is a rare but interesting occurrence (0.6%) of hyphema in feline sterilization procedures, when a tiletamine/zolazepam combination is used for anesthesia induction. It is self-limiting, with most animals returning to normal within about 20 hours [59].

Box 4.22 Anesthesia concerns/complications for reproductive procedures.

- *Pain*: A balanced analgesic plan is warranted for all patients undergoing reproductive procedures. This includes appropriate premedication, induction agents such as ketamine when not contraindicated to provide preemptive analgesia, and local blocks where applicable to reduce noxious stimulus transmission. Postoperatively, NSAIDs are administered when not contraindicated in addition to other take-home analgesics (e.g., gabapentin). Liposomal encapsulated bupivacaine in the tissue layers during closure of abdominal incisions provides a long-lasting analgesia into the discharge period.
- *Hemorrhage*: Major arteries perfuse the reproductive organs; inappropriate hemostasis from a slipped ligation or tearing of a pedicle requires aggressive volume support while the surgeon locates the hemorrhaging vessel.

Table 4.7 Cat total injectable intramuscular combinations.

Option 1: Drug dosage (mg/kg)	Option 2: Volume (for every 4 kg of cat)
Butorphanol 0.3 OR Buprenorphine 0.03	Butorphanol (10 mg/mL) 0.12 mL OR Buprenorphine (0.3 mg/mL) 0.4 mL OR Buprenorphine (0.6 mg/mL) 0.2 mL
Dexmedetomidine 0.005–0.015	Dexmedetomidine (0.5 mg/mL) 0.04–0.12 mL
Ketamine 7.5–10 OR Alfaxalone 2–5	Ketamine (100 mg/mL) 0.3–0.4 mL OR Alfaxalone (10 mg/mL) 0.8–2.0 mL

2. Anesthesia protocol: dog castration

Dogs for castration are premedicated, catheterized, intubated, and placed on maintenance anesthetic. It is common for premedication to include an opioid and sedative. Testicular block with local anesthetic attempts to provide a balanced technique (see Chapter 7). The opioid premedication is usually sufficient for intraoperative and postoperative analgesia. An injectable dose of a NSAID is administered postoperatively in the healthy patient, with oral NSAIDs to go home.

3. Anesthesia protocol: ovariohysterectomy

For both cat and dog spays, it is common to combine an opioid and sedative for premedication. Mu agonist opioids, such as morphine, hydromorphone, methadone, or buprenorphine, are appropriate opioid selections in dogs, although hydromorphone is avoided if possible in the cat. Sedation with an alpha-2 agonist also provides analgesia but drug selection is based on the patient's preanesthetic assessment. Consider incorporating incisional liposomal encapsulated bupivacaine (5.3 mg/kg diluted sufficiently to cover the length of the incision) to provide long-acting local analgesia. Postoperative analgesia includes repeating a dose of opioid for postoperative pain and at minimum a single dose of NSAIDs, with possibly additional NSAIDs for administration at home, if no contraindications exist. A lidocaine patch over the incision also provides additional analgesia when regular or liposomal encapsulated bupivacaine is not available. In cases of feline spay, there was no difference in postoperative pain score for either liposomal encapsulated bupivacaine or regular bupivacaine [60].

4. Anesthesia protocol: dystocia/cesarean section (C-section)

C-sections, either as emergencies or as scheduled procedures, are performed when fetal survival is prioritized (even if the owner elects to spay the animal after the neonates are delivered). Certain breeds, such as the Bulldog, Boston Terrier, and French Bulldog, have a high incidence of C-section [61], as do Great Danes [62]. There is often good success with C-sections, especially for nonurgent surgery, nonbrachycephalic dams, and smaller litters, which are statistically associated with live puppies at delivery. Radiographs provide a fetal head count, so the number of puppies for removal is quantified. A focal ultrasound is performed to see if any of the fetuses are viable in an emergency C-section. Viable fetuses may influence drug selection in the anesthetic protocol. The anesthetist takes into consideration drugs that will pass to the fetus and how these drugs impact the fetus. It is important to obtain preoperative BW in the mother (especially electrolytes, including ionized calcium and hydration status).

If the surgeon elects to perform an OVH where fetal survival is *not* intended or expected, the anesthetic plan follows a similar protocol for an OVH (see "Ovariohysterectomy"). A bupivacaine line block of 2 mg/kg can be performed before the incision is made and after the sterile preparation. For experienced anesthetists, who are capable of an expeditious epidural, the use of low-dose bupivacaine and an opioid profoundly reduces the requirements for intraoperative opioids, and is encouraged [63]. However, if the epidural takes a prolonged period of time, the neonates may be compromised (Boxes 4.23–4.25).

Box 4.23 Anesthesia complications related to pregnancy.

- *Delayed GI motility*: Decreased GI motility in the bitch and queen means that although the mother may not have eaten for a prolonged period of time, there may still be food in the stomach. In humans, Mendelson syndrome is one cause of maternal death; this syndrome is characterized by aspiration of GI contents by the pregnant mother during anesthesia. It is prudent to promptly inflate the cuff on the ET tube after the patient is intubated and prepare for suctioning of GI contents in these patients. If aspiration is suspected postoperatively, appropriate therapy for aspiration pneumonia is instituted. Preemptive GI protection, such as famotidine, is encouraged.
- *Effective circulating volume*: As noted earlier, these patients present often after having gone off food and water in preparation for the delivery of the young. If the patient appears dehydrated, preoperative volume loading with 10–30 mL/kg of crystalloids is warranted. Otherwise, placing the mother on twice maintenance fluid therapy (5 mL/kg/h) until the team is ready for induction is appropriate.
- *Hypocalcemia*: An ionized calcium level is assessed in the mother prior to beginning the procedure; supplementation with calcium in the fluids is used as needed.
- *Hypoventilation*: As the bitch or queen nears term, hypoventilation becomes a more significant problem due to the functional obstruction of diaphragmatic tone secondary to abdominal filling. Assisted ventilation is often necessary in these cases.

Box 4.24 Anesthesia protocol tips for C-sections (Table 4.8).

- *Obtain IV access*: This is usually accomplished without sedation, as high progesterone levels present in the pregnant animal facilitate handling. If IM sedation is required to obtain IV access, sedation (opioid or medetomidine) may be given, as long as it is reversible. Interestingly, one study found good puppy vigor and survival at 2 h and up to 7 days later when medetomidine was used and then reversed in the puppy [64]. Crystalloid fluids, ideally containing calcium (e.g., LRS), are started.
- *Minimize time* between induction and the OR suite.
- *Preparation*: The patient is provided supplemental oxygen via oxygen mask during preoperative preparation. Preparation includes clipping the surgical area and epidural area, as well as a dirty scrub before induction (try to allow patient to remain in sternal/standing position). The surgeon is scrubbed and has the table opened and ready. Opioid premedication is advised if an epidural is not planned following induction.
- *Induction*: Following preoxygenation, induce with propofol or alfaxalone IV to effect (ideally, in the OR) [65,66], with alfaxalone resulting in better puppy vitality for the first 60 minutes (although there was no difference in puppy survival between the two agents in the same study) [67]. If no IM sedation was necessary, a high dose of induction agent may be needed to intubate patient.
- *Maintenance and analgesia*: Gas inhalants are routinely used for maintenance, as evidence suggests CRI with drugs such as alfaxalone may delay maternal recovery and puppy vigor [68]. Without premedication, inhalant requirements are high which increases the potential for maternal hypotension risking decreased perfusion to the uterus and, in turn, hypoxemia in the fetus. Regional anesthetic techniques (i.e., line blocks, epidural) are helpful to minimize inhalant requirement. At closure, liposomal encapsulated bupivacaine (5.3 mg/kg diluted) can be used as an infiltrative block distributed in the tissue layer closures, avoiding the mammary tissue. Some anesthetists elect to administer a single dose of NSAID SQ to help a mother in recovery.
- *Recovery*: Recovering the mother involves providing adequate analgesia without significant sedation so the mother is capable of cleaning and nursing the newborns. As soon as possible after closure and cleaning of the surgery site, the neonates are encouraged to nurse to prevent hypoglycemia and allow passive transfer. A bitch or queen that is in pain may reject or even become aggressive toward young attempting to nurse. Therefore, it is recommended to manage the mother's pain appropriately.

Box 4.25 Fetal resuscitation (Table 4.9).

- *Fetal breathing*: If neonates are slow to vocalize, begin with intentional rubbing to stimulate respiration and ventilation. A bulb syringe is used to clear mucus from mouth and nares. Flow-by oxygen is used via mask to provide supplemental oxygen. Vigorous rubbing from caudal to cranial along the neonate's dorsum helps stimulate breathing and clearing of airway.
- *Drug reversal*: If the neonate is still slow to vocalize and sedatives or opioids were used in the mother, place a drop of reversal agent under the newborn's tongue. For opioids, naloxone is a common reversal; for benzodiazepines, flumazenil is used. Fetal and neonatal metabolism of drugs is inferior to that of an adult, due in large part to the immaturity of the liver and kidneys, where the majority of drugs are broken down and excreted, respectively. Therefore, minimizing the drugs administered to the mother by conservative dosing or the use of non-systemic drug routes is the best way to minimize the impact of drugs on the young. Where epidurals are not performed, opioids are administered during the perioperative period.
- *Contraindicated agents when focusing on puppy survival*: Conversely, agents such as ketamine, benzodiazepines, and thiopental are associated with decreased puppy vigor at birth [69]. Xylazine is also contraindicated [70], although an unusual study did not find this contraindication with medetomidine [64].
- *Setting up for puppies*: A warm area should be dedicated for the neonates until the mother is recovered from anesthesia. Circulating water blankets and/or air warming units are helpful in providing appropriate warmth.

Table 4.8   C-section with priority of puppy survival.

Step 1: Obtain IV catheter without sedation; use EMLA cream on clipped skin to facilitate placement. Clip and scrub abdomen and lumbosacral area for procedure and epidural (see Chapter 7), respectively. Some anesthetists will administer an opioid if the patient is difficult to handle, although opinions differ on this point.

Step 2: Fluid bolus 10–30 mL/kg over 10 min. Continue fluids at 5–15 mL/kg/h.

Step 3: Preoxygenate, maintain patient in sternal recumbency (avoid dorsal recumbency). Place monitoring equipment on patient.

Step 4: Alfaxalone 2–4 mg/kg IV or propofol 4–6 mg/kg IV to effect. During induction, an experienced anesthetist may perform an epidural, if expedient.

Step 5: Inflate cuff on ET tube as soon as possible and begin gas inhalant.

Step 6: Sterile prep. Incisional line block with bupivacaine 1–2 mg/kg.

Step 7: Encourage expedient removal of puppies. Support blood pressure for the mother to ensure perfusion to the uterus and therefore oxygenation to the remaining pups.

Step 8: Administer systemic opioids with low fat solubility (such as morphine) after removal of puppies, if this was not administered preemptively. Administer epidural postoperatively, if not given before. Liposomal encapsulated bupivacaine (5.3 mg/kg diluted) as an infiltrative block can be administered in the tissue layers during closing (avoiding mammary tissue) for prolonged analgesia.

Step 9: Recover and consider postoperative pain control with an NSAID.[a]

[a]NSAIDs are administered in patients where no other contraindications exist and patient did not experience hypotension intraprocedurally.

ET, endotracheal; IV, intravenous; NSAID, nonsteroidal antiinflammatory drug.

Table 4.9   Neonatal resuscitation supplies.

Supplies	Use
Small ET tubes (2.5 mm ID) or 18–16 G catheter with stylet removed	Intubate if neonate not breathing
Bulb syringe	Suction mouth and nares
Warming units (circulating hot water blankets, air warming units, incubators, etc.)	Keep neonates warm until mother recovers
Small oxygen mask or large enough mask to fit pup inside	Provide supplemental oxygen
Flow-by oxygen source	Provide supplemental oxygen
Reversal agents for any drugs used in mom (i.e., naloxone, flumazenil, atipamezole)	Increase neonate vigor by reversing drugs exposed to *in utero*
Glucose supplement	Hypoglycemia
Warm towels	For rubbing neonates to stimulate breathing

ET, endotracheal; ID, internal diameter.

5. Anesthesia protocol: pyometra (open vs closed)

Pyometra is a uterine infection in intact female dogs or cats (although it can occur in the uterine stump of patients where an ovarian remnant is left at the time of the animal's OVH). Patients with an open pyometra are usually less systemically affected [71]. In a closed pyometra, patients are often severely septic before they are diagnosed, making them a higher anesthetic risk.

A major concern for the anesthetist when anesthetizing a dog with a pyometra is endotoxemia or septicemia. One of the most common pathogens in pyometra is *Escherichia coli*, which releases endotoxins into the bloodstream (endotoxemia). As the disease progresses, the pathogens risk infecting the bloodstream (septicemia) as well as the primary organ. While both conditions sicken a patient significantly, septicemia is life-threatening. The animal presents in shock with significant vasodilation. While IV antibiotics may improve the situation, the patient is at significant risk because surgery is required to remove the primary source of infection (i.e., the uterus). Inhalant anesthetics, which are necessary for surgery, exacerbate vasodilation. Vasopressor support (epinephrine, ephedrine, or phenylephrine) is often necessary in addition to standard management for hypotension. Additionally, as sepsis worsens, diseases such as acute respiratory distress (ARD), systemic inflammatory response (SIRs), secondary multiorgan failure, and disseminated intravascular coagulation (DIC) develop.

The anesthetic protocol for an open pyometra is based on the patient's preanesthetic assessment. For a closed pyometra, one carefully examines the patient for signs of shock (and addresses this prior to induction, to the greatest extent possible) as well as the patient's BW to see if other organs are damaged. These cases are often an ASA 4–5; owners are informed there is a real risk the patient may die with anesthesia and are consulted regarding cardiopulmonary resuscitation (CPR) status. The severity of this disease necessitates a cautious approach to anesthesia, and there is the possibility of prolonged hospitalization for these dogs who may present with moderate to severe depression, pale mucous membranes, and leukopenia [72]. Often a neuroleptic induction with an opioid such as fentanyl and a benzodiazepine are used to facilitate intubation followed by a CRI such as fentanyl to keep the vaporizer at the lowest possible setting to prevent consciousness. Heavy BP support is required to keep the patient stable and a short surgical time is a must.

G. Thoracotomy procedures

Respiration is important for both oxygenation of the body and removal of CO_2. Gas exchange is based on normal lung anatomy and shape, which is maintained by negative pressure in the thorax. When the thorax is entered, intrathoracic pressure equalizes with atmospheric pressure (i.e., negative pressure is lost). This results in the lung collapsing to its residual volume, which is not compatible with adequate gas exchange. Thoracotomy in the feline carries a greater risk of mortality than in the canine patient [73,74], so special care is taken in the case of feline thoracotomies (Box 4.26).

Box 4.26 Anesthetic concerns/common complications for thoracotomy procedures.

- *Hypoxemia*: When alveoli have collapsed, there is no longer adequate surface area for normal gas exchange. A patient will have significant ventilation to perfusion (V/Q) mismatch. Coupled with the concurrent hypoventilation, there is profound risk for severe and prolonged hypoxemia if appropriate interventional steps are not taken. One such step is the use of a peak end-expiratory pressure (PEEP) valve; a PEEP valve maintains a residual amount of pressure in the airway, preventing the alveoli from collapsing completely. Not only does this allow for continued gas exchange, it also helps with reexpanding the alveoli once negative pressure is restored. These patients are always maintained on 100% oxygen. Monitoring with a pulse oximeter (see Chapter 2) is essential both intraoperatively and postoperatively. Additionally, arterial blood gas analysis is key to evaluation of hypoxemia and ventilation.
- *Hypoventilation*: Because adequate gas exchange is compromised when the lungs equalize with atmospheric pressure, CO_2 is not effectively removed. This results in hypercapnia (hypoventilation). Respiration is assisted (manually or with a mechanical ventilator, often based on the needs of the surgeon); see Chapter 2 for instructions on how to use a mechanical ventilator. $EtCO_2$ monitoring is critical for moment-to-moment information on hypoventilation, as well as determining the effectiveness of assisted ventilation. $EtCO_2$ compared to $PaCO_2$ is beneficial to assess ventilation.
- *Iatrogenic pneumothorax*: It is understood that a thoracotomy will result in a pneumothorax; while this is managed during the procedure, the majority of concern for this iatrogenic pneumothorax occurs postoperatively. Chest tubes are a vital part of the postoperative plan. Staff working with these patients postoperatively need appropriate instruction on how to manually evacuate the chest. If at any time there is concern that the patient is "not right," the chest is evacuated! It takes very little time for respiratory collapse to occur if there is a buildup of air or fluid in the thorax. Continued monitoring with pulse oximetry is warranted postoperatively.
- *Pain*: A thoracotomy is a particularly painful procedure, both intraoperatively and postoperatively. A 0.3 mL/kg total volume epidural with morphine and saline assists with pain management in some of these patients, with this maximal volume intended to move the drug closer to its target site. A variety of local nerve blocks are available to mitigate pain intra- and postoperatively, and should be included whenever possible. This includes things as recent as a serratus plane block [75], intercostal nerve blocks with local anesthetic, and surgeons performing intraoperative specific local infiltration of nerves (see Chapter 7 for more details). Additionally, intraoperative multimodal CRIs (such as opioid, lidocaine [dogs only], and ketamine) and postoperative NSAIDs (if not contraindicated) help balance an analgesic plan. There is some debate about intrapleural drug administration via the chest tube postoperatively [76]. It is the opinion of the author that other options be employed first. A lidocaine patch over the incision site may also help postoperatively when liposomal encapsulated bupivacaine as an infiltrative injection in the various tissue layers is not used during closing.

---

1. Anesthetic protocol: traditional thoracotomy

If catheterization is not possible without sedation, premedication includes a full agonist opioid IM. Hydromorphone may cause the patient to pant or vomit so this drug is avoided, if possible. Methadone (0.5 mg/kg IM) is a suitable alternative. Selecting a sedative will depend on the patient's preanesthetic assessment (PE, BW, and disposition) and is avoided if unnecessary. If an IV catheter is placed without sedation, an opioid with/without a benzodiazepine is ideal IV. Once the patient is induced, an arterial line (see Chapter 2) is placed to monitor IBP as well as to allow sampling for blood gas analysis. ECG, capnography, Doppler, temperature, and SpO$_2$ are also monitored. Upon recovery, chest tubes are left in place until negative pressure is consecutively obtained (usually for the first 24 hours after a procedure). Supplemental oxygen (see Table 3.8) is used for any patient that cannot maintain a pulse oximeter reading greater than 94%. Patients are placed in a setting where they are closely monitored for respiratory distress. It may be helpful to maintain the arterial catheter during the first 12–24 hours of recovery in dogs.

2. Anesthetic protocol: diaphragmatic hernia

Diaphragmatic hernias present either acutely (secondary to trauma, for example) in respiratory distress, or chronically (secondary to a congenital malformation; the patient usually presents for unrelated reasons). A recent, traumatically induced diaphragmatic hernia is a suitable candidate for immediate surgical correction. A patient with a congenital diaphragmatic hernia has often compensated quite well over time for this abnormality; a thorough abdominal palpation, presence of a "heave" line (hypertrophied abdominal musculature to assist with breathing), and thoracic radiographs may confirm its presence. However, the choice of surgical repair for these chronic cases necessitates excellent anesthesia support; indeed, of the two, the congenital diaphragmatic hernia is the more difficult case to manage. It is advised that the congenital diaphragmatic hernia is only corrected with the supervision of a board-certified anesthesiologist.

H. Urological procedures (cystotomy, perineal urethrostomy [PU])

A cystotomy is a simple procedure often used to remove urinary calculi or masses; however, care is taken in the pre-workup phase to ensure that there are no stones in the urethra, which may significantly complicate surgery and therefore warrant referral (Box 4.27). Caudal abdominal radiographs are performed to evaluate for the presence/number count of uroliths in patients where the calculi are radiopaque. A PU is commonly performed due to urethra obstruction in neutered male cats. Abdominal ultrasound assists with the evaluation of free fluid in the abdomen; if this free fluid is urine, intervention for a bladder rupture is warranted as soon as possible (see Appendix E). BW is performed to evaluate kidney function and electrolyte values (especially serum potassium). A preoperative ECG is monitored to evaluate for any bradyarrhythmia associated with elevated serum potassium.

1. Anesthetic plan (Table 4.10)

The protocol is targeted at avoiding or reducing the dosage for drugs excreted by the kidney (e.g., ketamine). Otherwise, drugs are selected based on the patient's preanesthetic assessment.

Box 4.27 Anesthetic concerns/common complications for urological procedures.

- *Hyperkalemia (see also Chapter 3 "Hyperkalemia")*: One of the greatest concerns with a ruptured bladder or a blocked cat is the presence of hyperkalemia. This is life-threatening as serum potassium values elevated above 7.5 mEq/L result in severe bradycardia that may progress to asystole. Table 3.14 details management of hyperkalemia.
- *Urinary diuresis or retention*: For surgeries involving an obstruction in the urinary tract, avoid large fluid boluses or drugs that cause diuresis (e.g., alpha-2 agonists) until the procedure is completed. Systemic and epidural morphine has been demonstrated to result in an increase in antidiuretic hormone (ADH) and thus increases urinary retention. Because these cases of urinary retention receive more notoriety when they receive an epidural as opposed to routine premedication, a morphine epidural is often avoided. An epidural with local anesthetic is acceptable, as it should not affect ADH release.
- *Postobstructive diuresis*: This occurs following the unblocking of an obstructed cat. The patient requires a higher fluid rate or risks becoming dehydrated if urologic surgery follows the unblocking of the animal.

Aggressive fluid therapy is only used once the bladder has been incised or a patent urinary catheter is in place.

II. Orthopedic/neurology procedures

Patients may require an orthopedic procedure secondary to trauma, malignancy, malformation or degeneration, or rupture of joints and ligaments. These surgeries involve manipulation of bone and produce a significant degree of somatic pain.

A. Orthopedic procedures on the head

These procedures include those that often involve bones of the skull, commonly including mandibulectomies and maxillectomies (Box 4.28).

1. Anesthetic protocol

No drugs are specifically contraindicated in most orthopedic procedures. A second IV catheter is placed due to the frequent need for transfusion [78]. It is important to create a protocol based on the patient's preanesthetic assessment, and follow a plan that optimizes analgesia.

Premedication includes a mu opioid agonist and alpha-2 agonists, if not contraindicated, as both of these drug families possess analgesic properties. Maropitant is encouraged preoperatively in all patients to reduce the incidence of vomiting and nausea, especially preemptively in patients receiving opioids. Induction with ketamine (if not contraindicated) provides a loading dose as a ketamine CRI is indicated (see later discussion); benzodiazepines facilitate muscle relaxation if ketamine is used as induction agent. If one chooses to use an alternative induction drug, a subanesthetic dose of ketamine (0.5 mg/kg) is included to help decrease wind-up and provide the loading dose for the CRI if desired.

Table 4.10 Suggested anesthesia protocol for cystotomy and PU.[a]

Opioid premed (mg/kg)	Sedative premed (mg/kg)	Induction (mg/kg)	Maintenance	Intraoperative analgesia (mg/kg)	Postoperative analgesia (mg/kg)
(a) Methadone 0.3 (IV)–0.5 (IM) OR (b) Hydromorphone[a] 0.1 (IV)–0.2 (IM) OR (c) Morphine 0.5 IM	(a) Acepromazine[b] 0.02	(a) Alfaxalone 1–2 (dogs), 2–3 (cats) OR (b) Propofol 2–4 OR (c) Ketam-ine[c] 5 and diazepam 0.25	Isoflurane or sevoflurane	(a) Epidural (lumbosacral or sacrococcygeal) with local anes-thetic only: (i) Preservative-free bupivacaine 0.5 AND (b) Opioid options: (i) Intermittent bolus: Methadone 0.3 IV OR (ii) Hydromorphone 0.05–0.1 IV OR (iii) Fentanyl 0.005 IV as needed OR (c) CRI (i) Fentanyl CRI 0.01–0.042 mg/kg/h IV	(a) Intermittent bolus: (i) Methadone 0.3 IV q 4–6 h OR (ii) Hydromorphone[a] 0.05–0.1 IV q 4 h OR (iii) Buprenorphine[d] 0.03 IV q 6–8 h

[a]Avoid hydromorphone in cats, if possible.

[b]Avoid alpha-2 agonists, especially if urinary obstruction, as these drugs cause diuresis and may increase chance of rupture.

[c]Avoid ketamine in cats with renal insufficiency.

[d]High-concentration formulation of buprenorphine is an alternative and potentially useful analgesic for these cases; see Chapter 7.

CRI, constant-rate infusion; IM, intramuscular; IV, intravenous.

Box 4.28 Anesthesia concerns/complications for orthopedic procedures on the head.

- *Aspiration*: When an orthopedic procedure is performed in the mouth, such as with a maxillectomy or mandibulectomy, there is a risk of aspirating blood or surgical flush. If the surgeon chooses to pack the pharyngeal region with gauze, the number of gauzes are counted and a prominent reminder note is placed to ensure removal of all packing material. Extubating with the cuff partially inflated helps minimize aspiration.
- *Hemorrhage*: Major arteries course through many of the approaches for orthopedic procedures. While every surgeon strives for adequate hemostasis, occasionally this is not achieved. A preoperative cross-match and blood type is recommended, as up to 42.7% of maxillectomies required a transfusion in one study [77,78]. The anesthetist notes if significant quantities of blood are present in the suction canister or there is a fair amount of soaked 4 × 4 gauze sponges (see Chapter 3 "Blood loss/hemorrhage"). This is unusual during an orthopedic procedure, and if hemorrhage becomes visually significant, it is quantified to see if intervention (i.e., blood transfusion) is required. A second catheter is placed to provide a port for transfusion, should it become necessary.
- *Noxious stimuli/pain*: These procedures warrant aggressive pain management from the start of the case, as pain is a common comorbidity [79]. Preemptive, multimodal analgesia is important as well as appropriate intraoperative analgesia to avoid wind-up pain. Multimodal analgesia involves the use of regional techniques (see Chapter 7) where possible, as well as systemic drugs. Frequent (q4h) reassessment of pain with a suitable pain scale (see Appendix A) is necessary for the first 24 hours, so that adjustments tailored to each patient can be implemented.
- *Postoperative swelling*: As with any surgery that manipulates the oral region, it is sensible to prepare for possible swelling leading to postoperative airway compromise. In one study, there was cervical swelling and self-limiting sublingual swelling in two out of 19 dogs [77]. Having additional drugs for reintubation, additional ET tubes and a laryngoscope is appropriate.

Maintenance with inhalant anesthetic plus a local block (see Chapter 7) is desirable. A local block will not simply modify pain transmission; it will prevent transmission from occurring. If a local block for the surgery site is not available or successful, a multimodal CRI such as opioid, ketamine, and lidocaine (avoid lidocaine CRI in felines) is a suitable alternative.

If hypotension was not a prevalent comorbidity during the procedure, postoperative administration of a NSAID is warranted, as well as continued administration of a full mu agonist opioid for at least the next 24 hours. When recovering patients that underwent an orthopedic procedure involving the facial bones near or around the mouth, one should ensure the patient can swallow and suction the back of mouth before extubating.

B. Thoracic limb orthopedic procedures

These procedures most commonly include arthroscopies, fractures, and angular limb deformity corrections involving the radius, ulna, and/or humerus (Box 4.29). Amputations are covered in the section on soft tissue procedures but many concepts overlap.

2. Anesthetic plan

There are no major contraindications regarding perianesthetic drugs specific to front limb orthopedic procedures. Maropitant is encouraged preoperatively in all patients to reduce

---

Box 4.29 Anesthetic concerns/common complications for thoracic limb orthopedic procedures.

- *Pain*: Procedures involving orthopedic repair are painful and require adequate analgesia. Thankfully, local regional analgesic techniques assist with preventing pain transmission in this region; see Chapter 7. Where local regional techniques cannot be used, CRIs of a mu opioid, ketamine and lidocaine (dogs only) are used. NSAIDs are used if not contraindicated. Liposomal encapsulated bupivacaine placed during incisional closure of each tissue layer is encouraged.
- *Patient access*: As the surgeon requires access to the cranial half of the body, it is most practical to place a catheter in the hindlimb for easier access, and to locate monitoring caudally in the patient when possible.

---

incidence of vomiting and nausea, especially preemptively in patients receiving opioids. Sedatives, when not contraindicated, have great advantages when included in the premedication (e.g., induction and inhalant reduction, sedation, potentially additive analgesia). No specific induction drugs are contraindicated by the procedure. If a ketamine induction is not desirable but a CRI is planned for intraoperative analgesia, a low dose can be administered during induction as the loading dose (0.5 mg/kg). Maintenance for these procedures generally involves inhalant anesthetics with supportive crystalloid fluid. Appropriate analgesia is key. Attention to pain management in continued into the postoperative phase, including the return to normalcy at home. Discharge analgesia often includes continuation of NSAIDs, where not contraindicated, and gabapentin.

C. Hindlimb orthopedic procedures

These include lateral suture, tibial plateau leveling osteotomy (TPLO), tibial tuberosity advancement (TTA), medial patella ligament repair (MPL), femoral head osteotomy (FHO), etc. (Box 4.30).

Box 4.30 Anesthetic concerns/common complications for hindlimb orthopedic procedures.

- *Pain*: Procedures involving the stifle and ligament repair are painful and require adequate analgesia; there is often a protracted course of the disease before it is finally addressed, so often the pain is both chronic and acute (i.e., the surgical intervention). Thankfully, hindlimb procedures have a variety of local regional analgesic techniques that can be employed; it is imperative to review Chapter 7 for the multitude of applicable blocks available to actually stop nociception for these patients. Where local regional techniques cannot be used, CRI of a mu opioid, ketamine and lidocaine (dogs only) are used. NSAIDs are used if not contraindicated; care is taken to ensure that the patient remains on the same NSAID after surgery as it was on before surgery. Liposomal encapsulated bupivacaine placed during incisional closure of each tissue layer is encouraged. In cases where this is the only local block used for TPLOs, there was a lower requirement for opioids postoperatively than when traditional bupivacaine was used during closure [80].
- *Mobility*: Postoperatively, patients requiring hindlimb procedures may not be completely ambulatory, especially when local regional blocks are performed. Sling walk assistance is encouraged.

---

1. Anesthetic plan

There are no major contraindications specific to hindlimb orthopedic procedures regarding perianesthetic drugs. Maropitant is encouraged preoperatively in all patients to reduce the incidence of vomiting and nausea, especially preemptively in patients receiving opioids. Sedatives, when not contraindicated, have great advantages when included in the premedication (e.g., induction and inhalant reduction, sedation, potentially additive analgesia). No specific induction drugs are contraindicated by the procedure. Selection is based on the individual patient. If a ketamine is not desirable but a CRI is planned for intraoperative analgesia, a low dose of ketamine can be administered during induction (0.5 mg/kg). Maintenance for these procedures generally involves inhalant anesthetics with supportive crystalloid fluid. Appropriate analgesia is key (see section above, Pain). Attention to pain management is continued into the postoperative phase, including the return to normalcy at home. Discharge analgesia often includes continuation of NSAIDs, where not contraindicated, and gabapentin.

D. Dorsal hemilaminectomy

Patients requiring a dorsal hemilaminectomy have a herniated disk with spinal cord compression in the thoracic or lumbar spine (Box 4.31). While some animals (e.g., dachshunds) exhibit an inherent tendency toward a ruptured disk (type I disk disease), a slow protrusion of the disk over time causes compression (type II disk disease), generally in older, large-breed dogs. Diagnosing the location of the protrusion requires a neurologic examination, +/− spinal radiographs, computed tomography (CT), and/or magnetic resonance imaging (MRI), depending on the surgeon's preference or experience.

Box 4.31 Anesthesia concerns/common complications for hemilaminectomy procedures.

- *Bradycardia and hypotension*: Bradycardia and hypotension are common in these procedures, with up to 70% of dogs experiencing bradycardia and anywhere from 33.9% to 57% of dogs experiencing hypotension [81,82]. Although hypotension likely did not worsen neurologic outcome [83], It can certainly compromise other organ systems in the body, such as the kidney. In addition to the association between hypotension and hypothermia (see below), hypotension was associated with an increased administration of drugs to resolve bradycardia, demonstrating the role heart rate plays in cardiac output, with improving bradycardia resulting in less hypotension.
- *Dehydration*: Immobile patients commonly present slightly dehydrated with an increased PCV and TP. It is helpful to restore volume by placing a catheter and administering maintenance fluids to the patient while the anesthetist prepares for anesthesia. Care is taken to make sure the animal does not have a distended bladder, as their neurologic dysfunction means these patients often cannot urinate (palpate and express, if necessary, or consider a single-pass urinary catheter).
- *Hypothermia*: This is the most complication (63.8% incidence) associated with anesthesia for dorsal hemilaminectomies [81]. Dogs which underwent an MRI to diagnosis the disk herniation as well as those which had hypotension were at increased risk of hypothermia. Dogs which received alpha-2 agonists or were at an increased body weight had a reduced risk of hypothermia. Presumably, dogs who received alpha-2 agonists underwent a CT instead of an MRI for diagnostic purposes, which would shorten the time spent in the diagnostic phase and reduce the incidence of hypothermia.

- *Hyperthermia*: On the other end of the spectrum, about 20% of patients actually experienced hyperthermia during dorsal hemilaminectomy [81]. Use of alpha-2 agonists and increased duration of general anesthesia were associated with this. This suggests that vigilant temperature monitoring is necessary and as the patient begins to warm, aggressive patient warming is reduced.
- *Noxious stimuli/pain*: Manipulation of tissues around the spinal cord is intensely stimulating, and pain management for these patients is key, both for short-term benefits to the animal as well as for long-term sequelae. Up to 15% of these patients may develop a chronic pain syndrome [84], which is more complex to manage than acute pain. As this pain becomes more widely recognized, the veterinary community continues to develop advanced local anesthetic techniques to address these patients' pain. For example, an erector spinae plane (ESP) block used for hemilaminectomies reduced opioid consumption and additional CRIs necessary perioperatively. The ESP block also reduced the associated bradycardia secondary to the use of opioids [85]. As an aside, however, this is a technically advanced block; readers who perform dorsal hemilaminectomies routinely are encouraged to attend advanced CE training in how to perform ESP blocks. However, straightforward techniques such as periincisional infiltration of bupivacaine administered presurgically reduced perioperative opioid administration [86]. There is mixed evidence about topical analgesia, such as morphine, applied epidurally before closure of the surgical site, with possible benefits when using this as part of multimodal analgesia [87,88].
  Finally, it bears mentioning that alternative therapies such as acupuncture or pulsed electromagnetic field may provide benefits to dogs undergoing surgery for thoracolumbar disk disease [89–92].
- *Progressive spinal cord degeneration*: The animal will gradually and progressively lose neurologic function. Initially, the animal may lack conscious proprioception, in which case the patient is often managed medically. As the disease worsens to include loss of motor function and ability to urinate, the supervising clinician may decide to proceed to surgery. It is important for the anesthetist to help with bladder expression (to avoid bladder atony), as this is often easily performed once the patient is asleep. When deep pain is lost, the decision to proceed to surgery is often an urgent attempt to remove compression and restore motor function. These patients are considered true emergencies and anesthesia is prioritized for them.
- *Regurgitation*: Approximately one out of every 20 dogs (4.9%) which underwent dorsal hemilaminectomy had regurgitation as a complication [81]. This suggests it is imperative to administer GI protection (e.g., famotidine) to increase the pH of stomach contents as soon as it is confirmed the patient will go to surgery. Please see Chapter 3, for a more thorough discussion on regurgitation.

1. Anesthetic plan

The anesthetic protocol is based on patient presentation. No drugs are specifically contraindicated, although including GI protection is strongly encouraged. The classic "back dog" is usually healthy otherwise but it is always important to do a complete PE and routine BW. Premedication includes a full mu agonist +/- an alpha-2 agonist if not contraindicated (*note*: if surgeon preference is a CT for imaging confirmation of disk site, this premedication may provide heavy enough sedation where general anesthesia is unnecessary for CT). Intraoperatively, opioid, lidocaine (for dogs), ketamine [73], alpha-2 agonists [74] or their combinations, when administered as CRIs, work nicely to manage noxious stimuli. Before the use of steroids or NSAIDs, the anesthetist must ensure these drugs have not been previously administered. Ensure that pharmacologic options are available to increase heart rate (e.g., atropine or glycopyrrolate) and support blood pressure (e.g., dopamine or dobutamine). Methods to maintain normothermia must also be available, as well as the technology to continuously monitor body temperature for increases or decreases. Liposomal encapsulated bupivacaine may provide a benefit during incisional closing, as lidocaine patches do not provide additional analgesia for this procedure in dogs [75]. Postoperative opioid and lidocaine (dogs) CRIs are often warranted.

E. Ventral slot

When disk herniation occurs in the cervical spine, the surgical approach is performed ventrally. This requires the surgeon to work around many delicate and important structures, including the trachea, esophagus, carotid arteries, and jugular vessels to access the spinal cord (Box 4.32).

1. Anesthetic protocol

The drug protocol is tailored to the patient's preanesthetic assessment. Premedication includes a full mu agonist opioid. Drugs that cause vomiting are avoided (i.e., hydromorphone or morphine IM). Maropitant (and GI protection) is encouraged preoperatively in all patients to reduce the incidence of vomiting and nausea, especially preemptively in patients receiving opioids. It is ideal to avoid hyperextension of the neck during intubation. Intraoperatively, opioid, lidocaine (for dogs), ketamine, or their combinations, when administered as CRIs, work nicely to manage noxious stimuli. Before the use of steroids or NSAIDs, the anesthetist must ensure these drugs have not been previously administered. Liposomal encapsulated bupivacaine may provide a benefit during incisional closing. Postoperative opioid and lidocaine (dogs) CRIs are often warranted.

Box 4.32 Anesthetic concerns/complications for ventral slot procedures.

- *Aspiration pneumonia*: Dogs undergoing cervical intervertebral disk decompression surgery are at risk for aspiration pneumonia [93]. Avoid drugs that cause regurgitation or vomiting (i.e., hydromorphone, morphine, alpha-2 agonists) postoperatively [40]. Sadly, evidence does not support a reduction in the incidence of aspiration pneumonia from simple interventions such as a metoclopramide CRI [41]. If oxygen saturation is inappropriate after extubation, thoracic films are warranted.
- *Hemorrhage*: Hemorrhage is one of the most common complications of a ventral slot procedure [94]. This occurs secondary to venous sinus proximity as well as vascular disruption and may be profound. Intraoperative blood loss is watched closely. A preoperative crossmatch and blood typing is recommended. A second catheter is placed to provide a port for transfusion, should it become necessary.
- *Noxious stimuli/pain*: These patients often experience persistent pain postoperatively, so good preemptive analgesia is warranted [94]. A full agonist opioid (morphine, hydromorphone, fentanyl), ketamine, and lidocaine (in dogs) CRI is ideal intraoperatively and continued postoperatively. Avoid extending or flexing the neck, especially during restraint and intubation.
- *Occlusion of the ET tube*: As the surgeon distracts tissue to access the vertebrae, it is possible to occlude the ET tube, if it was not placed distal to the point of distraction. The anesthetist must measure the ET tube to beyond the thoracic inlet to avoid the surgeon possibly occluding the ET tube during the surgical approach. $EtCO_2$ monitoring is essential. Some anesthetists prefer the use of wire-guarded ET tubes to prevent occlusion.

III. Scoping procedures

Scoping procedures are minimally invasive means to visualize internal structures and obtain cultures or biopsies. A scope is also useful to assist with therapeutic interventions, such as the placement of feeding tubes or removal of a foreign body, in order to avoid more invasive approaches.

A. Bronchoscopy and bronchial alveolar lavage (BAL) (Box 4.33)

1. Anesthetic protocol

This procedure is not painful. The anesthetic protocol is selected based on drugs that result in minimal respiratory depression, are reversible, and have a short duration. IV access is an absolute necessity. Placement of monitoring equipment is completed in the cooperative patient before induction. While this procedure is not painful, it is often helpful to select a full mu agonist for premedication in case an opioid CRI is necessary to reduce the amount of maintenance drug required for anesthesia. Propofol or alfaxalone are the induction agents of choice and are suitable for maintaining anesthesia when administered as CRIs. Additionally, administering midazolam during induction will reduce the amount of propofol required (this is avoided in cases of laryngeal exam). If available, jet ventilation is ideal for these patients; however, many institutions do not have a jet ventilator. This means the patient is extubated before the procedure begins; however, it is wise to begin with induction and intubation of the patient to allow the anesthetist to get all monitoring in order and fully saturate the patient with oxygen. If the clinician wishes to collect cultures, a sterile ET tube is required for intubation.

Once the anesthetist is comfortable that the patient's monitoring equipment is functional and the patient is stable, then the patient is extubated and the scoping procedure begins. If the scope will fit through the ET tube, there is an adapter available with a port that has a diaphragm, through which the scope enters (Figure 4.2). The diaphragm allows closure of the anesthesia

---

Box 4.33 Anesthetic concerns/complications for a BAL procedure.

- *Airway*: This procedure performed in small patients is a challenge to the anesthetist because the diameter of the scope may exceed the internal diameter of the ET tube (which is not the case for larger patients). In small patients, this means it is not possible to have the patient intubated while performing the bronchoscopy. This is problematic because it both compromises the patient's gas exchange and requires an alternative to gas inhalant for maintaining anesthesia. Without connection to an anesthesia circuit, the anesthetist cannot manually ventilate for the patient and thus, hypoventilation will ensue. Additionally, without supplemental oxygenation delivered through the circuit, the patient may rapidly desaturate and become hypoxemic. Respiratory and, subsequently, cardiac arrest may occur in these cases. Maintenance of anesthesia is often accomplished with TIVA. See "Head and neck procedures" for additional information concerning loss of access and trigeminal vagal response.

    Additionally, it is good practice to know if the clinician performing the bronchoscopy would like to be present at induction for an airway exam.
- *Respiratory compromise*: Often times, this procedure is performed because the patient has a degree of respiratory compromise or distress. Stress is minimized to avoid worsening respiratory distress.

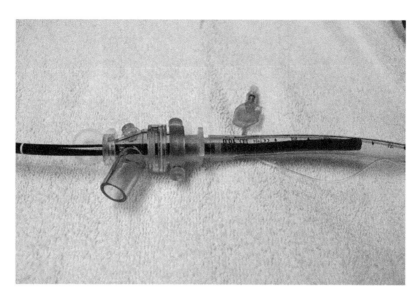

Figure 4.2   Supplies for oxygen insufflation during a BAL. *Source:* Courtesy of Patricia Queiroz-Williams.

circuit so the anesthetist can ventilate the patient. In a patient that is not intubated, supplemental oxygen is administered through the scope or by red rubber catheter attached to the fresh gas outlet on the anesthesia machine. In these patients, reintubation occurs when the patient desaturates, and immediately following the bronchial lavage. The patient is allowed to recover with supplemental oxygen, before reintroducing the scope. Special attention is paid to the pulse oximetry reading, and the procedure is transiently aborted when the SpO_2 drops below 93%.

In recovery, it is ideal to have supplemental oxygen available following extubation. Albuterol is available to assist in bronchodilation.

B. Rhinoscopy and biopsy (Box 4.34)

1. Anesthetic protocol

In some cases, the stimulation from the procedure is so intense that the patient may move and shake their head. Additional boluses of induction agent or fentanyl can help minimize this movement. A quiet recovery is desirable to avoid dislodging any clots following biopsies. A low dose of acepromazine, if not given as a premedication, may be administered IV following extubation, where not otherwise contraindicated. The ET tube cuff is left partially inflated for extubation to help minimize chances of aspiration of blood surrounding the ET tube.

C. Gastroscopy (upper/lower GI) (Box 4.35)

1. Anesthetic protocol

The anesthetic protocol is tailored to the patient's preanesthetic assessment and underlying diseases. The premedication choice of atropine and morphine may make passage of the

---

Box 4.34 Anesthetic concerns/complications for rhinoscopy and biospy procedures.

- *Hemorrhage*: The nasal passage is well perfused and thus rhinoscopy may result in hemorrhage; a small number of these cases will have marked and significant hemorrhage [95]. Coagulation panels are assessed preoperatively to ensure that a patient will adequately clot if biopsies are performed. Nasal phenylephrine and ice packing are common therapies to control continued hemorrhage. In case of profound hemorrhage, the patient may need a cross-match and/or blood typing in order to provide a transfusion. A second catheter is indicated if hemorrhage occurs, so the transfusion occurs through a separate port.

  Aspiration of blood is also a risk, so ensure the ET tube cuff is inflated. Before biopsies are performed often it is advised to place an oral pharyngeal pack to help protect the integrity of the airway at extubation. If a pharyngeal pack is placed, make sure a prominent reminder to remove it is in place. This pack must be removed before the start of recovery or discontinuation of maintenance anesthesia.
- *Noxious stimulation/pain*: Rhinoscopy and biopsies are very stimulating procedures, often necessitating rapid changes in anesthetic plane. There is evidence that inclusion of a local block may reduce the level of responsiveness for patients undergoing these procedures [96–98].
- See "Head and neck procedures" for additional information concerning loss of access and trigeminal vagal response.

Box 4.35 Anesthetic concerns/complications for gastroscopy procedures.

- *Distension of the stomach*: Pain fiber upregulation occurs in the GI tract with visceral organ distension; therefore, insufflating the stomach significantly leads to discomfort for the patient. Fortunately, visualization for the individual performing the endoscopy is usually adequate without hyperinflating the stomach. The anesthetist palpates the stomach at the edge of the ribs prior to beginning the procedure; this allows for a comparison as the stomach is inflated.
- *Hypoventilation*: Hyperdistending the stomach also leads to hypoventilation by compression on the thorax and negatively impacts venous return (and thus BP). If hyperinflation is suspected or confirmed by palpation, the anesthetist communicates this to the person performing the endoscopy with the request to desufflate the abdomen marginally. At the end of the procedure, it is necessary to desufflate the entire stomach to prevent problems in recovery.
- *Vagal event*: As the stomach is distended, it is possible that profound parasympathetic upregulation will occur; bradycardia can ensue quickly. It is recommended to draw up a 0.04 mg/kg dose of atropine in advance to administer IV if this occurs.

---

endoscope through the pyloric sphincter more difficult [99], so these drugs are avoided prior to passing the scope into the stomach. Whatever induction combination is chosen, additional induction drug is available, as one of the hallmark characteristics of these procedures is periods of intense stimulation intermittently in an otherwise minimally stimulated patient, resulting in an abrupt change of the anesthetic plane. Recovery is a concern because the procedure has often disrupted a patient that was previously stable; that is, there is now gas in the stomach. These patients warrant close postanesthetic monitoring although not for the sole purpose of ensuring adequate analgesia, as they often are only mild to moderately painful.

www.wiley.com/go/shelby/anesthesia2

Please go to the companion website for access to videos relating to the book

References

1. Ovbey DH, Wilson DV, Bednarski RM, et al. Prevalence and risk factors for canine post-anesthetic aspiration pneumonia (1999–2009): a multicenter study. Vet Anaesth Analg. 2014;41(2):127–36.
2. Brosnan R, Pypendop B, Siao K, Stanley S. Effects of remifentanil on measures of anesthetic immobility and analgesia in cats. Am J Vet Res. 2009;70(9):1065–71.
3. Herrera M, Mehl M, Kass P, Pascoe P, Feldman E, Nelson R. Predictive factors and the effect of phenoxybenzamine on outcome in dogs undergoing adrenalectomy for pheochromocytoma. J Vet Intern Med. 2008;22(6):1333–9.
4. Zublena F, De Gennaro C, Corletto F. Retrospective evaluation of labetalol as antihypertensive agent in dogs. BMC Vet Res. 2020;16(1):256.
5. Merlin T, Veres-Nyeki K. Anaesthetic management and complications of canine adrenalectomies: 41 cases (2007–2017). Acta Vet Hung. 2019;67(2):282–95.
6. Woods KS, Brisson BA, Defarges AM, Oblak ML. Congenital duplex gallbladder and biliary mucocele associated with partial hepatic cholestasis and cholelithiasis in a cat. Can Vet J. 2012;53(3):269–73.
7. Bennett SL, Milne M, Slocombe RF, Landon BP. Gallbladder mucocoele and concurrent hepatic lipidosis in a cat. Aust Vet J. 2007;85(10):397–400.
8. Parkanzky M, Grimes J, Schmiedt C, Secrest S, Bugbee A. Long-term survival of dogs treated for gallbladder mucocele by cholecystectomy, medical management, or both. J Vet Intern Med. 2019;33(5):2057–66.
9. Rogers E, Jaffey JA, Graham A, et al. Prevalence and impact of cholecystitis on outcome in dogs with gallbladder mucocele. J Vet Emerg Crit Care. 2020;30(1):97–101.
10. Jaffey JA, Pavlick M, Webster CR, et al. Effect of clinical signs, endocrinopathies, timing of surgery, hyperlipidemia, and hyperbilirubinemia on outcome in dogs with gallbladder mucocele. Vet J. 2019;251:105350.
11. Allerton F, Swinbourne F, Barker L, et al. Gall bladder mucoceles in Border terriers. J Vet Intern Med. 2018;32(5):1618–28.
12. Hattersley R, Downing F, Gibson S, et al. Impact of intra-operative hypotension on mortality rates and post-operative complications in dogs undergoing cholecystectomy. J Small Anim Pract. 2020;61(10):624–9.
13. Burns BR, Hofmeister EH, Brainard BM. Anesthetic complications in dogs undergoing hepatic surgery: cholecystectomy versus non-cholecystectomy. Vet Anaesth Analg. 2014;41(2):186–90.

Chapter 4

14. Beck JJ, Staatz AJ, Pelsue DH, et al. Risk factors associated with short-term outcome and development of perioperative complications in dogs undergoing surgery because of gastric dilatation-volvulus: 166 cases (1992–2003). J Am Vet Med Assoc. 2006;229(12):1934–9.

15. Zonca A, Ravasio G, Gallo M, et al. Pharmacokinetics of ketamine and propofol combination administered as ketofol via continuous infusion in cats. J Vet Pharmacol Ther. 2012;35(6):580–7.

16. Goksin I, Adali F, Enli Y, et al. The effect of phlebotomy and mannitol on acute renal injury induced by ischemia/reperfusion of lower limbs in rats. Ann Vasc Surg. 2011;25(8):1118–28.

17. Lewis RM, Rice JH, Patton MK, et al. Renal ischemic injury in the dog: characterization and effect of various pharmacologic agents. J Lab Clin Med. 1984;104(4):470–9.

18. Yatsu T, Arai Y, Takizawa K, et al. Effect of YM435, a dopamine DA1 receptor agonist, in a canine model of ischemic acute renal failure. Gen Pharmacol. 1998;31(5):803–7.

19. Halpenny M, Markos F, Snow HM, et al. Effects of prophylactic fenoldopam infusion on renal blood flow and renal tubular function during acute hypovolemia in anesthetized dogs. Crit Care Med. 2001;29(4):85–60.

20. Boscan P, Pypendop BH, Siao KT, et al. Fluid balance, glomerular filtration rate, and urine output in dogs anesthetized for an orthopedic surgical procedure. Am J Vet Res. 2010;71(5):501–7.

21. Kummeling A, Teske E, Rothuizen J, Van Sluijs FJ. Coagulation profiles in dogs with congenital portosystemic shunts before and after surgical attenuation. J Vet Intern Med. 2006;20(6):1319–26.

22. Dancker C, MacFarlane PD, Love EJ. The effect of neuraxial morphine on postoperative pain in dogs after extrahepatic portosystemic shunt attenuation. Vet Anaesth Analg. 2020;47(1):111–18.

23. Burgoyne LL, Billups CA, Jirón JL, et al. Phantom limb pain in young cancer-related amputees: recent experience at St Jude children's research hospital. Clin J Pain. 2012;28(3):222–5.

24. Yamauchi Y, Izumi Y, Hashimoto K, et al. Needle-tract seeding after percutaneous cryoablation for lung metastasis of colorectal cancer. Ann Thorac Surg. 2011;92(4):e69–71.

25. Sanchez A, Valverde A, Sinclair M, et al. Antihistaminic and cardiorespiratory effects of diphenhydramine hydrochloride in anesthetized dogs undergoing excision of mast cell tumors. J Am Vet Med Assoc. 2017;251(7):804–13.

26. Abbo LA, Ko JC, Maxwell LK, et al. Pharmacokinetics of buprenorphine following intravenous and oral transmucosal administration in dogs. Vet Ther. 2008;9(2):83–93.

27. Ko JC, Maxwell LK, Abbo LA, Weil AB. Pharmacokinetics of lidocaine following the application of 5% lidocaine patches to cats. J Vet Pharmacol Ther. 2008;31(4):359–67.

28. Credie L de F, Luna SP, Futema F, et al. Perioperative evaluation of tumescent anaesthesia technique in bitches submitted to unilateral mastectomy. BMC Vet Res. 2013;9:178.

29. Moreira CM, Oliveira RL, Costa GA, Corgozinho KB, Luna SP, Souza HJ. Evaluation of tumescent local anesthesia in cats undergoing unilateral mastectomy. Vet Anaesth Analg. 2021;48(1):134–41.

30. Vullo C, Tambella AM, Falcone A, Marino G, Catone G. Constant rate infusion of lidocaine, tumescent anesthesia and their combination in dogs undergoing unilateral mastectomy. Animals. 2021;11(5).

31. Portela DA, Romano M, Briganti A. Retrospective clinical evaluation of ultrasound guided transverse abdominis plane block in dogs undergoing mastectomy. Vet Anaesth Analg. 2014;41(3):319–24.

32. Yilmaz OT, Toydemir TS, Kirsan I, Dokuzeylul B, Gunay Z, Karacam E. Effects of surgical wound infiltration with bupivacaine on postoperative analgesia in cats undergoing bilateral mastectomy. J Vet Med Sci. 2014;76(12):1595–601.

33. McNally E, Robertson S, Pablo L. Comparison of time to desaturation between preoxygenated and nonpreoxygenated dogs following sedation with acepromazine maleate and morphine and induction of anesthesia with propofol. Am J Vet Res. 2009;70(11):1333–8.

34. Gruenheid M, Aarnes TK, McLoughlin MA, et al. Risk of anesthesia-related complications in brachycephalic dogs. J Am Vet Med Assoc. 2018;253(3):301–6.

35. Doyle CR, Aarnes TK, Ballash GA, et al. Anesthetic risk during subsequent anesthetic events in brachycephalic dogs that have undergone corrective airway surgery: 45 cases (2007–2019). J Am Vet Med Assoc. 2020;257(7):744–9.

36. Lindsay B, Cook D, Wetzel JM, Siess S, Moses P. Brachycephalic airway syndrome: management of post-operative respiratory complications in 248 dogs. Aust Vet J. 2020;98(5):173–80.

37. Brodbelt D. Perioperative mortality in small animal anaesthesia. Vet J. 2009;182(2):152–61.

38. Jeffery ND, Talbot CE, Smith PM, Bacon NJ. Acquired idiopathic laryngeal paralysis as a prominent feature of generalised neuromuscular disease in 39 dogs. Vet Rec. 2006;158(1):17.

39. Bahr KL, Howe L, Jessen C, Goodrich Z. Outcome of 45 dogs with laryngeal paralysis treated by unilateral arytenoid lateralization or bilateral ventriculocordectomy. J Am Anim Hosp Assoc. 2014;50(4):264–72.

40. Wilson D, Monnet E. Risk factors for the development of aspiration pneumonia after unilateral arytenoid lateralization in dogs with laryngeal paralysis: 232 cases (1987–2012). J Am Vet Med Assoc. 2016;248(2):188–94.

41. Milovancev M, Townsend K, Spina J, et al. Effect of metoclopramide on the incidence of early postoperative aspiration pneumonia in dogs with acquired idiopathic laryngeal paralysis. Vet Surg. 2016;45(5):577–81.

42. Naan EC, Kirpensteijn J, Kooistra HS, Peeters ME. Results of thyroidectomy in 101 cats with hyperthyroidism. Vet Surg. 2006;35(3):287–93.

43. Reagan JK, Selmic LE, Fallon C, et al. Complications and outcomes associated with unilateral thyroidectomy in dogs with naturally occurring thyroid tumors: 156 cases (2003–2015). J Am Vet Med Assoc. 2019;255(8):926–32.

44. Coleman KA, Smeak DD. Complication rates after bilateral versus unilateral total ear canal ablation with lateral bulla osteotomy for end-stage inflammatory ear disease in dogs: 79 ears. Vet Surg. 2016;45(5):659–63.

45. Wainberg SH, Selmic LE, Haagsman AN, et al. Comparison of complications and outcome following unilateral, staged bilateral, and single-stage bilateral ventral bulla osteotomy in cats. J Am Vet Med Assoc. 2019;255(7):828–36.

46. Vlasin M, Artingstall R, Mala B. Acute upper airway obstruction as a life-threatening complication of ventral bulla osteotomy: report of two consecutive cases. JFMS Open Rep. 2021;7(1):20551169211005923.

47. Carter JE, Motsinger-Reif AA, Krug WV, Keene BW. The effect of heart disease on anesthetic complications during routine dental procedures in dogs. J Am Anim Hosp Assoc. 2017;53(4):206–13.

48. Herring IP, Bobofchak MA, Landry MP, Ward DL. Duration of effect and effect of multiple doses of topical ophthalmic 0.5% proparacaine hydrochloride in clinically normal dogs. Am J Vet Res. 2005;66(1):77–80.

49. Binder DR, Herring IP. Duration of corneal anesthesia following topical administration of 0.5% proparacaine hydrochloride solution in clinically normal cats. Am J Vet Res. 2006;67(10):1780–2.

50. Norgate DJ, Nicholls D, Geddes RF, Dawson C, Adami C. Comparison of two protocols for insulin administration and fasting time in diabetic dogs anaesthetised for phacoemulsification: a prospective clinical trial. Vet Rec. 2021;188(11):e81.

51. Batista CM, Laus JL, Nunes N, Patto Dos Santos PS, Costa JL. Evaluation of intraocular and partial CO_2 pressure in dogs anesthetized with propofol. Vet Ophthalmol. 2000;3(1):17–19.

52. Hofmeister EH, Williams CO, Braun C, Moore PA. Propofol versus thiopental: effects on peri-induction intraocular pressures in normal dogs. Vet Anaesth Analg. 2008;35(4):275–81.

53. Hasiuk MM, Forde N, Cooke A, Ramey K, Pang DS. A comparison of alfaxalone and propofol on intraocular pressure in healthy dogs. Vet Ophthalmol. 2014;17(6):411–16.

Chapter 4

54. Costa D, Leiva M, Moll X, Aguilar A, Pena T, Andaluz A. Alfaxalone versus propofol in dogs: a randomised trial to assess effects on peri-induction tear production, intraocular pressure and globe position. Vet Rec. 2015;176(3):73.

55. Gunderson EG, Lukasik VM, Ashton MM, Merideth RE, Madsen R. Effects of anesthetic induction with midazolam-propofol and midazolam-etomidate on selected ocular and cardiorespiratory variables in clinically normal dogs. Am J Vet Res. 2013;74(4):629–35.

56. Levy JK, Bard KM, Tucker SJ, Diskant PD, Dingman PA. Perioperative mortality in cats and dogs undergoing spay or castration at a high-volume clinic. Vet J. 2017;224:11–15.

57. Gates MC, Littlewood KE, Kongara K, Odom TF, Sawicki RK. Cross-sectional survey of anaesthesia and analgesia protocols used to perform routine canine and feline ovariohysterectomies. Vet Anaesth Analg. 2020;47(1):38–46.

58. Williams V, Lascelles B, Robson M. Current attitudes to, and use of, peri-operative analgesia in dogs and cats by veterinarians in New Zealand. N Z Vet J. 2005;53(3):193–202.

59. Schenk AP, McGrath AM, Beatty CA, et al. Feline post-sterilization hyphema. Vet Ophthalmol. 2020;23(3):588–91.

60. Gordon-Evans WJ, Suh HY, Guedes AG. Controlled, non-inferiority trial of bupivacaine liposome injectable suspension. J Feline Med Surg. 2020;22(10):916–21.

61. Evans KM, Adams VJ. Proportion of litters of purebred dogs born by caesarean section. J Small Anim Pract. 2010;51(2):113–18.

62. Alonge S, Melandri M. Effect of delivery management on first-week neonatal outcome: how to improve it in Great Danes. Theriogenology. 2019;125:310–16.

63. Martin-Flores M, Anderson JC, Sakai DM, et al. A retrospective analysis of the epidural use of bupivacaine 0.0625–0.125% with opioids in bitches undergoing cesarean section. Can Vet J. 2019;60(12):1349–52.

64. De Cramer KGM, Joubert KE, Nothling JO. Puppy survival and vigor associated with the use of low dose medetomidine premedication, propofol induction and maintenance of anesthesia using sevoflurane gas-inhalation for cesarean section in the bitch. Theriogenology. 2017;96:10–15.

65. Alef M. [Anaesthesia for canine caesarean section – an evidence-based approach]. Tierarztl Prax Ausg K Kleintiere Heimtiere. 2017;45(1):27–38.

66. Metcalfe S, Hulands-Nave A, Bell M, et al. Multicentre, randomised clinical trial evaluating the efficacy and safety of alfaxalone administered to bitches for induction of anaesthesia prior to caesarean section. Aust Vet J. 2014;92(9):333–8.

67. Doebeli A, Michel E, Bettschart R, Hartnack S, Reichler IM. Apgar score after induction of anesthesia for canine cesarean section with alfaxalone versus propofol. Theriogenology. 2013;80(8):850–4.

68. Conde Ruiz C, Del Carro AP, Rosset E, et al. Alfaxalone for total intravenous anaesthesia in bitches undergoing elective caesarean section and its effects on puppies: a randomized clinical trial. Vet Anaesth Analg. 2016;43(3):281–90.

69. Moon-Massat P, Erb H. Perioperative factors associated with puppy vigor after delivery by cesarean section. J Am Anim Hosp Assoc. 2002;38(1):90–6.

70. Moon P, Erb H, Ludders J, Gleed R, Pascoe P. Perioperative risk factors for puppies delivered by cesarean section in the United States and Canada. J Am Anim Hosp Assoc. 2000;36(4):359–68.

71. Jitpean S, Ambrosen A, Emanuelson U, Hagman R. Closed cervix is associated with more severe illness in dogs with pyometra. BMC Vet Res. 2017;13(1):11.

72. Jitpean S, Strom-Holst B, Emanuelson U, et al. Outcome of pyometra in female dogs and predictors of peritonitis and prolonged postoperative hospitalization in surgically treated cases. BMC Vet Res. 2014;10:6.

73. Moores AL, Halfacree ZJ, Baines SJ, Lipscomb VJ. Indications, outcomes and complications following lateral thoracotomy in dogs and cats. J Small Anim Pract. 2007;48(12):695–8.

Chapter 4

74. Majeski SA, Steffey MA, Mayhew PD, et al. Postoperative respiratory function and survival after pneumonectomy in dogs and cats. Vet Surg. 2016;45(6):775–81.
75. Asorey I, Sambugaro B, Bhalla RJ, Drozdzynska M. Ultrasound-guided serratus plane block as an effective adjunct to systemic analgesia in four dogs undergoing thoracotomy. Open Vet J. 2021;10(4):407–11.
76. Dabir S, Parsa T, Radpay B, Padyab M. Interpleural morphine vs bupivacaine for postthoracotomy pain relief. Asian Cardiovasc Thorac Ann. 2008;16(5):370–4.
77. de Mello Souza CH, Bacon N, Boston S, Randall V, Wavreille V, Skinner O. Ventral mandibulectomy for removal of oral tumours in the dog: surgical technique and results in 19 cases. Vet Comp Oncol. 2019;17(3):271–5.
78. MacLellan RH, Rawlinson JE, Rao S, Worley DR. Intraoperative and postoperative complications of partial maxillectomy for the treatment of oral tumors in dogs. J Am Vet Med Assoc. 2018;252(12):1538–47.
79. Matthiesen DT, Manfra Marretta S. Results and complications associated with partial mandibulectomy and maxillectomy techniques. Probl Vet Med. 1990;2(1):248–75.
80. Reader RC, McCarthy RJ, Schultz KL, et al. Comparison of liposomal bupivacaine and 0.5% bupivacaine hydrochloride for control of postoperative pain in dogs undergoing tibial plateau leveling osteotomy. J Am Vet Med Assoc. 2020;256(9):1011–19.
81. Bruniges N, Rioja E. Intraoperative anaesthetic complications in dogs undergoing general anaesthesia for thoracolumbar hemilaminectomy: a retrospective analysis. Vet Anaesth Analg. 2019;46(6):720–8.
82. Fenn J, Laber E, Williams K, et al. Associations between anesthetic variables and functional outcome in dogs with thoracolumbar intervertebral disk extrusion undergoing decompressive hemilaminectomy. J Vet Intern Med. 2017;31(3):814–24.
83. Dixon A, Fauber AE. Effect of anesthesia-associated hypotension on neurologic outcome in dogs undergoing hemilaminectomy because of acute, severe thoracolumbar intervertebral disk herniation: 56 cases (2007–2013). J Am Vet Med Assoc. 2017;250(4):417–23.
84. Zidan N, Medland J, Olby N. Long-term postoperative pain evaluation in dogs with thoracolumbar intervertebral disk herniation after hemilaminectomy. J Vet Intern Med. 2020;34(4):1547–55.
85. Portela DA, Romano M, Zamora GA, et al. The effect of erector spinae plane block on perioperative analgesic consumption and complications in dogs undergoing hemilaminectomy surgery: a retrospective cohort study. Vet Anaesth Analg. 2021;48(1):116–24.
86. McFadzean WJM, Macfarlane P, Granger N, Murrell JC. Influence of peri-incisional epaxial muscle infiltration with bupivacaine pre- or post-surgery on opioid administration in dogs undergoing thoraco-lumbar hemilaminectomy. Vet J. 2021;270:105622.
87. Aprea F, Cherubini GB, Palus V, Vettorato E, Corletto F. Effect of extradurally administered morphine on postoperative analgesia in dogs undergoing surgery for thoracolumbar intervertebral disk extrusion. J Am Vet Med Assoc. 2012;241(6):754–9.
88. Barker JR, Clark-Price SC, Gordon-Evans WJ. Evaluation of topical epidural analgesia delivered in gelfoam for postoperative hemilaminectomy pain control. Vet Surg. 2013;42(1):79–84.
89. Machin H, Taylor-Brown F, Adami C. Use of acupuncture as adjuvant analgesic technique in dogs undergoing thoracolumbar hemilaminectomy. Vet J. 2020;264:105536.
90. Laim A, Jaggy A, Forterre F, Doherr MG, Aeschbacher G, Glardon O. Effects of adjunct electroacupuncture on severity of postoperative pain in dogs undergoing hemilaminectomy because of acute thoracolumbar intervertebral disk disease. J Am Vet Med Assoc. 2009;234(9):1141–6.
91. Alvarez LX, McCue J, Lam NK, Askin G, Fox PR. Effect of targeted pulsed electromagnetic field therapy on canine postoperative hemilaminectomy: a double-blind, randomized, placebo-controlled clinical trial. J Am Anim Hosp Assoc. 2019;55(2):83–91.

Chapter 4

92. Zidan N, Fenn J, Griffith E, et al. The effect of electromagnetic fields on post-operative pain and locomotor recovery in dogs with acute, severe thoracolumbar intervertebral disc extrusion: a randomized placebo-controlled, prospective clinical trial. J Neurotrauma. 2018;35(15):1726–36.

93. Posner LP, Mariani CL, Swanson C, Asakawa M, Campbell N, King AS. Perianesthetic morbidity and mortality in dogs undergoing cervical and thoracolumbar spinal surgery. Vet Anaesth Analg. 2014;41(2):137–44.

94. Rossmeisl JH Jr, White C, Pancotto TE, Bays A, Henao-Guerrero PN. Acute adverse events associated with ventral slot decompression in 546 dogs with cervical intervertebral disc disease. Vet Surg. 2013;42(7):795–806.

95. Lent SE, Hawkins EC. Evaluation of rhinoscopy and rhinoscopy-assisted mucosal biopsy in diagnosis of nasal disease in dogs: 119 cases (1985–1989). J Am Vet Med Assoc. 1992;201(9):1425–9.

96. Cremer J, Sum SO, Braun C, Figueiredo J, Rodriguez-Guarin C. Assessment of maxillary and infraorbital nerve blockade for rhinoscopy in sevoflurane anesthetized dogs. Vet Anaesth Analg. 2013;40:432–9.

97. Fizzano KM, Claude AK, Kuo LH, et al. Evaluation of a modified infraorbital approach for a maxillary nerve block for rhinoscopy with nasal biopsy of dogs. Am J Vet Res. 2017;78(9):1025–35.

98. Chohan AS, Pascoe PJ. Comparison of the efficacy and duration of desensitization of oral structures following injection of a lidocaine-bupivacaine mixture via lateral percutaneous and modified infraorbital approaches in dogs. Am J Vet Res. 2021;82(1):22–7.

99. Donaldson LL, Leib MS, Boyd C, Burkholder W, Sheridan M. Effect of preanesthetic medication on ease of endoscopic intubation of the duodenum in anesthetized dogs. Am J Vet Res. 1993;54(9):1489–95.

Chapter 4

Chapter 5

Anesthesia in patients with concurrent disease

Sharon Tenenbaum Shih

This chapter addresses anesthetic considerations and protocols for patients with specific diseases. The pathophysiology of the disease, its influence on anesthesia, recommended drug protocols, expected or common complications, and preventive or treatment methods for these complications are reviewed. While some drugs may be ideal for a particular disease, the anesthetic protocol is often based on the anesthetist's familiarity, availability, and cost-effectiveness of these drugs. As with other chapters, many of these recommendations are a reflection of the author's personal preference.

I. Cardiovascular disease

Cardiovascular disease involves either a disturbance of the conduction system (which may manifest as an abnormal rhythm) or an alteration of the structure of the heart itself. Structural abnormalities are broadly categorized into systolic, diastolic, and obstructive dysfunction. Cardiac patients usually compensate for their disease and may display only limited clinical signs (CS), such as exercise intolerance, coughing, or an increased RR while sleeping. Unfortunately, anesthesia disrupts the physiologic balance even in a healthy patient. Therefore, the compensated patient stands a reasonable chance of decompensation during an anesthetic event.

To minimize the impact of this occurring, a thorough understanding of the patient's current disease is necessary. This is obtained by a preanesthetic physical exam (PE), blood work (BW), a thorough history of which cardiac medications the patient receives, and a cardiovascular workup (ECG and echocardiogram). A preoperative blood pressure (BP) is also obtained as a baseline. This is important both because drugs such as ACE inhibitors (e.g., enalapril or benazepril, alone or in combination with aldosterone receptor antagonists such as spironolactone) are commonly prescribed to these patients, and because of the growing awareness of cardiovascular–renal axis disorders [1]. For example, dogs which receive enalapril prior to their anesthetic event are more likely to experience moderate to severe hypotension than those which do not [2]. Ultimately, that hypotension may negatively impact renal function.

Small Animal Anesthesia Techniques, Second Edition. Edited by Amanda M. Shelby and Carolyn M. McKune.
© 2023 John Wiley & Sons, Inc. Published 2023 by John Wiley & Sons, Inc.
Companion website: www.wiley.com/go/shelby/anesthesia2

Most cardiac protocols share common goals: use of reversible drugs, avoiding hypoxemia, maintaining cardiac output (CO) (by maintaining a normal heart rate and blood pressure), avoiding extreme changes in vascular tone (i.e., vasoconstriction or vasodilation), minimizing hypothermia to avoid postoperative shivering, minimizing anesthesia time, and creating a stress-free recovery.

A. Conduction and rhythm disturbances

The conduction system (electrical component) of the heart triggers the heart's mechanical actions (contraction component, i.e., forward flow of blood). When conduction disruptions occur while a patient is anesthetized, this may result in a worsened forward flow versus when a patient is awake and compensates appropriately. Arrhythmias are classified in many ways, but a broad category would be whether it is a bradyarrhythmia (a slow abnormal rhythm) or a tachyarrhythmia (a fast abnormal rhythm). A thorough discussion of cardiac arrhythmias is found in Chapter 3.

1. Anesthesia concerns/common complications

(a) Bradyarrhythmias: Because CO is equal to heart rate (HR) multiplied by stroke volume (SV), a slow HR will decrease CO. Due to the reduction of CO secondary to the use of general anesthesia (inhalants, as well as other injectable agents), there is a risk of severely compromising perfusion to vital tissues including the brain, kidney, and liver.

(b) Tachyarrhythmias: Perfusion to the heart occurs during diastole. When a tachyarrhythmia occurs, the heart spends very little time in diastole, resulting in compromised myocardial perfusion. This significantly worsens ventricular arrhythmias as the ventricle is the largest heart muscle body to perfuse.

2. Anesthesia protocol

A patient which is scheduled for an elective procedure but has an arrhythmia on PE must have at minimum an ECG analyzed before anesthesia proceeds. An echocardiogram is highly recommended to rule out any structural abnormalities. In emergent cases where the procedure and anesthesia are unavoidable, the goals are to stabilize and/or reduce the impact of the arrhythmia. This means using cardiac-friendly drugs for premedication (i.e., opioids and benzodiazepines), induction (i.e., alfaxalone or etomidate with a benzodiazepine, or neuroleptic anesthesia [fentanyl and a benzodiazepine]), and reducing the amount of inhalant administered (i.e., through the use of opioids for their MAC-sparing effect, as well as local blocks if possible). Adding some local lidocaine on the larynx will aid with intubation. Additionally, with bradyarrhythmias, it is necessary to increase HR, either through the use of anticholinergics, isoproterenol, or a temporary pacemaker. In cases of tachycardia, it is essential to know whether the tachycardia is ventricular (below the AV node) or supraventricular (above the AV node) in origin. Ventricular arrhythmias may slow in response to lidocaine; see Chapter 3 for treatment of arrhythmias.

Chapter 5

B. Structural abnormalities

1. Systolic dysfunction

Systolic dysfunction includes diseases such as valvular insufficiencies (mitral regurgitation [MR] or tricuspid regurgitation [TR] and dilated cardiomyopathy [DCM]). One of the most common complications secondary to this disease, under anesthesia, is hypotension. In patients with DCM, arrhythmias are a common sequela (ex. atrial fibrillation) and some necessitate treatment. Pimobendan is a drug with a unique mechanism of action that includes positive inotropy (an increase in contractility of the heart) and is also an inodilator (which causes vasodilation by calcium sensitization and phosphodiesterase inhibition) [3]. Studies suggest that dogs administered pimobendan demonstrate a significantly longer life span when they have myxomatous mitral valve disease [4].

(a) Anesthesia concerns/common complications:

- Maintain HR with normal heart rate as the target goal (and within 25% of resting HR as a point of absolute treatment), with an anticholinergic as needed (atropine or glycopyrrolate); if the anesthetist must choose between slightly below or slightly above resting HR, these cases often benefit from a slightly elevated HR. In the case of mitral or tricuspid regurgitation, this slight tachycardia will help with forward flow and prevent back flow into the atria. However, one must also try to avoid severe tachycardia.
- Avoid peripheral vasoconstriction as this will increase afterload and decrease SV, both of which compromise CO. Slight vasodilation may help improve forward flow and decrease flow back into the atria.
- Maintain myocardial contractility by ensuring the patient receives pimobendan prior to their procedure if they are currently prescribed this drug, and by using inotropic agents, such as dopamine or dobutamine (see Table 10). Dopamine and dobutamine are also used to correct hypotension.
- Avoid volume overload with a conservative fluid therapy plan (usually 2–3 mL/kg/h for canine patients or 1–2 mL/kg/h for feline patients). Do not administer fluid boluses for hypotension unless there is true volume loss or evidence of hypovolemia.
- Minimize stress during the perioperative period as well as the postoperative recovery period.
- Keep inhalant to minimum alveolar concentration (MAC) or less during anesthesia. For example, end-tidal isoflurane concentration would stay below 1.25%.
- Prevent hypothermia to decrease postoperative shivering, which will increase myocardial oxygen requirement.

(b) Anesthetic protocol (Table 5.1): Premedications facilitate IV catheterization with minimal stress and reduce drug and inhalant requirement. When selecting drugs for the anesthetic protocol, reversible drugs are ideal in the cardiac patient. Opioids, given in higher doses, will help reduce the need for sedatives that may impact the cardiovascular system. However, high doses of opioids may cause bradycardia; this is usually treated with an anticholinergic (which may be included in the premedication). Patients with mild MR might benefit from a low dose of acepromazine (0.01 mg/kg) to reduce afterload and provide additional sedation. Benzodiazepines are also suitable based on the patient's temperament, but may cause agitation and excitement at times. The use of eutectic mixture of local anesthetic (EMLA) cream helps reduce stress during catheter placement [5–7]. Dexmedetomidine is contraindicated in these

Chapter 5

Table 5.1 Systolic dysfunction.

Premedication (mg/kg)	Induction (mg/kg)	Maintenance	Intraoperative analgesia[a] (mg/kg)	Postoperative analgesia[a] (mg/kg)
Opioid (select one) (a) Methadone 0.3–0.5 IM, 0.2–0.3 IV OR (b) Hydromorphone 0.1 IM, 0.05 IV OR (c) Fentanyl 0.002–0.005 IV OR (d) Buprenorphine 0.01–0.03 IM or IV OR (e) Butorphanol 0.1–0.4 IM or IV Sedative (if needed) (a) Midazolam 0.1 IM OR (b) Acepromazine 0.005–0.02 IV (MR only) +/– (c) Alfaxalone 1–3 IM	(a) Etomidate 1–2 IV +/– midazolam 0.1–0.2 IV OR (b) Alfaxalone 1–2 to effect IV +/– midazolam 0.1–0.3 IV OR (c) Propofol 2 + Ketamine 2 ("ketofol") to effect +/– midazolam 0.2 OR (d) Fentanyl 0.01 and midazolam 0.2	(a) Sevoflurane OR (b) Isoflurane AND CRI for reduction of inhalant requirement	(a) Appropriate local regional block (b) MAC-sparing CRI (mg/kg/h) (i) Fentanyl 0.012–0.042 OR (ii) Hydromorphone 0.03 OR (iii) Remifentanil 0.012–0.042 +/– (iv) Ketamine 0.6 mg/kg/h +/– (v) (dogs only) Lidocaine 1–3 mg/kg/h, loading dose 1–2 mg/kg IV required Fluids: Crystalloids 2–3 mL/kg/h (canine) or 1–3 mL/kg/h (feline)	(a) CRI: (i) Fentanyl 0.002–0.005 mg/kg/h OR (ii) Hydromorphone 0.01 mg/kg/h OR (b) Intermittent bolus: (i) Methadone 0.3 IV q 4–6 h OR (ii) Hydromorphone 0.05–0.1 IV q 4–6 h AND (c) NSAID where not contraindicated +/– (d) Liposomal encapsulated bupivacaine infiltrative block 5.3 mg/kg

"AND" means that multiple choices from this column are selected, "+/–" means that it is up to the anesthetist if they would like to combine multiple choices, "OR" means that the anesthetist will choose one or the other selection. For example, the postoperative analgesia column would be interpreted as including an opioid and an NSAID, with an optional long-acting local anesthetic block. An anticholinergic IM is ideal if HR is low following premedication, prior to induction. Lidocaine is avoided in cats.

[a] Analgesia requirements should adequately address the level or degree of anticipated pain and are dependent on the procedure being performed.

CRI, constant-rate infusion; IM, intramuscular; IV, intravenous; MAC, minimum alveolar concentration; MR, mitral regurgitation; NSAID, nonsteroidal antiinflammatory drug.

patients due to severe vasoconstriction and reflex bradycardia. Preoxygenation for a minimum of 5–10 minutes prior to induction is appropriate until the patient is intubated. Monitoring equipment is placed on the patient prior to induction if possible. A preoperative ECG and BP are obtained at this time as a baseline.

Historically, etomidate (after an effective premedication and typically with a benzodiazepine) was considered the ideal induction agent for these cases, as it minimally affects HR and BP. However, alfaxalone is cardiac friendly [8–10]. In the author's experience, it also produces a smoother induction than etomidate. Premedications are used to reduce the dose of the induction agent needed and to decrease inhalant requirement. A benzodiazepine is also considered as part of the induction to reduce the amount of induction agent needed [11]. Inhalants are routinely used to maintain anesthesia but constant-rate infusions (CRIs) such as fentanyl, or other opioids, are used to reduce the MAC requirement of inhalants, thus minimizing negative cardiovascular side-effects. Local blocks are included where appropriate. Positive inotropes such as dopamine or dobutamine are used to support BP by increasing contractility and therefore increasing the cardiac output. Dopamine at higher doses causes vasoconstriction; these higher doses are avoided.

Monitoring includes an ECG, CO_2, temperature, pulse oximetry, Doppler and ideally invasive blood pressure (IBP), if obtainable. In extremely critical cardiovascular patients, central venous pressure (CVP) is performed to closely monitor preload (venous return and fluid status). Fluid therapy is conservative (2–3 mL/kg/h) with minimal to no administration of fluid boluses.

In recovery, patients may require supplemental oxygen, depending on the procedure and severity of cardiovascular disease. Continuous pulse oximetry monitoring is important during the recovery phase. Patients with mild to moderate cardiovascular disease tolerate anesthesia with minimal complications, provided the protocol is appropriate for them [12].

(c) Key points: Dilated cardiomyopathy is one of the most difficult cardiac diseases to manage for the anesthetist. Knowing how severely the patient's ejection fraction (i.e., the patient's ability to provide forward flow) is impacted will give the anesthetist an idea of how seriously the patient is compromised; an echocardiogram is necessary for this information. In addition to the above goals, the best possible management of these patients is to minimize anesthesia time, and only undergo elective procedures when they are "stable." This often includes management of any concurrent arrhythmias as well as the use of drugs such as pimobendan (a positive inotrope). A dobutamine CRI is also considered in DCM patients to help increase myocardial contractility; however, it is not without increases in myocardial O_2 consumption, increased coronary blood flow requirements and decreased myocardial mechanical efficiency in these patients [13]. However, in the face of hypotension (which has its own deleterious effects), it is a suitable choice.

2. Diastolic dysfunction

Diastolic dysfunction includes diseases such as hypertrophic cardiomyopathy (HCM) and pericardial disease, where there is limited filling of the ventricle due to small chamber size. HCM is associated with a higher all-cause mortality in cats due to the increased cardiovascular death and its contributions to noncardiovascular death, so special care is taken with these cats [14].

(a) Anesthesia concerns/common complications:
- Avoid excessive peripheral vasodilation or constriction.
- Maintain HR within 25% of baseline; if the anesthetist must choose between slightly below or slightly above resting HR, these cases often benefit from a slightly decreased HR to allow more filling time.
- Avoid increases in myocardial contractility and myocardial oxygen consumption. This includes avoiding drugs such as ketamine and positive inotropes. Atropine is avoided due to the potential for tachycardia. Glycopyrrolate is used instead to help increase HR, when needed, as the heart rate increase is more often moderate, rather than profound. Severe hypothermia is avoided, since it causes shivering postoperatively and increases myocardial oxygen demand significantly.
- Maintain adequate circulating volume without causing fluid overload (conservative fluid rates of 1–2 mL/kg/h).
- If BP is compromised, one should assess the depth of anesthesia and try to reduce the inhalant concentration to help decrease vasodilation. The use of local blocks also helps to reduce the inhalant concentration. If this does not correct the BP, phenylephrine is used at 0.03–0.06 mg/kg/h to tighten vascular tone [15]. The goal is to return vascular tone back to its baseline prior to the impact of inhalant anesthesia (which reduces SVR). Phenylephrine works directly on alpha receptors to promote vasoconstriction; this can become profound at higher doses. It is difficult to know if this occurs with routine monitoring, but invasive cardiovascular monitoring equipment and measuring of lactate levels (which should remain below 2.0 mmol/L) provides general information on adverse effects due to the use of phenylephrine. If lactate levels increase, it is possible there is compromised perfusion secondary to vasoconstriction. If this occurs, phenylephrine is decreased or discontinued. It is most prudent, as blood pressure returns to normal, for phenylephrine to be gradually but expeditiously removed from the support measures.

(b) Anesthetic protocol (Table 5.2): If sedation is needed in patients with HCM, low doses of dexmedetomidine facilitate the goals of decreasing HR to allow more time in diastole as well as reducing MAC of inhalants. An opioid is included to help reduce the dose of dexmedetomidine and also provide analgesia. Alfaxalone can be administered IM in situations where a patient is extremely fractious. In a study on cats with HCM, systolic anterior motion and left ventricular outflow tract obstruction, medetomidine (an alpha-2 agonist similar to dexmedetomidine) was used for sedation and helped improve forward flow [16]. Benzodiazepines may be used as part of the premedication but may result in agitation. For cardiac patients, it is good practice to administer drugs that are reversible and which have minimal cardiovascular effects.

Patients are preoxygenated before induction and up to the point of intubation. Inductions with etomidate or alfaxalone with the addition of midazolam are ideal. If the patient is cooperative, monitoring equipment is placed prior to induction. Isoflurane or sevoflurane at low concentrations are used routinely for maintenance.

Table 5.2 Diastolic dysfunction.

Premedication (mg/kg)	Induction (mg/kg)	Maintenance	Intraoperative analgesia[a] (mg/kg)	Postoperative analgesia[a] (mg/kg)
Opioid (select one)	Sedative (if needed)	(a) Sevoflurane OR	(a) Local regional block	(a) CRI:
(a) Methadone 0.3–0.5 IM, 0.2–0.3 IV	(a) Midazolam 0.1 IM OR	(b) Isoflurane AND	AND	(i) Fentanyl 0.002–0.005 mg/kg/h
OR	(b) Dexmedetomidine 0.001–0.003 IM or IV	CRI for reduction of inhalant requirement	(b) Opioid CRI (mg/kg/h)	OR
(b) Fentanyl 0.002–0.005 IV	+/–		(i) Fentanyl 0.012–0.042	(ii) Hydromorphone 0.01 mg/kg/h
OR	(c) Alfaxalone 1–3 IM			OR
(c) Buprenorphine 0.01–0.03 IV or IM			Fluids: Crystalloid 1–2 mL/kg/h (cats) or 2–3 mL/kg/h (dogs)	(b) Intermittent bolus:
OR	(a) Etomidate 1–2 IV +/– midazolam 0.1–0.2 IV			(i) Methadone 0.3 IV q 4–6 h
(d) Butorphanol 0.1–0.4 IM or IV	OR			OR
	(b) Alfaxalone 1–3 IV to effect +/– midazolam 0.1 IV			(ii) Hydromor-phone 0.05–0.1 IV q 4–6 h
				AND
				(c) NSAID where not contraindicated
				+/–
				(d) Liposomal encapsu-lated bupivacaine infil-trative block 5.3 mg/kg

"AND" means that multiple choices from this column are selected, "+/–" means it is up to the anesthetist if they would like to combine multiple choices, "OR" means that the anesthetist will choose one or the other selection. For example, the postoperative analgesia column would be interpreted as including an opioid and an NSAID, with an optional long-acting local anesthetic block. Lidocaine is contraindicated in cats.

[a] Analgesic selection should be appropriate for the duration of procedure and level of anticipated pain.

CRI, constant-rate infusion; IM, intramuscular; IV, intravenous; NSAID, nonsteroidal antiinflammatory drug.

Recovery should occur in a stress-free environment. Supplemental oxygen should be available if necessary and continuous pulse oximetry is used.

3. Obstructive dysfunction

Obstructive dysfunction includes diseases such as fulminant heartworm disease or valvular stenosis (pulmonic or aortic). Cardiac diseases with obstructive dysfunction have reduced CO and limited cardiac reserve. In addition, the ventricular chambers begin to hypertrophy in response to pushing volume against an obstruction. As with other types of cardiovascular disease, these patients often compensate until heart failure develops. Anesthetizing these animals carries the risk of decompensation.

(a) Anesthesia concerns/common complications:
* Maintain HR within 25% of resting HR; if the anesthetist must choose between slightly below or slightly above resting HR, these cases often benefit from a decreased HR, allowing hypertrophied cardiac muscles time in diastole to perfuse.
* Avoid severe peripheral vascular tone changes, such as anesthesia-induced peripheral vasodilation. Depending on the disease, different inotropes and vasopressors are considered for BP interventions. Phenylephrine CRI is the agent of choice. Caution is exercised when using this pressor, and lactate levels are measured if this drug is used at higher dose intervals for an extended period of time.
* Avoid volume overload by using a conservative fluid therapy (usually 1–2 mL/kg/h in cats or 2–3 mL/kg/h in dogs) [17].
* Avoid severe increases in myocardial contractility and oxygen consumption by avoiding drugs like ketamine and positive inotropes.
* Minimize stress during the perioperative and postoperative recovery periods.
* A propofol or alfaxalone CRI is used for patients that are heartworm positive as total intravenous anesthesia. An opioid CRI is used in addition to help reduce the dose of propofol or alfaxalone needed.

(b) Anesthetic protocol (Table 5.3): In general for cardiac patients, it is good practice to administer drugs that are reversible and have minimal cardiovascular effects (i.e., an opioid and benzodiazepine). The goal of premedication is to provide sufficient sedation to minimize stress, facilitate IV catheterization and reduce the amount of drugs necessary for induction and maintenance. If the patient is cooperative, IV catheterization is performed with the assistance of EMLA cream in the nonsedated patient [7,18]. It is important to preoxygenate these patients. Placement of monitoring equipment prior to induction is ideal (Doppler, ECG, noninvasive blood pressure [NIBP] and, when obtainable, IBP). Rapid access to the airway is important to minimize oxygen desaturation. Neuroleptic anesthesia (opioid + benzodiazepine), etomidate with midazolam, or alfaxalone with midazolam are ideal for induction. Low doses of propofol may be used following bolus of opioid, benzodiazepine, and/or lidocaine.

MAC-sparing CRIs and local blocks are indicated to reduce inhalants; extremely critical canine patients may require minimal to no inhalant when placed on high doses of opioid

Table 5.3 Obstructive heart disease.

Premedication (mg/kg)	Induction (mg/kg)	Maintenance	Intraoperative analgesia[a] (mg/kg)	Postoperative analgesia[a] (mg/kg)
Opioid[a] (select one) (a) Methadone 0.3–0.5 IM, 0.2–0.3 IV OR (b) Hydromorphone (canine) 0.1 IM, 0.05 IV OR (c) Fentanyl 0.002–0.005 IV OR (d) Buprenorphine 0.01–0.03 IV or IM OR (e) Butorphanol 0.1–0.4 IV or IM	Sedative (a) Midazolam 0.1 IM +/– (b) Alfaxalone 1–3 IM (a) Etomidate 1–2 IV to effect +/– midazolam 0.1–0.2 IV OR (b) Alfaxalone 1–2 IV to effect +/– midazolam 0.1–0.2 IV OR (c) Fentanyl 0.005–0.01 and midazolam 0.2 (canine)	(a) Sevoflurane OR (b) Isoflurane OR (c) TIVA: (i) Alfaxalone 4–6 mg/kg/h (ii) Propofol (for use with patients with heartworm disease) 6–24 mg/kg/hr AND CRI for reduction of inhalant requirement	(a) Local regional block AND (b) Opioid CRI (mg/kg/h) (i) Fentanyl 0.012–0.042 OR (ii) Hydromorphone 0.01–0.03 OR (iii) Remifentanil 0.012–0.042 Fluids: Crystalloid 1–2 mL/kg/h (cats) or 2–3 mL/kg/h (dogs)	(a) CRI: (i) Fentanyl 0.002–0.005 mg/kg/h OR (ii) Hydromorphone 0.01 mg/kg/h OR (b) Intermittent bolus: (i) Methadone 0.3 IV q 4–6 h OR (ii) Hydromorphone 0.05–0.1 IV q 4–6 h AND (c) NSAID where not contraindicated +/– (d) Liposomal encapsulated bupivacaine infiltrative block 5.3 mg/kg

"AND" means that multiple choices from this column are selected. "+/–" means it is up to the anesthetist if they would like to combine multiple choices, "OR" means that the anesthetist will choose one or the other selection. For example, the postoperative analgesia column would be interpreted as including an opioid and an NSAID, with an optional long-acting local anesthetic block.

[a]Analgesic selection should be appropriate for the duration of procedure and level of anticipated pain.

CRI, constant-rate infusion; IM, intramuscular; IV, intravenous; NSAID, nonsteroidal antiinflammatory drug; TIVA, total intravenous anesthesia.

Chapter 5

CRIs. Monitoring includes at least IBP, ECG, Doppler, SpO_2, and capnography. In recovery, be prepared to provide oxygen supplementation. Recovery should occur in a stress-free environment where the patient is closely monitored.

II. Endocrine diseases

A. Diabetes insipidus

Diabetes insipidus (DI) is rare in veterinary patients. This disease occurs either centrally or at the level of the kidney (nephrogenically); the patient either does not secrete or does not respond to (respectively) antidiuretic hormone (ADH). The lack of ADH effect results in an animal that urinates large volumes and thus must drink large volumes to accommodate its polyuria. It is important to stabilize these patients (especially correcting dehydration) prior to anesthesia. Animals with confirmed DI are not anesthetized for elective procedures until their DI is managed, through the use of desmopressin. For nonelective procedures, volume status is of critical importance prior to anesthesia. Generally speaking, these patients have a free water deficit that is corrected as best as possible prior to anesthesia.

1. Anesthesia concerns/common complications

- Water is not restricted at any point for these patients. These patients are considered dehydrated, both systemically and cerebrally.
- Monitor electrolytes (especially sodium) throughout anesthesia and into recovery; use of fluid therapy assists with keeping sodium in the patient's target range, which should match their sodium on blood work. See Chapter 3 p.80 for management of hypernatremic patients, as rapid changes in sodium have severe neurologic consequences.
- Fluid choice is based on matching the sodium in the fluid to as close to the patient's blood sodium as possible. For example, if the patient's sodium is 160 mEq/L, 0.9% NaCl is the closest match at 154 mEq/L.

2. Anesthetic protocol

No anesthetic is specifically contraindicated for patients with DI; however, it is important to select drugs based on patient presentation and preanesthetic assessment. Judicious fluid therapy is warranted. In order to minimize the time to return of a patient's full function (and thus drinking on its own), it is wise to use reversible drugs whenever possible. Premedication is tailored to level of invasiveness of the procedure, with invasive procedures warranting full mu agonist opioids and minimally invasive procedures warranting mildly depressive drugs such as butorphanol. Induction with propofol is smooth and the drug is metabolized quickly. Alfaxalone is also considered but has a longer metabolism. Maintenance anesthesia with inhalants also includes the use of an opioid CRI, such as fentanyl or remifentanil, which reduces MAC of inhalant. Postoperative analgesia is tailored to the level of invasiveness of the procedure.

B. Diabetes mellitus

Diabetes mellitus (DM) is characterized by either relative or absolute insulin deficiency. DM is classified into two main categories. Type 1 diabetes is more common in dogs and is a true lack of insulin production. Type 2 diabetes is more commonly seen in cats and results in an insulin resistance. However, the cat (unsurprisingly as it is a cat) may have transient diabetes, noninsulin-dependent diabetes, or traditional insulin-dependent diabetes. Most commonly, in anesthesia cases, the patient is insulin dependent. Ultimately, the body's inability to regulate glucose with insulin leads to osmotic diuresis and excessive urination. If insulin is not exogenously administered, the body will attempt to utilize other energy sources, which results in ketone formation and, especially with any perpetuating factors (such as stress), ketoacidosis.

Ketoacidosis is a life-threatening emergency that is addressed before anything else but the most crucial of surgeries. Therefore, the anesthetist is typically confronted with the managed (although infrequently regulated) diabetic. Routine BW including a complete blood count (CBC) and chemistry is performed; knowing electrolytes is essential. A urinalysis to assess for ketonuria is warranted. Special attention is paid to the hydration status of the patient. Diabetic patients may have an enlarged liver and weakened abdominal muscles, which will contribute to inadequate ventilation during anesthesia. Pancreatitis is also seen in DM patients. Therefore, gastroprotectants (such as maropitant, pantoprazole, and famotidine) are often included in the anesthetic protocol.

Phacoemulsification is a common procedure performed on patients with DM for the removal of cataracts. Due to the nature of the procedure, the eye must remain in a central position using neuromuscular blocking agents such as atracurium and rocuronium. While some studies have shown that these patients may require higher rocuronium infusion dosing than patients that do not have DM [19], others show no difference when using atracurium [20].

Overall, the diabetic patient may be quite difficult to manage under anesthesia, especially when the diabetes is not controlled. Hypotension is moderate to severe in patients that have DM undergoing phacoemulsification. This may be attributed to the hypovolemia that these patients may exhibit due to the hyperglycemia [21].

1. Anesthesia concerns/common complications

- *Timing*: The focus of the anesthetic protocol is minimizing time out of the patient's routine feeding schedule. Elective procedures are scheduled in the morning so the patient recovers by the evening, and the patient is offered food as soon as they are fully recovered from anesthesia. During that time of fasting, glucose is monitored and supplemented if needed. Additionally, short-acting, reversible drugs are used where appropriate to minimize the "hangover" effects.
- *Fasting*: In managed diabetics, patients are fasted for 2–4 hours after a pâté consistency food is given, with half dose of their regular insulin given in the morning [22]. BG is measured at admission to ensure the patient is not hypoglycemic.
- *Blood glucose monitoring*: Monitor BG every 30–60 min, beginning immediately after induction. A sampling line (either an arterial line or a large-bore catheter) is convenient for this purpose. Normal glucose is 80–120 mg/dL but knowing a diabetic patient's level of regulation will indicate their "normal." A poorly regulated patient,

stress from hospitalization, fasting, and certain drugs that may be administered (ex. dexmedetomidine) will alter this blood glucose state. Typical diabetic patients have a BG of 200–250 mg/dL; a glucose drop below 200 mg/dL may prompt intervention. If glucose is less than 120 mg/dL in any diabetic patient, give dextrose 2.5–5% at regular surgical rate of 5 mL/kg/h in the canine and 3 mL/kg/h in the feline. This is often accomplished with a buretrol or smaller bag of fluids, as the patient's requirements for dextrose may fluctuate over the anesthetic period. If a dextrose bolus is needed, 0.5–1 mL/kg of 50% dextrose is given slowly over 10 minutes after it is diluted with saline in a 1:3 ratio.

If glucose levels exceed the patient's "normal" BG based on BW (or more generically, over 300 mg/dL), regular insulin at 0.1–0.2 IU/kg IV or SQ is administered. Alternatively, a CRI of regular insulin at 0.05 IU/kg/h, if continually monitored, may assist in regulation. It is prudent for the anesthetist to remember, however, that the patient is better off "sweet than sour" and therefore *aggressively* lowering BG is inappropriate.

- *Fluid resuscitation*: Dehydration is common in these patients; this is corrected prior to anesthesia if possible. Dehydration may contribute to hypotension (see below).
- *Hypotension*: Diabetic dogs were more likely than their nondiabetic counterparts to experience moderate to severe hypotension, which may be due to hypovolemia secondary to osmotic diuresis [21]. Monitoring blood pressure is necessary in these dogs, and it is prudent to begin with a fluid bolus to correct hypotension, when it becomes evident.
- *Electrolyte abnormalities*: It has been reported that life-threatening hyperkalemia could occur in an uncontrolled diabetic patient under anesthesia (possibly due to an insulin deficiency and blood hyperosmolarity) [23]. It is prudent to have access to blood sampling, through a second IV catheter or an arterial line, in order to evaluate blood electrolytes intraoperatively.

2. Anesthetic protocol (Table 5.4)

Dexmedetomidine results in a transient hyperglycemia and is avoided when possible. Selection of premedication and induction drugs is based on patient presentation with a preference given to titratable drugs (i.e., propofol, alfaxalone, etomidate). Most induction agents are relatively short-acting and will be metabolized quickly. Inhalants are routinely used. CRIs are used to provide analgesia and reduce inhalant requirements. The patient receives continued glucose checks at 30–60 min intervals until they resume eating, including time spent in recovery. Glucose supplementation (2.5–5%) in crystalloid fluids may be required throughout the recovery phase at 2–5 mL/kg/h. Appropriate and balanced postoperative analgesia is necessary in cases of invasive procedures so the patient resumes normal function as quickly as possible. Local blocks are contraindicated if there is peripheral neuropathy present.

C. Hyperadrenocorticism (Cushing disease)

Hyperadrenocorticism is an increase in corticosteroids, either exogenously due to supplementation or from the adrenal glands themselves (secondary to a primary adrenal mass or pituitary gland tumor causing stimulation of the adrenal gland). While the term "Cushing disease"

Table 5.4 Diabetes mellitus.

Premedication (mg/kg)	Induction (mg/kg)	Maintenance	Intraoperative analgesia (mg/kg/h)	Postoperative analgesia (mg/kg)
Opioid (a) Methadone 0.3–0.5 IM, 0.2–0.3 IV OR (b) Hydromorphone 0.1 IM, 0.05 IV OR (c) Buprenorphine 0.01–0.03 IV, IM OR (d) Butorphanol 0.1–0.4 IV, IM **Other drugs:** (a) Sedative (if needed) 　(i) Acepromazine 0.01–0.02 　OR 　(ii) Midazolam 0.1 IM 　OR 　(iii) Alfaxalone 1–3 IM AND (b) GI protection: 　(i) Famotidine 1 mg/kg IV or SC 　AND 　(ii) Maropitant 1 mg/kg IV or SC	(a) Propofol 1–4 to effect +/– midazolam 0.2 OR (b) Alfaxalone 1–3 IV +/– midazolam 0.1–0.2 IV OR (c) Propofol 2 + Ketamine 2 ("ketofol") to effect +/– midazolam 0.2	(a) Sevoflurane OR (b) Isoflurane +/– CRI for reduction of inhalant requirement	(a) Opioid CRI (select one) 　(i) Fentanyl 0.012–0.042 　OR 　(ii) Hydromorphone 0.03 　OR 　(iii) Remifentanil 0.012–0.042 +/– (b) Adjunctive CRI 　(i) Lidocaine CRI 1.5–3 +/– (c) Local regional block **Fluids:** Crystalloids +/– 2.5–5% dextrose 2–5 mL/kg/h	(a) CRI: 　(i) Fentanyl 0.002–0.005 mg/kg/h 　OR 　(ii) Hydromorphone 0.01 mg/kg/h +/– 　(iii) Lidocaine 1.5 mg/kg/h OR (b) Intermittent bolus: 　(i) Methadone 0.3 IV q 4–6 h 　OR 　(ii) Hydromorphone 0.05–0.1 IV q 4–6 h AND (e) NSAID where not contraindicated +/– (d) Liposomal encapsulated bupivacaine infiltrative block 5.3 mg/kg

"AND" means that multiple choices from this column are selected, "+/–" means that the anesthetist will choose one or the other selection. For example, the postoperative analgesia column would be interpreted as including an opioid from the options (either as a CRI or intermittently given) and an NSAID, with an optional lidocaine CRI and optional long-acting local anesthetic block.

In patients who received pantoprazole for greater than 36 hours, pantoprazole will replace famotidine.

Lidocaine is contraindicated in cats; alternatively, lidocaine patches are an option alongside incision for both the cat and dog.

CRI, constant-rate infusion; GI, gastrointestinal; IM, intramuscular; IV, intravenous; NSAID, nonsteroidal antiinflammatory drug; SC, subcutaneous.

Chapter 5

153

actually indicates the pituitary form of hyperadrenocorticism, it is often used interchangeably for all forms of hyperadrenocorticism. Hyperadrenocorticism is confirmed or suggested based on a variety of methods, including history of supplementation, ACTH stimulation, low-dose dexamethasone suppression test, high-dose dexamethasone suppression test, and urine cortisol to creatinine ratio.

Clinical signs of this disease include polyuria and polydipsia (PU/PD), polyphagia, thin hair and skin, especially on the flank and abdomen, along with pyoderma, a "pot belly" appearance, panting, muscle weakness, and lethargy. On PE, hepatomegaly is present. Potential concurrent disease processes which merit investigation include hypertension, hypercoagulability, renal disease, and diabetes mellitus. Characteristic BW abnormalities include a stress leukogram, increases in RBC counts, increase in platelets, BG, ALP, ALT, triglycerides, and cholesterol, and a decrease in phosphate. Urinalysis reveals a decreased urine specific gravity (USG), proteinuria, and possibly bacterial infection. In one study, the mortality rate was as high as 14.6% for patients undergoing an adrenalectomy to address the primary adrenal mass resulting in Cushing disease [24]; the anesthetic protocol is carefully planned as the outcome of the procedure has been associated with the anesthetic management [24].

1. Anesthesia concerns/common complications

- *Fragile skin*: Care is taken when clipping these patients. Their skin is prone to bruising and lacerations. The hair that is clipped does not grow back as quickly or aesthetically as the hair of a normal patient, so minimizing the clipped areas is indicated.
- *Concurrent medications*: As with all patients, a thorough understanding of all medications or supplements a hyperadrenocortical patient receives is important for the anesthetist. A patient which has iatrogenic adrenocortical disease (i.e., is on glucocorticoid supplementation) is *not* abruptly taken off glucocorticoids prior to anesthesia, as an Addisonian crisis may result (see p.157). Some patients with the pituitary form of Cushing disease are treated with selegiline HCl (Anipryl,® Zoetis). This drug is an irreversible monoamine oxidase inhibitor (MAOI), meaning that until new MAOs are formed, monoamines are not oxidized and therefore increase in circulation. While this is useful in certain disease states, too much monoamine may result in *serotonin syndrome*, characterized by hyperthermia, tachycardia, hypertension and muscle tremors, which range in severity from mild to fatal. Additional drugs that increase the availability of monoamines are contraindicated (e.g., tramadol, metoclopramide, trazodone). During the anesthetic period, meperidine, fentanyl, and pentazocine are avoided for patients receiving MAOIs. It appears morphine is the most suitable opioid, although neurologic depression may accompany administration of morphine in a patient on selegiline HCl. Some authors suggest avoiding ketamine as it may exacerbate the symptoms of a serotonergic crisis, but there is little, if any, nonanecdotal information for this recommendation.
- *Hypoventilation*: This results from muscle weakness and abdominal distension secondary to hepatomegaly and fat redistribution; mechanical ventilation is warranted.
- *Management of concurrent diseases*: The possibility of a pulmonary thromboembolism (PTE) secondary to hypercoagulability is something the anesthetist should be vigilant to monitor for; this is suggested by a large difference between $EtCO_2$ and

arterial CO_2 (see Chapter 3, p.69, "Pulmonary thromboembolism"). The use of reversible drugs is recommended to ensure the patient is able to wake up quickly. Most clinicians also request the patient has frequent walks in the postoperative period to reduce the formation of blood clots.

* *Survival*: In patients undergoing an adrenalectomy to address their Cushing disease, the survival rate was better statistically when patients received hydrocortisone intra-operatively [24]. The anesthetist should discuss this with the surgeon prior to the procedure.

2. Anesthetic protocol (Table 5.5)

Premedication reduces stress and facilitates IV catheterization; oftentimes, a sedative is unnecessary, but the anesthetist can include acepromazine in low doses or midazolam as necessary. Care is taken when clipping the site of the IV catheter to prevent abrasions and bruising. Morphine, hydromorphone, and methadone are safe choices that provide appropriate analgesia for invasive procedures. Following IM premedication, patients are watched for respiratory depression. Preoxygenation is recommended for at least 5–10 minutes. If the patient is cooperative, monitoring equipment such as Doppler, ECG, and NIBP are placed prior to induction. Induction is accomplished with many options depending on the patient's anesthetic assessment and drug availability. Etomidate results in adrenocortical suppression, although whether this is beneficial is unknown. Inclusion of a benzodiazepine helps reduce the amount of etomidate necessary; however, even small amounts of etomidate will result in adrenocortical suppression [25]. A neuroleptic induction may work well for extremely critical patients. Propofol and alfaxalone are also acceptable choices for induction in combination with a benzodiazepine to reduce the amount of true induction agent needed. Inhalants are used to maintain anesthesia. A CRI of opioids (i.e., fentanyl, hydromorphone) and/or lidocaine helps provide analgesia and reduce MAC requirements of the inhalant.

Diligent monitoring of ventilation, invasive blood pressure, acid–base status, and electrolyte analysis is performed throughout the procedure, and possibly into recovery. Patients are extubated only when they are able to adequately ventilate themselves and monitored after extubation for trouble ventilating. Supplemental oxygen is provided to patients which need it.

D. Hypoadrenocorticism (Addison's disease) [26]

A deficiency of glucocorticoid and/or mineralocorticoid from the adrenal glands is called hypoadrenocorticism (Addison disease). The atypical Addisonian will only have deficiency in glucocorticoids, not mineralocorticoids. The adrenal gland's outermost layer, the zona glomerulosa, is responsible for secreting mineralocorticoids (with aldosterone as one of the most important). When the zona glomerulosa no longer secretes aldosterone, electrolyte excretion and water regulation become dysfunctional. The subsequent layer, the zona fasciculata, is responsible for cortisol (glucocorticoid) production and when this is impaired, many normal functions of the body (such as metabolism, cardiovascular stability, and response to stress) are compromised.

156

Table 5.5 Cushing disease.

Premedication (mg/kg)	Induction (mg/kg)	Maintenance	Intraoperative analgesia (mg/kg/h)	Postoperative analgesia (mg/kg)
Opioid (select one) (a) Methadone 0.3–0.5 IM, 0.2–0.3 IV OR (b) Hydromorphone 0.1 IM, 0.05 IV OR (c) Morphine 0.1–0.5 IM OR (d) Buprenorphine 0.01–0.03 IV, IM OR (e) Butorphanol 0.1–0.4 IV, IM	(a) Propofol 2–4 IV to effect +/- midazolam 0.2 IV OR (b) Alfaxalone 1–3 IV +/- midazolam 0.1–0.2 IV OR (c) Propofol 2 + Ketamine 2 ("ketofol") to effect +/- midazolam 0.2 OR (d) Etomidate 1–2 IV +/- midazolam 0.1–0.2 IV	Sevoflurane OR Isoflurane AND CRI for reduction of inhalant requirement Fluids: Balanced, isotonic electrolyte solution	(a) Opioid CRI (i) Fentanyl 0.012–0.042 OR (ii) Hydro-morphone 0.03 OR (iii) Remifentanil 0.012–0.042 +/- (b) Lido-caine CRI 1.5–3 +/- (c) Local regional block	(a) Opioid CRIs: (i) Fentanyl 0.002–0.005 mg/kg/h OR (ii) Hydromorphone 0.01 mg/kg/h OR (b) Intermittent bolus: (i) Methadone 0.3 IV q 4–6 h OR (ii) Hydromor-phone 0.05–0.1 IV q 4–6 h +/- (c) Lidocaine 1.5 mg/kg/h +/- (d) Liposomal encapsulated bupivacaine infiltrative block 5.3 mg/kg

Sedative (if needed) — (a) Acepromazine 0.01–0.02 IV, IM / OR / (b) Midazolam 0.1 IM, IV / +/-

"AND" means that multiple choices from this column are selected, "+/-" means it is up to the anesthetist if they would like to combine multiple choices, "OR" means that the anesthetist will choose one or the other selection. For example, the postoperative analgesia column would be interpreted as including an opioid from the options (either as a CRI or intermittently given), with an optional lidocaine CRI and optional long-acting local anesthetic block.

Lidocaine is contraindicated in cats; alternatively, lidocaine patch can be placed alongside incisions in cats and dogs. Preoxygenate patients. In patients on Anipryl®, meperidine is avoided, as are fentanyl and remifentanil.

CRI, constant-rate infusion; IM, intramuscular; IV, intravenous.

Addison disease is often referred to as "the great pretender" because the clinical signs of this disease are vague; they include weakness, lethargy, inappetence, chronic vomiting and diarrhea, pre-renal azotemia (sometimes mistaken for renal failure and not present with atypical Addison), and occasionally PU/PD. The patient may be hypotensive with abnormalities related to hyperkalemia (bradycardia and ECG changes including loss of P waves, wide and bizarre QRS waves, and tall, tented T waves). Suspected Addison disease is confirmed by testing the adrenocortical reserve with ACTH stimulation. Elective procedures in an unmanaged Addisonian patient are postponed until the patient is stabilized.

Even in the managed Addisonian patient, it is recommended that a CBC and chemistry are performed. Common abnormalities on the CBC include absence of stress leukogram – this is unusual for an animal presenting as ill or "not doing right." Anemia is likely present but may be masked by hypovolemia, resulting in a relatively normal PCV. Abnormalities on the chemistry include a host of electrolyte abnormalities, such as hypoglycemia, hyperkalemia with hyponatremia (ratio Na:K <27, although this may vary by lab analyzer), hypochloremia, and hypercalcemia, as well as azotemia and acidosis (which are secondary to hypovolemia). A urinalysis may reveal a low USG. When Addison disease is confirmed, traditional management usually includes desoxycorticosterone pivalate (DOCP) for mineralocorticoid supplementation and a corticosteroid for glucocorticoid (such as prednisone) supplementation.

In the managed Addisonian patient, it is the author's preference to schedule elective procedures after recent administration of DOCP, rather than close to the next date of administration (as it is administered every 25 days per the manufacturer). Additionally, it is imperative that any maintenance glucocorticoid is given on schedule, and in some cases, an additional dose is administered preemptively.

1. Anesthesia concerns/common complications

- *Addisonian crisis*: An Addisonian crisis manifests as life-threatening hypovolemic shock and hyperkalemia in patients acutely removed from glucocorticoids. Patients must receive large volumes of 0.9% NaCl for volume resuscitation and may require treatment for hyperkalemia (see Chapter 3, p.78). When recognized, supplementation with dexamethasone after volume resuscitation will benefit the patient without interfering in an ACTH stimulation test for confirmation of hypoadrenocorticism.
- *Effective circulating volume*: Fluid stabilization with 0.9% NaCl is necessary prior to any procedure; aggressiveness of stabilization is based on how well managed the Addisonian patient is. Unstable cases may require up to 90 mL/kg (shock dose/blood volume of a dog) of 0.9% NaCl for the first hour. Goal-directed therapy is important; giving aliquots of fluid and assessing the patient will help better titrate the correct amount and avoid volume overload.
- *Hyperkalemia*: Preinstrumentation, especially an ECG, is warranted if the patient allows. Arrhythmias associated with hyperkalemia, and their treatments, are discussed in Chapter 3. Hyperkalemia is one of the most life-threatening electrolyte abnormalities. It requires aggressive and timely treatment.
- *Hypoglycemia*: Hypoglycemic patients may require a 2.5–5% dextrose supplementation. A dextrose bolus may be needed. A dose of 0.5–1 mL/kg of 50% dextrose may be given slowly and diluted in a 1:3 ratio with saline.

Chapter 5

- *Hypotension*: Obtain a BP measurement prior to induction. Hypotension is difficult to manage in these cases, but heavily relies on volume support. IBP measurement is optimal. Inotropes, such as dobutamine, might also be useful for BP support as well as helping to lower potassium concentration, once volume status is optimized.
- *Stress*: These patients compensate poorly for stress; of all patients, minimizing stress is a top priority in the Addisonian patient.
- *Supplementation*: Ensure any managed Addisonian has received their corticoid supplementation for the day, and their mineralocorticoid supplementation within the last month (DOCP). Unmanaged cases receive hydrocortisone 2–4 mg/kg IV prior to induction. It is best to increase their glucocorticoid supplementation during their stay in the hospital.

2. Anesthetic protocol (Table 5.6)

These patients usually require lower drug dosages than the standard patient; when possible, use reversible, short-acting drugs. Premedication with an opioid and application of EMLA cream will reduce the stress associated with IV catheterization. A neuroleptic anesthesia premed/induction will often facilitate intubation. Propofol or alfaxalone to effect, with midazolam 0.2 mg/kg to reduce the amount of primary induction agent necessary, is used as well. Etomidate is contraindicated in these patients due to its inhibition of steroidogenesis and decreasing cortisol production for 4–6 hours postoperatively. Inhalant anesthetics are routinely used for anesthesia maintenance. Opioid CRIs are used to reduce the MAC requirement of inhalant anesthetics. Provide MV if necessary; however, the anesthetist must be cognizant of the negative impacts MV will have on BP and discontinue it in the face of hypotension. These patients require aggressive fluid therapy. It is ideal to monitor CVP and IBP. Additionally, $EtCO_2$, blood gas analysis, BG, and electrolytes are closely monitored throughout anesthesia and recovery.

E. Hyperthyroidism

Hyperthyroidism results in excessive thyroid hormone production, increasing a patient's metabolic state. While relatively rare in dogs (generally secondary to a thyroid tumor which is functional; most are not), hyperthyroidism is extremely common in the aging cat. Clinical signs consist of weight loss (often in the face of increased appetite), vomiting, increased activity, and PU/PD. On PE, the patient is thin/has poor body condition with muscle wasting and at least one palpably enlarged thyroid gland. These patients are often agitated and easily stressed; stress evokes respiratory changes such as dyspnea and hyperventilation. Cardiovascular changes include hypertension, tachycardia, arrhythmias, and increased oxygen requirements. Often times, a gallop murmur is auscultated. Further investigation of the cardiac system may reveal cardiac enlargement and heart failure, which in cats manifests as pulmonary edema or pleural effusion.

While azotemia may be present, an absence of renal problems is not uncommon; even if the beginning stages of renal failure exist in the cat, the kidney is heavily perfused secondary to the hypermetabolic state so that renal values remain normal. This is important information for the anesthetist, because it is unwise to assume these patients have adequate kidney reserve.

Table 5.6   Addison's disease.

Premedication (mg/kg)	Induction (mg/kg)	Maintenance	Intraoperative analgesia (mg/kg/h)	Postoperative analgesia (mg/kg)
Opioid (select one)	Sedative (if needed)	(a) Sevoflurane	(a) Opioid CRI	(a) Opioid CRIs:
(a) Methadone 0.3 IM, 0.2 IV	(a) Midazolam 0.1 IM	OR	(i) Fentanyl 0.012–0.042	(i) Fentanyl 0.002–0.005 mg/kg/h
	(a) Alfaxalone 1–3 +/– midazolam 0.2	(b) Isoflurane		
OR	(b) Acepromazine 0.01–0.02 IM	+/–	OR	OR
(b) Hydromorphone 0.05 IM, 0.05 IV	OR	CRI for reduction of inhalant requirement	(ii) Hydromorphone 0.03	(ii) Hydromorphone 0.01 mg/kg/h
	(b) Propofol 2 + ketamine 2 ("ketofol") to effect +/– midazolam 0.2			
OR			OR	OR
(c) Morphine 0.1–0.5 IM		Fluids: Balanced, isotonic crystalloid solution	(iii) Remifentanil 0.012–0.042	(b) Intermittent bolus:
	OR			(i) Methadone 0.3 IV q 4–6 h
OR	(c) Propofol to effect +/– midazolam 0.2		+/–	
(d) Buprenorphine 0.01–0.03 IV, IM			(b) Lidocaine CRI 1.5–3 (dogs only)	OR
				(ii) Hydromorphone 0.05–0.1 IV q 4–6 h
OR			+/–	
(e) Butorphanol 0.1–0.4 IV, IM			(c) Local regional block	+/–
				(c) Lidocaine 1–3 mg/kg/h
				+/–
				(d) Liposomal encapsulated bupivacaine infiltrative block 5.3 mg/kg

"AND" means that multiple choices from this column are selected, "+/–" means that it is up to the anesthetist if they would like to combine multiple choices, "OR" means that the anesthetist will choose one or the other selection. For example, the postoperative analgesia column would be interpreted as including an opioid from the options (either as a CRI or intermittently given), with an optional lidocaine CRI and optional long-acting local anesthetic block.

Preoxygenate. Give hydrocortisone 2–4 mg/kg IV at induction if unsure of glucocorticoid supplementation. Lidocaine is contraindicated in cats; alternatively, lidocaine patch is used alongside incision in both dogs and cats.

CRI, constant-rate infusion; IM, intramuscular; IV, intravenous.

This is also important to note in any patients that have received radioiodine treatment for their hyperthyroidism. A decrease in blood volume and velocity at the level of the kidney may occur in patients post treatment, as shown by contrast enhanced ultrasound [27]. Changes in BW include an elevated T4 level, increased RBC count, and increased liver enzymes (ALT, ALP, AST).

1. Anesthesia concerns/common complications

- *Client communication*: If it is necessary to anesthetize an uncontrolled hyperthyroid cat, the owner must be thoroughly counseled regarding the increased anesthetic risk, as well as intraoperative and postoperative risks (including sudden death). The CPR status of the cat is confirmed with the anesthetist. In cats that are euthyroid, this risk is greatly diminished (although not eliminated). It is recommended that a patient receives treatment (methimazole) prior to undergoing an elective procedure. A T4 analysis is performed prior to the procedure to confirm normal levels.
- *Cooperativeness*: Hyperthyroid patients cope even more poorly than a normal cat with restraint, putting both personnel and the cat at risk. Gabapentin 100 mg orally on the morning of the procedure is ideal to reduce stress.
- *Adequate premedication is a necessity*. Cardiac arrest has been experienced clinically due to stress induced from restraint. It is not uncommon for these cats to exhibit dyspnea and panting from even minimal handling and restraint.
- *Hypertension*: The vast majority of these cats are hypertensive. A BP is obtained prior to induction, if possible, without causing too much stress to the patient. If it is not possible to obtain a BP without a premedication, a BP is attempted when the patient is more sedated, knowing that this may be altered by the medications. The anesthetist should be aware of any drugs that are used to control the hypertension (ACE inhibitors, Ca+ channel blockers, etc.). Depending on the response to the medication, these drugs may be withheld on the day of surgery (i.e., if the patient is very responsive to BP medication, it may be withheld to prevent intraoperative hypotension; see next) (see Appendix F).
- *Hypoventilation*: If respiratory muscles are weak, hypoventilation will be evident under anesthesia. As long as cardiovascular parameters are within normal limits, mechanical ventilation is initiated for these patients.
- *Multiorgan involvement*: Given the number of organ systems impacted by hyperthyroidism, minimizing time under anesthesia and maintaining adequate tissue perfusion (i.e., preventing hypotension) are critical to success in these patients.
- *Tachycardia*: Patients who are severely hypertensive and tachycardic are stabilized on beta-blockers prior to anesthesia; this may also decrease the incidence of arrhythmias. Intraoperatively, cats with heart rates over 220 bpm may benefit from esmolol at an initial bolus of 0.1–0.5 mg/kg IV slowly followed by CRI of 6–12 mg/kg/h [28].
- *Hypothermia*: In an underweight patient, thermoregulation is difficult due to increased body surface area and use of a nonrebreathing system in small patients.
- *Thyroid storm*: This complication is life-threatening and is characterized by rapid release of thyroid hormones into systemic circulation (usually in response to stress). Clinical signs include tachycardia and hyperthermia; a patient which experiences this can develop pulmonary edema and decompensate rapidly. While this occurs most

commonly postoperatively, it can occur intraoperatively. Treatment involves control-ling the symptoms. Cool the patient with cool IV fluids and high fresh gas flow rates, and use abdominal lavage for open abdominal procedure.

- *Surgical planning*: If a subtotal thyroidectomy is performed, damage to the recurrent laryngeal nerves and swelling can contribute to airway obstruction at extubation. The proximity of the thyroid gland to the parathyroid glands makes hypocalcemia a pos-sible postoperative complication if a bilateral thyroidectomy is performed. Close attention needs to be paid to calcium levels postoperatively, with supplementation provided as necessary. The patient is placed on a seizure watch postoperatively and monitored for any neurologic signs.

2. Anesthetic protocol

It is important the anesthetist thoroughly understands all systems affected and the level of involvement of each system, and whether all of these conditions are managed. Premedication with opioids alone in the hyperthyroid cat tends to make most cats euphoric; this may or may not alleviate agitation to facilitate IV catheterization, although inclusion of eutectic mixture of lidocaine and prilocaine cream may help in this regard [29]. High doses of opioids will result in dysphoria [30,31]. Alfaxalone IM is considered as a premedication in fractious cats. In the case of significantly unmanageable patients, inclusion of dexmedetomidine may render the patient more manageable and decrease the HR. Smooth, short-acting induction agents such as propofol or alfaxalone IV given slowly to effect are warranted. The anesthetist includes a benzodiazepine to reduce the amount of induction agent needed. Cats which show structural cardiac changes are induced with etomidate or alfaxalone and a benzodiazepine. Anesthetics causing sympathetic stimulation are avoided (i.e., ketamine). Unfortunately, there are very few options to allow for a reduction in MAC in cats, but an opioid CRI will provide analgesia even in light of a vaporizer setting that is not reduced. Local blocks, such as an epidural, if warranted, are considered.

An ECG is vital to detect arrhythmias, and an arterial line gives continuous information on blood pressure. Caution is taken when placing arterial lines in the feline patient, due to a decrease in collateral blood supply and a higher risk of necrosis occurring after placement. It is also important to monitor body temperature closely.

F. Hypothyroidism

Hypothyroidism, manifested as a deficiency in thyroid hormone, is one of the most common diseases seen in older dogs. The function of the thyroid gland is to maintain a normal meta-bolic state, and therefore hypothyroidism results in a decreased metabolic state. Common clinical signs include lethargy, depression, intolerance of cold, and obesity. Cardiovascular changes secondary to hypothyroidism include bradycardia and decreased CO due to decreased myocardial contractility. A decreased metabolic rate makes patients more sensitive to anes-thetics, as the drugs are not metabolized as quickly. Common BW abnormalities include a nonregenerative anemia, elevation in cholesterol, triglycerides, and a decrease in total T4. For a full discussion on diagnosis of hypothyroidism utilizing thyroid assays, the reader is referred to other texts.

Chapter 5

1. Anesthesia concerns/common complications

- *Delayed gastric emptying*: With the overall slowdown in metabolism, the GI tract does not empty in a timely manner. Even with fasting, the anesthetist is prepared for regurgitation. Gastroprotectants are included in the anesthesia protocol to help decrease the risk of vomiting and nausea.
- *Drug dosages*: Use lower drug doses, drugs to "effect" or reversible, short-acting drugs when possible.
- *Hypotension*: Patients which have not returned to normal T4 levels have multiple cardiovascular issues, but hypotension frequently manifests itself under anesthesia, due to the increased drug sensitivity coupled with an already decreased CO and decrease in intravascular volume. These patients are minimally responsive to traditional management of hypotension with positive inotropes due to alteration in beta-adrenergic receptors. This leads to a decrease in response to catecholamines and anticholinergics. It is advised that hypothyroid patients are managed for their disease prior to elective procedures, because of the uncertainty in blood pressure management.
- *Hypothermia*: Core temperature is poorly maintained in these patients due to a decrease in metabolism. Heat support is provided perioperatively.
- *Prolonged recovery*: Slow drug metabolism and hypothermia both prolong recovery in these patients.

2. Anesthetic protocol

The modifications to a routine anesthesia protocol depend on how well a patient's hypothyroid disease is controlled; in patients that are fully stabilized, minimal changes are necessary. It is recommended that a patient be on treatment for several weeks prior to anesthesia for an elective procedure and a T4 checked prior to anesthesia.

Patients with a degree of unmanaged hypothyroidism will present the anesthetist with some challenges. Lower drugs doses are generally given due to the decrease in metabolic rate. Preferentially, the anesthetist selects drugs that are short-acting and reversible. Often times, only a low dose of an opioid (no sedative) is required for premedication, although this is often combined with an anticholinergic to prevent opioid-induced bradycardia. Preoxygenation and preinstrumentation are important for these patients.

Ketamine is considered the induction agent of choice, if not otherwise contraindicated, to increase HR and stimulate release of any catecholamines present. This will also help with a transient increase in BP. This agent is combined with a benzodiazepine for muscle relaxation. A CRI of ketamine will balance the anesthesia technique. Gas inhalants are used but kept as low as possible due to the patient's sensitivity to anesthetic drugs; studies in patients with induced hypothyroidism did not show a decreased requirement in isoflurane MAC concentration [32]. A short-acting opioid CRI such as remifentanil or fentanyl is included to allow the anesthetist to keep the inhalant levels low. High doses of opioids are avoided due to the bradycardia that might ensue which may be less responsive to interventions with anticholinergics and catecholamines. Ephedrine is useful in management of intraoperative hypotension and bradycardia.

Close monitoring of the patient is warranted throughout the prolonged recovery period.

G. Pheochromocytoma

Pheochromocytomas arise from the chromaffin cells of the adrenal medulla and are catecholamine-producing adrenal tumors. Often these tumors are found incidentally. Patients frequently have indistinct signs and it is not until a patient is anesthetized that the ramifications of these tumors come to light. Clinical signs include lethargy and weakness, inappetence and weight loss, vomiting, and PU/PD. On PE, panting, pale mucous membranes (secondary to vasoconstriction), tachycardia, and a possibly a fever are present. BW changes include anemia, a stress leukogram, increased liver enzymes (ALP, ALT, AST), azotemia, and electrolyte alterations. If there is a suspicion of an adrenal tumor, a complete workup before anesthesia is indicated, including an abdominal ultrasound and/or CT to determine the degree of vascular involvement before surgical planning.

1. Anesthesia concerns

- *Hemorrhage*: This tumor is highly invasive and any attempts to remove it may result in massive hemorrhage. It is prudent to blood type and cross-match these patients and ensure that blood products are available. Two large-bore IV catheters are placed in case blood products are necessary.
- *Hypertension and tachycardia*: The secretion of epinephrine (canine) or norepinephrine (feline) results in profound vasoconstriction (via stimulation of the alpha-adrenergic receptors), as well as tachycardia. The body compensates for this unrelenting increase in vascular tone by decreasing circulating volume. The only relief for the vascular system is stimulation of the beta receptors by catecholamine release, which results in some small degree of vasodilation. When these patients are anesthetized, the ensuing vasodilation in light of the decreased effective circulating volume may result in cardiovascular collapse. To reduce this possibility, a patient with a pheochromocytoma is administered alpha-adrenergic-blocking drugs such as phenoxybenzamine prior to their anticipated anesthesia, with the intention of allowing them relief of vasoconstriction in order to restore effective circulating volume. This has significantly improved outcome [7]; ideally, this is done for 14 days prior to anesthesia. It is inappropriate to administer a beta-blocker (i.e., esmolol) to reduce tachycardia if the patient is not alpha-blockaded, as the beta-blockade may worsen hypertension by blocking the beta smooth muscle effects.
- *Impaired venous return*: This tumor is very invasive into surrounding vasculature, including the vena cava. In addition to possible intraoperative blood loss, there is also concern regarding the degree of impairment on venous return to the heart and compounding compromise to CO.

2. Anesthesia protocol

Premedication with a full mu agonist opioid (hydromorphone, methadone) will provide sedation, preoperative analgesia and a reduction in the drugs necessary for induction and maintenance of anesthesia. If a sedative is necessary, benzodiazepines have the lowest number of cardiovascular side-effects. As much monitoring and support equipment as possible is

Chapter 5

pre-placed in the awake patient, using things such as EMLA cream to facilitate arterial line placement and a large-bore second catheter. Minimizing time under anesthesia is critical.

The only induction agent contraindicated is ketamine. Due to its very safe profile, a neuroleptic induction with fentanyl and a benzodiazepine is often chosen in these cases. Additional alfaxalone or propofol are titrated only to effect in order to intubate the patient. Lidocaine is used on the larynx to help with intubation. Maintenance with inhalant and a balanced technique with an opioid and lidocaine (dogs only) CRI is suitable. Intraoperatively, in a patient which has received phenoxybenzamine, esmolol is used to address tachycardia, and nitroprusside is administered to reduce hypertension. Magnesium is also considered for tachycardia and blood pressure management as nitroprusside may be extremely expensive and is somewhat difficult to dose in smaller patients. Acepromazine is avoided due to the alpha-blockade already in place with phenoxybenzamine. Blood for transfusion must be available.

The patient will continue to have high levels of circulating catecholamines for several days, so the postoperative period is a critical time for these patients; as much monitoring as possible is continued (i.e., arterial line is left in). Glucose is monitored postoperatively as hypoglycemia is a possible complication. Continuous ECG and blood pressure monitoring is advised.

H. Insulinoma

Insulinoma is a functional tumor of the beta cells of the pancreas that secrete insulin. In a normal patient, a glycemic feedback mechanism allows for proper secretion of insulin due to a higher concentration of glucose in the body. An insulinoma secretes insulin regardless of this glycemic feedback mechanism, therefore hypoglycemia will ensue. This usually occurs in middle-aged to older dogs.

Signs are usually neurologic due to the severe hypoglycemia, including trembling, confusion, hunger, and nervousness to more extreme neurologic signs, such as seizures. Mild signs usually resolve without intervention. With extremely severe hypoglycemia, cardiac and respiratory arrest can occur. There are usually no major abnormalities noted on PE, but BW will show hypoglycemia. A fasting hypoglycemia with inappropriate high serum insulin concentrations will diagnose an insulinoma. A full workup includes abdominal ultrasound, thoracic radiographs, and possibly a CT for surgical planning.

Insulinomas have a high risk of metastasis at the time of diagnosis. Therefore, hypoglycemia and neurologic signs often continue even after surgery or several months postoperatively. Surgery is rarely curative and long-term medical treatment is usually necessary to prevent hypoglycemic crises from occurring.

1. Anesthesia concerns

- *Hypoglycemia*: Avoiding severe hypoglycemia is extremely important. These patients should not be fasted overnight; instead, small, frequent meals are given until 6 hours before surgery.
- *Additional medication*: Prednisone is administered to antagonize insulin and therefore decrease hypoglycemia. Diazoxide, a benzothiadiazide, may also be administered as it prevents K-ATP channels on beta plasma cell membranes from closing. This prevents the cells from depolarizing and reduces the amount of insulin secreted.

- *Target blood glucose*: These patients have usually adapted to lower BG concentrations that run between 40 and 60 mg/dL, while the patient remains asymptomatic. It is not recommended to push these patients to "normal" blood glucoses (>80 mg/dL) with dextrose or dextrose CRIs as this may result in the release of insulin, therefore making hypoglycemia worse. Dextrose is reserved if neurologic signs are noted, or if BG drops below the normal insulin level for the specific patient undergoing anesthesia (i.e., there is no "one size fits all" guideline). Glucose is monitored frequently in these patients.

2. Anesthesia protocol

Glucose monitoring intraoperatively occurs every 30–60 minutes. Any balanced isotonic crystalloid fluid is used; dextrose at 2.5–5% is added only if the patient has a fall in BG compared to their resting BG. The goal is to maintain the BG roughly at 50–60 mg/dL, keeping in mind some patients tolerate BG as low as 30–40 mg/dL. Glucagon CRI at 5–40 ng/kg/min (bolus of 50 ng/kg IV) is another treatment option. It is important to measure the BG when surgical manipulation of the tumor is occurring as this may cause release of insulin and therefore worsen hypoglycemia. Drugs that increase cerebral metabolic rate are avoided.

Premedication with full mu opioids are a reasonable choice and will help decrease sympathetic stimulation (which can cause an increase in BG, therefore releasing insulin, thus leading to a further decrease in BG). Gastroprotectants (maropitant and famotidine or pantoprazole) are also included. Induction with propofol or alfaxalone combined with a benzodiazepine or neuroleptanesthesia are all acceptable for these patients.

If possible, monitoring equipment is placed while the patient is preoxygenated. A sampling line is also appropriate due to frequent BG monitoring. An opioid CRI will help to reduce inhalant requirement. Some anesthetists will also include an alpha-2 agonist as it may suppress insulin secretion and increase plasma glucose [33]. Adequate perfusion to the pancreas throughout the procedure is important to help prevent pancreatitis. The MAP is kept over 60 mmHg and hypoxemia is avoided. BG monitoring should continue postoperatively, and the patient is monitored for neurologic signs and seizures.

III. Hepatic function diseases

Hepatic function is of critical importance to the anesthetist. It is responsible for protein synthesis, drug metabolism, glycogen storage, and production of coagulation factors. Certain disease states will alter hepatic leakage enzymes; these disease states must be very advanced to alter hepatic function, however. Therefore, the focus of this section is on disease that impairs hepatic function.

Portosystemic shunts (PSS) are prototypical examples of such alterations, but things like end-stage cirrhosis or liver damage secondary to drug (i.e., NSAID) overdose result in similar changes. On PE, the patient with PSS is dull, small in size and may have a history of seizures. Dullness is often due to hepatic encephalopathy; medical management is warranted prior to anesthesia to resolve hepatic encephalopathy. On BW, anemia, an increase in ammonia and bile acids, and a decreased BUN, BG, albumin, cholesterol, and prolonged coagulation times are present. Urinalysis may reveal ammonium biurate crystals, which result in uroliths.

1. Anesthetic concerns/common complications

- *Congenital abnormalities*: In any animal presenting with a congenital abnormality such as a PSS, a particularly thorough PE is warranted to ensure there are no congenital abnormalities of other body systems, such as the cardiovascular, respiratory, and renal systems.
- *Drug metabolism*: Select drugs that are extrahepatically metabolized or short-acting/reversible. Drugs dependent on the liver for metabolism have a more profound effect for a longer duration in patients with insufficiencies. Barbiturates are contraindicated. If the patient has neurologic hepatic encephalopathy due to a PSS, benzodiazepines are controversial, due to an increase in endogenous benzodiazepines and altered central nervous system receptors to benzodiazepines. By giving more benzodiazepines, the patient may become more dysphoric or even comatose for a prolonged duration. Lidocaine may rapidly accumulate in patients with extreme liver insufficiencies.
- *Hemorrhage (see Chapter 3 "Hemorrhage," p.64)*: The liver is extremely vascular. Liver biopsies and PSS ligations all have the potential for significant hemorrhage. This is compounded by the concurrent coagulation disorders of PSS. Two IV catheters (one large gauge) are recommended; the patient is blood typed and/or cross-matched before surgery. Coagulation times may be performed based on clinician preference; many cases of PSS are presumed to have coagulopathies.
- *Hypoglycemia*: Monitor BG every 30–60 min. Supplement fluids with 2.5–5% dextrose as necessary.
- *Hypotension*: Maintain hepatic profusion (i.e., blood pressure). These patients are commonly hypotensive when maintained under general anesthesia. Monitoring IBP is ideal, but as clotting times are increased, an arterial catheter may be contraindicated. Hypotension from anesthetics is compounded by the reduction in oncotic pressure secondary to the decrease in protein production; often, plasma is the fluid of choice for patients where albumin is low (give plasma if albumin is less than 2.0 g/dL). Alternatively, a hetastarch bolus of 2–5 mL/kg is an option. However, hetastarch may worsen coagulopathies if given at higher doses; a total dose of 0.8 mL/kg/h is not exceeded. Positive inotropes and reducing MAC requirements with fentanyl or remifentanil CRIs will help reduce the risk of hypotension.
- *Hypothermia*: The small size of these patients and the use of a nonrebreathing circuit make thermoregulation very difficult for the anesthetist. Circulating warm water blankets, forced air warming devices, and plastic wrap may reduce the degree of hypothermia, but the patient is unlikely to be normothermic if anesthetized for a procedure involving an open abdomen. Warming the patient after premedication is extremely important in these cases and warm abdominal lavage is utilized.
- *Mentation*: Patients which present clinically with hepatic encephalopathy are medically managed prior to anesthesia. If the patient is not medically managed, recovery in these patients is often markedly prolonged and may require mechanical ventilation. If the patient has seizures, antiseizure medication (such as levetiracetam) is recommended prior to surgery.

2. Anesthetic protocol (Table 5.7)

Agents metabolized by the liver (e.g., barbiturates and phenothiazine tranquilizers), highly protein-bound agents (e.g., diazepam and barbiturates), and hepatotoxic agents (e.g., halothane) are avoided because of poor hepatic function and hypoalbuminemia. Use reversible, short-acting, extrahepatically metabolized drugs when possible. An opioid appropriate for the level of pain anticipated +/− an anticholinergic (as necessary) are administered as a premedication. Inductions with propofol or alfaxalone are smooth and both have extrahepatic metabolism [34]. Although isoflurane is considered the inhalant of choice in patients with liver disease due to its low liver metabolism, in reality sevoflurane is only marginally more metabolized by the liver and the two are likely comparable. Remifentanil, if available, is metabolized by plasma esterase and therefore is not dependent on the liver for termination of effect, making it a suitable choice to reduce inhalant levels and provide analgesia. In practicality, fentanyl CRIs are often used but this drug does require liver metabolism. Check blood glucose periodically throughout surgery and supplement with dextrose as needed.

The patient's mentation and degree of hypothermia will affect recovery, which is likely to be prolonged.

IV. Neurological disorders: Intracranial disease

The calvarium is a fixed space and as such, there is a balance of tissue (the brain itself) and fluid (i.e., blood and cerebral spinal fluid [CSF]) within that space. If one of the components increases, another must decrease or an increase in intracranial pressure (ICP) will result. The concern for patients with intracranial disease is the increase of ICP causing herniation of brain tissue, resulting in death. Unfortunately, anesthetizing these patients disrupts cerebral blood flow, one of the three major components in the calvarium, and this becomes critical in patients which already have a disrupted balance (i.e., intracranial disease).

A thorough history and neurologic exam as part of a complete PE helps to identify the presence, frequency and duration of seizures, trauma or a neurotoxin in cases of intracranial disease of unknown cause. The following are signs of increased ICP: altered levels of consciousness, miosis, mydriasis, anisocoria, decreased pupillary reflex, papilledema, and Cushing reflex which includes bradycardia, hypertension, and breathing disturbances. CBC, chemistry, and urinalysis may be normal but will help to identify any contributing comorbidities.

1. Anesthetic goals/special considerations

- *Autoregulation*: Inhalant anesthesia will disrupt the brain's normal ability to autoregulate its own perfusion pressure; inhalants allow for a dose-dependent increase in cerebral blood flow (CBF) by causing vasodilation, which is detrimental to these patients. Thus, a reduction in inhalant requirement is a primary goal.
- *Cerebral metabolic rate (CMRO$_2$)*: One of the anesthetist's goals for these patients is to reduce CMRO$_2$. In general, anesthesia does this. The anesthetist, however, is careful to avoid dissociative anesthetics (ketamine) which may increase the CMRO$_2$. Allowing the patient to become mildly hypothermic (95–96.8 °F) will also reduce CMRO$_2$.

Table 5.7 Hepatic disease.

Premedication (mg/kg)	Induction (mg/kg)	Maintenance	Intraoperative analgesia (mg/kg/h)	Postoperative analgesia (mg/kg)

Other medications: Avoid sedatives, if possible, reduce doses if necessary
 	
(a) GI protection:
  (i) Famotidine 1 IV or SC
  AND
  (ii) Maropitant 1 IV or SC
 	
Opioid (select one)
(a) Methadone 0.3 IM, 0.2 IV
OR
(b) Morphine 0.5 IM
OR
(c) Hydromorphone 0.05–0.1 IV, IM
OR
(d) Fentanyl 0.002–0.005 IV
OR
(e) Butorphanol 0.1–0.4 IM, IV
OR
(f) Buprenorphine 0.01–0.03 IV, IM
	(a) Propofol 2–4 IV to effect
	OR
	(b) Alfaxalone 1–3
		(a) Isoflurane
		OR
		(b) Sevoflurane
		AND
		Opioid CRI for reduction of inhalant requirement
			(a) Opioid CRI
			  (i) Fentanyl 0.012–0.042
			  OR
			  (ii) Remifentanil 0.012–0.042
			+/–
			(b) Local regional block
				(a) Fentanyl CRI 0.002–0.005 mg/kg/h OR
				(b) Intermittent bolus:
				  (i) Methadone 0.5 IM q 4–6 h
				  OR
				  (ii) Buprenorphine 0.01–0.03 IV, IM
				+/–
				(c) Liposomal encapsulated bupivacaine infiltrative block 5.3 mg/kg

"AND" means that multiple choices from this column are selected, "+/–" means it is up to the anesthetist if they would like to combine multiple choices, "OR" means that the anesthetist will choose one or the other selection. For example, the postoperative analgesia column would be interpreted as including an opioid from the options (either as a CRI or intermittently given), with an optional long-acting local anesthetic block.

In patients who received pantoprazole for greater than 36 hours, pantoprazole will replace famotidine.

CRI, constant-rate infusion; GI, gastrointestinal; IM, intramuscular; IV, intravenous; SC, subcutaneous.

- *Glycemic control*: Hyperglycemia worsens neurologic outcomes in people, but hypoglycemia is not beneficial either [35]. Little information on animals is available in this regard. It is best for the anesthetist to monitor BG, with a target goal of maintaining euglycemia through the use of regular insulin if necessary. The BG range should be maintained between 80 and 180 mg/dL.
- *Hypoxemia*: PaO_2 below 60 mmHg will trigger more blood flow to the brain in order to maintain perfusion. If hypoxemia is present, careful steps are taken to determine the underlying cause and begin treatment (see Chapter 3 "Hypoxemia," p.66).
- *Cushing reflex*: This reflex occurs in response to significant increases in ICP, and heralds impending brain herniation; as such, it is a life-threatening emergency. It is easily recognized by profound bradycardia and significant hypertension. Any anesthetic utilized is immediately discontinued. Treatment involves reducing ICP by giving 4 mL/kg hypertonic saline over 2–5 min or mannitol 0.5–1.5 g/kg over 10–20 min. The patient is repositioned with the head raised at 30° above the heart, and the head is packed with ice packs. Ventilation targets an $EtCO_2$ of 30–35 mmHg throughout anesthesia. Severe hypocarbia (<30 mmHg) is also avoided as this reduces perfusion to the brain which leads to ischemic injury. Any compression around the neck (e.g., positioning devices) is removed. Anticholinergics are avoided as a decrease in HR is the physiologic response to the massive increase in mean arterial blood pressure. Giving anticholinergics will cause a tachycardia (and possibly worsen hypertension) that will mask if a true Cushing reflex is occurring. A neurologist may also choose to include corticosteroids in the treatment plan and is consulted in this regard.
- *ICP*: The target goal of maintaining as normal ICP as possible is achieved through several practical steps.
    - Avoid vomiting. This is done by choosing opioids such as methadone, and avoiding opioids such as hydromorphone or morphine, as well as alpha-2 agonists. Gastroprotectants (such as maropitant) are included in the protocol to help decrease the risk of vomiting. An increased risk of aspiration pneumonia has been associated with neurosurgery and neurologic disease in dogs [36]. This is also similar in cats, with 7% of cats with neurologic disease developing aspiration pneumonia [37]. The risk of pneumonia in patients which underwent multiple anesthetic procedures for radiation treatment was reduced by several changes in the anesthetic protocol including decreased use of anticholinergics, decreased use of pure mu opioids, changing the patient's position (both during intubation and during recovery), when the cuff of the ET tube was inflated, as well as using an aseptic technique with the equipment used for intubation [38].
    - Avoid jugular compression.
    - Avoid coughing or gagging, especially when the patient is intubated. Lidocaine is applied topically to help decrease the sensitivity of the larynx.
    - Avoid fluid overload.
    - Position patient with the head elevated (ideally 30° degrees above heart).
- *Seizures*: Seizures are detrimental in that they increase $CMRO_2$. Seizures may occur at any time during anesthesia and will go unnoticed in the adequately anesthetized patient. Diazepam or midazolam 0.5–1 mg/kg IV are used as treatment.
- *Ventilation*: Changes in $EtCO_2$ will also impact CBF. As CO_2 increases, so does CBF. Unfortunately, too low CO_2 may result in cerebral ischemia. Maintain $PaCO_2$ between 32 and 38 mmHg and $EtCO_2$ between 30 and 35 mmHg. Mechanical ventilation is often necessary for this maneuver.

2. Anesthetic protocol (Table 5.8)

Sedation is often unnecessary for IV catheterization; however, if IM premedication is needed, avoid drugs that cause vomiting and extreme respiratory depression. Methadone 0.2–0.5 mg/kg IV or IM (lower doses needed for IV dosing) with midazolam 0.1 mg/kg if needed are used for premedication. If an IV catheter is placed, a fentanyl bolus at 0.0025–0.005 mg/kg is given IV and a fentanyl CRI is continued throughout the procedure. Preoxygenate all patients prior to induction.

The induction drugs of choice are propofol or alfaxalone given slowly IV to effect, but etomidate will reduce CBF as well. However, etomidate is avoided in patients with a seizure history. Anesthesia is maintained with a propofol or alfaxalone CRI with/without lidocaine CRI. Alfaxalone CRIs are considered for patients with cardiac disease or in cats. A rougher recovery has been noted with patients recovering from alfaxalone CRIs [39,40]. If mechanical ventilation is utilized, an opioid CRI such as remifentanil or fentanyl will reduce the amount of drug necessary to maintain immobility. If it is not possible to maintain the patient solely on an opioid and propofol or alfaxalone CRI, inhalants are added but kept at less than 1 MAC. It is ideal to monitor blood gas analysis to ensure $PaCO_2$ is within optimal range (32–38 mmHg); however, it is often more practical to monitor $EtCO_2$. IBP is preferred so a Cushing reflex is detected early and reliably.

3. Key points

In cases of traumatic brain injury, complications arise both from the direct injury itself and the brain's response to this injury (swelling and inflammation, vasospasm, etc.). These cases are not anesthetized unless absolutely necessary; indeed, a large portion of things that would normally require anesthesia are performed without anesthesia due to the degree of obtundation of the patient. Mannitol is avoided in these patients as they often have a disrupted blood–brain barrier and therefore mannitol may worsen cerebral edema; hypertonic saline may be a better choice for these patients. Oxygen support is provided to these patients.

V. Renal insufficiencies

From the perspective of the anesthetist, the kidney serves to eliminate fluids and drugs after they are metabolized by the liver; however, the kidney's role physiologically is much broader and the reader is referred to other texts for a more thorough discussion on the many functions of the kidney.

Renal disease is a broad term indicating dysfunction of the kidney; the scope of this dysfunction ranges from renal insufficiency to true renal failure. Indeed, clinical signs (CS) and BW changes are slow to manifest because of the kidney's incredible reserve. By the time renal failure is diagnosed, over 75% of the kidney's functional capacity has been lost (which is when BUN and creatinine begin to elevate). Renal failure results from a number of causes, including toxins, parathyroid disease and concurrent hypercalcemia, infectious disease, sepsis, and idiopathic renal failure. Disturbingly, feline patients which have undergone anesthesia within the previous *year* have an increased risk of developing CKD [41,42], highlighting the need to perform high-quality anesthesia in our feline patient population.

Table 5.8 Intracranial disease.

Premedication (mg/kg)		Induction (mg/kg)	Maintenance (mg/kg/h)	Intraoperative analgesia (mg/kg)	Postoperative analgesia (mg/kg)
Opioid (select one) (a) Methadone 0.3 IM, 0.2 IV OR (b) Butorphanol 0.2–0.4 IV, IM OR (c) Buprenorphine 0.01–0.03 IV, IM	Other drugs: Sedative (if needed) (a) Midazolam 0.1 IM, IV AND (b) GI protection: (i) Famotidine 1 IV or SC AND (ii) Maropitant 1 IV or SC +/– (c) Mannitol 0.5–1.5 g/kg over 15–20 min	(a) Propofol 2–4 IV +/– Midazolam 0.1–0.2 IV OR (b) Alfaxalone 1–3 IV +/– Midazolam 0.1–0.2 IV	(a) Propofol CRI 12–24 OR (b) Alfaxalone CRI 4.2–9 OR (c) Isoflurane <1 MAC OR (d) Sevoflurane <1 MAC +/– CRI for reduction of inhalant requirement	(a) Intermittent bolus: (i) Methadone 0.3 IV q 4–6 h OR (ii) Fentanyl, 0.005 IV as needed OR (b) Fentanyl or remifentanil CRI 0.01–0.02	(a) Intermittent opioid bolus: (i) Methadone 0.1–0.5 IM q 4–6 h OR (ii) Buprenorphine 0.01–0.03 IM, IV OR (c) Fentanyl CRI 0.002–0.005

"AND" means that multiple choices from this column are selected, "+/–" means it is up to the anesthetist if they would like to combine multiple choices, "OR" means that the anesthetist will choose one or the other selection. For example, the postoperative analgesia column would be interpreted as including an opioid from the options either as a CRI or intermittently given.

In patients who received pantoprazole for greater than 36 hours, pantoprazole will replace famotidine.

Continuously observe patient after premedication. Because steroids may be necessary to reduce swelling, avoid NSAIDs. Preoxygenate patients. Lidocaine CRI is contraindicated in cats.

CRI, constant-rate infusion; GI, gastrointestinal; IM, intramuscular; IV, intravenous; MAC, minimum alveolar concentration; SC, subcutaneous.

Renal failure may be acute or chronic. It is unusual for the anesthetist to be presented with a patient in acute renal failure, as this condition is possibly reversible and thus anesthesia (which will worsen renal perfusion) is contraindicated in these patients. The one exception to this is the patient with a ureteral obstruction, which is discussed under anesthetic considerations.

This section will focus on chronic renal failure, a permanent and ultimately fatal disease. Clinical signs of chronic renal failure include depression, weight loss, vomiting, and PU/PD. As uremia (a systemic disease resulting from the accumulation of toxins) develops, mentation becomes dull (uremic encephalopathy) and there is an odor to the pet's breath. On PE, kidneys are palpably small and oral ulcerations are often present.

On auscultation, cardiac arrhythmias are present in some of these patients; indeed, veterinary medicine is beginning to appreciate the pathologic interplay between the two organ systems [1]. This connection between these systems occurs in both healthy patients and those with disease. In human medicine, the pathophysiology of these two systems is named the "cardiorenal system" [1]. For both systems, it is important that blood pressure is evaluated prior to inducing anesthesia. BW often reveals an anemia, azotemia (elevations in BUN and creatinine), acidosis, hypoproteinemia, hyperamylasemia, electrolyte changes (including hypokalemia, hyperphosphatemia, hypocalcemia, hypermagnesemia), and a possible hyperglycemia.

1. Anesthesia concerns/common complications

- *Acidosis*: A venous or arterial blood gas provides the patient's current pH. If pH is below 7.1, therapy is warranted. Acidosis alters many of the anesthetic drugs administered, changing their availability due to the level of ionized versus nonionized forms. In order to provide treatment, the anesthetist must first identify if the acidosis is primarily metabolic (common in chronic renal failure) or respiratory in nature; please see Chapter 3, p.72 for more information.
- *Drugs selection*: Drugs dependent on renal elimination for termination of their effect are minimized or avoided in these patients. This includes ketamine in cats (which excrete norketamine, an active metabolite, unchanged) and some muscle relaxants (e.g., vercuronium). Midazolam does not have active metabolites reliant on renal excretion and so may be a more suitable choice than diazepam. Etomidate results in hemolysis, which is difficult for the kidney, and is therefore avoided in renal failure patients unless absolutely necessary due to severe cardiac disease. Regardless of which drug is selected, it is prudent to decrease the dosage or titrate the drug to effect, as many of the anesthetic agents are protein bound and renal failure patients are often hypoproteinemic. Uremic patients, possibly due to their neurologic changes, also appear particularly sensitive to anesthetic drugs.
- *Fluid balance*: These patients often do not tolerate changes in volume well. Placement of a urinary catheter allows for measurement of urine output, which is anticipated to decrease with anesthesia. It is often helpful to hospitalize patients undergoing anesthesia for an elective procedure the night prior to anesthesia for diuresis with maintenance IV fluids.
- *Renal function*: General anesthesia is likely to result in a transient decrease in renal function via indirect mechanisms such as changes in renal perfusion and sympathetic

stimulation secondary to surgery, regardless of agent and management. Appropriate management limits the impacts and hopefully prevents permanent damage.

- *Renal perfusion*: While several drugs are utilized to support the kidney, arguably the best strategy for preventing further kidney deterioration is maintaining renal perfusion. Because the kidney's ability to autoregulate its own perfusion is lost in response to anesthesia, maintaining normal BP is of the utmost importance in these animals. Dopamine or dobutamine may help maintain renal perfusion by providing inotropic support. Mannitol and fenoldopam are also considered for patients with renal disease. Fenoldopam is a selective DA-1 receptor agonist which can help increase renal blood flow (RBF) and natriuresis and possibly provide renal protection against acute renal injury [43, 44].
- *Vascular access*: Cats with chronic renal failure (CRF) have vessels that are friable, often bleeding profusely when the tip of an IV catheter comes into contact with them. It is prudent for experienced personnel to attempt catheterizing these challenging vessels.
- *Urethral obstruction*: This is not considered a true renal insufficiency or chronic renal disease, but rather a postrenal azotemia. However, if not treated, it can lead to acute or chronic renal impairment [45]. This is an emergency that may present most commonly in male cats (and sometimes dogs). These patients must be sedated or anesthetized (after they are stabilized) in order to unblock the urethra. These patients usually present with some degree of azotemia, electrolyte abnormalities (hyperkalemia being the most life-threatening), and a firm bladder on palpation with the inability to excrete urine. Other presenting signs may include cardiovascular collapse, dehydration, hypovolemia, and a metabolic acidosis [46]. These patients require immediate intervention, especially the correction of abnormal electrolytes (see Chapter 3, "Treatment of hyperkalemia," p.79). Both surgical and medical interventions have a high morbidity and mortality rate in cats. An increase in the patient's age, a higher ASA status, preoperative bicarbonate administration, hyperkalemia, and an increase in creatinine were associated with increased anesthetic risk. The most common anesthetic complications included bradycardia, hypotension, and hypothermia [46]. These patients are not given any sedative or cardiodepressive drugs until they are stabilized and their potassium is within normal range.

2. Anesthetic protocol

Avoiding sedatives as part of the premedication is appropriate in these patients. In the patient where an opioid alone will not facilitate handling, midazolam (if the temperament is appropriate) does not rely on the kidney for elimination of active metabolites and is added. Acepromazine is considered for sedation in small doses since slight vasodilation may increase RBF in the canine patient. Induction drug selection is often based on the lesser of all evils; alfaxalone is probably the best choice, but slowly titrating the drug is key to preventing worsened kidney disease. If midazolam was not used for a premedication, it is used as part of the induction to help decrease the dose of alfaxalone needed. This helps decrease the hypotension seen with induction agent administration.

Isoflurane is the inhalant of choice for maintenance of anesthesia. The breakdown of sevoflurane results in the release of inorganic fluoride ions that are toxic in high levels. Compound

A, another renal toxic degradation product of sevoflurane (when in the presence of soda lime), is present in laboratory animals (rats). However, other species failed to demonstrate significant production. Therefore, if only sevoflurane is available, this is an acceptable alternative. Reducing the amount of inhalant necessary through the use of an opioid, such as fentanyl, CRI is warranted. Opioid epidural is controversial due to the possibility of urine retention. The author finds performing an opioid epidural is appropriate for painful abdominal procedures, including those that involve patients with questionable renal function, and inclusion of a local anesthetic in the epidural is rarely contraindicated. Epidurals greatly reduce MAC requirements of inhalant anesthetics. Alternatively, a transversus abdominis plane (TAP) block is performed without concerns for urinary retention and still provides sufficient analgesia for abdominal procedures.

The choice anesthetic for fluid maintenance is a balanced isotonic solution, which is buffered and should not worsen acidosis. Due to skeletal muscle weakness and sensitivity to respiratory depressants, the anesthetist supports ventilation. Fenoldopam may have a renal protective effect, but currently is an expensive agent for routine use [44]. Use of dopamine may help renal perfusion in our canine patients; there is controversy about the presence of dopamine receptors in the cat kidney [47], although dopamine for positive inotropic support is often utilized in this species.

VI. Respiratory/pulmonary disease

A. Upper airway disease

Upper airway disease involves the nasal passages, pharynx, and larynx. The most classic example of upper airway disease is the dog with brachycephalic airway syndrome, but laryngeal paralysis, tumors of the upper airway, foreign bodies, and swelling from trauma or snake bite all result in upper airway disease. See Chapter 4 for specific concerns for procedures involving the upper airway.

1. Anesthesia concerns/common complications

- *Minimize stress*: These patients are often maximally compensating for their airway disease; additional stress will significantly worsen the obstruction and may lead to respiratory arrest.
- *Obstruction*: An obstruction of the airway can occur preoperatively or postoperatively (Figure 5.1). In certain patients (i.e., brachycephalic patients), the animal may live their whole life with an obstruction. However, premedication and sedation worsen this obstruction. Postoperatively, while these patients are recovering, sedation contributes to their inability to maintain a patent airway. Obstruction increases work of breathing, which will eventually exhaust respiratory muscles. Hypoxemia also results from airway obstruction. Preoxygenation is always warranted in these cases, as is prolonged extubation.
- *Securing an airway*: Depending on what type of upper airway disease is present, routine intubation is a challenge for the anesthetist (i.e., in the patient with a tumor of the pharyngeal region). If this is suspected prior to anesthesia (usually based on

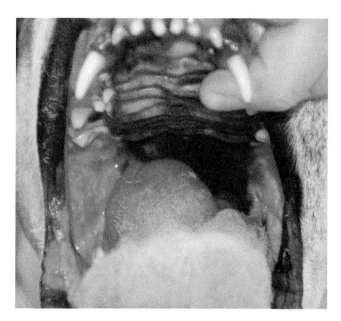

Figure 5.1   Airway obstruction. *Source:* Courtesy of Anderson da Cunha.

stridorous noises), having a variety of ET tube sizes, stylets, retrograde intubation equipment (Table 5.9) and possibly an endoscope may assist the anesthetist in obtaining a difficult airway.

Once the ET tube is placed, presence of $EtCO_2$ is used to verify accurate placement. A tracheotomy may also be indicated in certain cases.

Table 5.9   Retrograde intubation.

Materials: Clippers, scrub, sterile gloves, 18 G needle, guidewire, endotracheal (ET) tubes, laryngoscope

Technique:

1. Clip and prep an area of the skin over the trachea, approximately halfway between the mandible and thoracic inlet. Once the anesthetist is appropriately gloved, ensure the guidewire will fit through the 18 G needle. Another assistant positions the patient and opens their mouth appropriately.
2. Induce the patient.
3. Insert an 18 G needle between tracheal cartilages, directing the bevel cranially.
4. Advance the guidewire through the needle; the wire should course cranially and exit between the arytenoids.
5. Advance the wire out of the mouth and place an ET tube on the wire; the anesthetist will need enough length protruding from the mouth so the guidewire exits the connection on the ET tube.
6. Advance the ET tube down the guidewire. When the ET tube is successfully placed, remove the needle and guidewire. Place a light wrap if desired.

2. Anesthesia protocol

The objective of premedication is to provide enough sedation to minimize restraint for IV catheterization, while avoiding excessive relaxation that may predispose the patient to airway obstruction. Alpha-2 agonists are avoided for this reason (e.g., sedation is too profound). Low doses of acepromazine are beneficial to facilitate IV catheterization: however, an opioid without a sedative is a suitable option in manageable patients, provided appropriate antiemetic medication has been administered (i.e., maropitant or ondansetron). Hydromorphone may increase panting and cause vomiting so methadone is often a better choice. Gastroprotectants (such as famotidine 60 min prior to the procedure, or pantoprazole administered regularly for at least 36 h prior to the procedure) are added to reduce the risk of vomiting and the possible consequences if vomiting occurs (i.e., aspiration pneumonia). Preoxygenate the patient prior to induction for at least 5–10 min. Apply ECG and other monitoring equipment if the patient will allow prior to induction.

The goal of induction is rapid airway access (rapid-sequence induction). Proper use of a laryngoscope and having several sizes of ET tubes readily available assist with this. Inhalants (isoflurane or sevoflurane) are routinely used, although propofol or alfaxalone CRIs (forms of total intravenous anesthesia [TIVA]) are suitable in cases where extubation is anticipated. Opioid, ketamine, and lidocaine CRIs decrease MAC and provide analgesia when appropriate. These animals may require mechanical ventilation.

Recovery takes place in a quiet location where the patient is continuously monitored for respiratory distress. Respiratory distress is more likely to occur in brachycephalic breeds due to bronchospasm, laryngospasm, airway obstruction by the soft palate or swelling laryngeal tissue from traumatic intubation. Corticosteroids are beneficial in treating postoperative complications due to swelling and edema, so NSAIDs are often withheld until after the patient is completely recovered (i.e., the following day), and removed from the plan altogether if corticosteroids were included. Patients are placed in sternal recumbency with head and neck comfortably supported and extended. Leaving the ET tube in place as long as possible (*note: this may be hours*) is advised with continuous pulse oximetry monitoring. Only after the patient is strongly protesting, able to lift and support the head independently, and can swallow is the ET tube is removed. Continue to monitor SpO$_2$ and respiratory effort. Be prepared with laryngoscope, smaller ET tubes than originally used, additional induction agent and 100% oxygen to reintubate. In some cases supplemental oxygen via mask is all that is needed.

For extremely prolonged recoveries, reversal of drugs (i.e., opioids, benzodiazepines) given during the procedure is required. Usually, patience and time is the best method of recovery for brachycephalic breeds.

3. Key points

Brachycephalic patients without corrective surgery for brachycephalic syndrome (see Chapter 4, p.104) present an upper airway management challenge for the anesthetist, regardless of the reason for anesthesia (Figure 5.2).

Brachycephalic patients have a higher perianesthetic and postanesthetic risk compared to nonbrachycephalic breeds. Factors that increased brachycephalic complications perioperatively included a long duration of anesthesia, soft tissue procedures (as opposed to orthopedic or diagnostic procedures), use of ketamine plus a benzodiazepine (as opposed to propofol) for anesthetic induction, and invasive procedures [48].

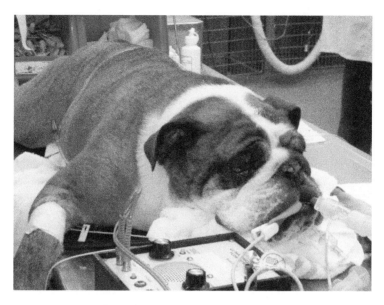

Figure 5.2   Brachycephalic patient. *Source:* Courtesy of Anderson da Cunha.

B. Lower airway disease

Lower airway disease encompasses structures below the level of the larynx (i.e., trachea, bronchi, lungs). Tracheal and large bronchial disease compromise the delivery of oxygen to the lungs; this includes diseases such as tracheal collapse or trauma, foreign bodies, and tumors. Gas exchange takes place in the lungs; diseases resulting in V/Q mismatch or diffusion barrier impairment (e.g., pulmonary edema, pneumonia, and asthma) are lower airway diseases which concern the anesthetist, as hypoxemia and increased work of breathing result. As is true for most patients with compromising disease, a complete PE and diagnostic workup are recommended. Diagnostic workup involves thoracic radiographs, pulse oximetry, and possible blood gas analysis. Depending on the severity of the disease, the patient may need supplemental oxygen even to complete a physical exam.

1. Anesthesia concerns/common complications

- *Bronchodilation*: Anticholinergics are simple bronchodilators the anesthetist already has at their disposal. Anticholinergics result in smooth muscle relaxation through muscarinic antagonism and therefore a degree of bronchodilation [49]. Additionally, bronchodilation is achieved with beta-2 agonists, which are administered either aerosolized or as an injection. Albuterol or terbutaline are two routinely used bronchodilators. Isoflurane is considered a potent bronchodilator but sevoflurane has mixed results in patients with asthma [50]. Dobutamine (and dopamine at higher doses) are beta-2 agonists that may exhibit some degree of bronchodilation, though more research needs to be performed in this area.
- *Minimize stress*: Although this is ideal for all patients, patients with respiratory disease are maximally compensating. Additional stress may result in decompensation and respiratory arrest.

- *NSAIDs*: NSAIDs are avoided (unless directly indicated) in patients with airway disease, as steroids may be necessary to address inflammation that is present or iatrogenically induced.
- *Elective procedures*: All elective procedures are postponed until the lower airway disease is managed, or resolved.
- *Mechanical ventilation (MV)*: MV reduces the work of breathing, which reduces the respiratory fatigue these animals are experiencing. When setting up the ventilator, it is important to allow for adequate duration of inspiration to maximize time for gas exchange.
- *Recovery*: The patient is recovered in a location where continuous monitoring is possible, and in a quiet, stress-free environment. Sadly, these two requirements are often mutually exclusive. Supplemental oxygen is provided and the pulse oximeter is continually monitored until the patient maintains a reading of 94–96% or greater without oxygen support.

2. Anesthesia protocol

Premedication includes an opioid and an anticholinergic. If the patient is severely stressed, acepromazine is added to the premedication to help with sedation. While it is prudent to avoid opioids that result in histamine release, opioids as a class decrease tracheal sensitivity, reduce stress, and are antitussive.

All patients with respiratory disease are continually observed after administration of premedication. If the animal is tolerant, begin preoxygenation at least 5–10 minutes prior to induction, and throughout the course of induction. If the patient is cooperative, instrumentation is placed prior to induction (i.e., ECG, NIBP, Doppler). Propofol or alfaxalone are the induction agents of choice for a smooth, controlled induction; however, there are no injectable induction drugs specifically contraindicated in these cases. The addition of a benzodiazepine will reduce the amount of induction agent necessary. Additional induction agent is kept available by the anesthetist, as are the laryngoscope and spare ET tubes of appropriate size, in case the patient requires reintubation during recovery. Maintenance of the patient on inhalants, +/− opioid CRIs, is common. These patients are not extubated unless absolutely required, and if so, are rapidly reintubated if pulse oximeter drops below 94%.

Specialized monitoring equipment includes spirometry loops for volume loop assessment. Otherwise, monitoring for these patients includes monitoring ventilation and oxygenation closely with SpO_2 and $EtCO_2$ as well as arterial blood gases if possible. Monitoring equipment is left on the patient until it is completely recovered and oxygenating well on its own.

3. Key points

Pulmonary edema in small animal patients is often secondary to cardiovascular disease (i.e., congestive heart failure [CHF]); these patients must have their cardiac disease thoroughly worked up, as well as CHF managed, prior to anesthesia for any elective procedure.

- *Diuretics*: Diuretics, such as furosemide, reduce circulating volume and therefore reduce the amount of pulmonary edema present. Although the patient may already receive diuretics as part of its maintenance therapy, additional diuretics are occasionally necessary intraoperatively due to changes in volume status subsequent to anesthesia. If the patient is already on diuretics such as furosemide, BW to assess electrolytes (particularly potassium) is warranted prior to anesthesia.

- *Fluid therapy*: Fluid therapy is kept to no more than 3 mL/kg/h during anesthesia, to prevent volume overload from worsening this disease.
- *Ventilation*: Intermittent positive pressure ventilation (IPPV) is indicated in these patients, as it might help move fluid out of the tracheobronchial tree as well as recruit compromised alveoli, ultimately increasing lung volume and the area for gas exchange. Sigh breaths (manually administered supramaximal pressures of 25–30 cmH_2O every 4–6 breaths) also assist with this recruitment. Patients in which alveolar recruitment maneuvers are used (increase tidal volume, sigh breaths, positive end-expiratory pressure [PEEP]) had an increase in PaO_2 and improved lung compliance [51].

Tracheal rupture appears more commonly in the cat than in the dog, and is often associated with previous intubations with a high-pressure, low-volume cuffed ET tube. This, coupled with negligent handling (rotating the cat without disconnecting it from the circuit, etc.), may result in a tracheal tear [52]. These patients often present with subcutaneous emphysema after an anesthetic procedure. Further diagnostics to rule out a pneumothorax or pneumomediastinum is warranted; in case of pneumothorax, a chest tap is warranted (see Table 3.10, p.71).

Often times, these patients are medically managed, but if the case is surgical, there are several management steps.

- *Intubation*: The level of the tear is important for the anesthetist, who will preferentially intubate past this tear. Unfortunately, this is sometimes difficult in cases of intrathoracic tracheal rupture. *The key lesson here is to never intubate beyond the thoracic inlet in your own patients.* When a tracheal tear knowingly occurs, communication between the anesthetist and surgeon is critical as well as quick intervention to correct the positioning of the ET tube [53].
- *Mechanical ventilation*: Leakage of air from the tracheal rupture will alter respiratory compliance, significantly increasing work of breathing and chance of hypoxemia for these patients. MV reduces the work of breathing, and offers recruitment options for compromised alveoli.

C. Space-occupying respiratory disease

Air, fluid (e.g., chyle, blood, pus, or transudates) or tissue (see Chapter 4 "Thoracotomy," p.123) accumulation affects the ability of the lungs to expand within the thoracic cavity. Thoracic masses (primary lung tumors such as carcinomas or mediastinal masses such as thymomas or lymphoma) also affect the ability of the lungs to expand, resulting in patients showing signs of respiratory distress. Underlying causes include a traumatic event (e.g., hit by car [HBC]), pathology (e.g., cancer or infectious agents) or idiopathic disease. This is also iatrogenically induced in procedures such as thoracoscopy or a thoracotomy (see Chapter 4, p.123). A thorough PE includes evaluation of respiratory effort and auscultation of the chest for lung sounds; however, in the case of acute respiratory disease, such as HBC, there may not be time to perform such an exam before respiratory arrest ensues.

Chapter 5

In the case of trauma, if an animal appears to have difficulty oxygenating (pale, often blue-gray mucous membrane color [MMC], increased RR, and obtunded mentation), a thoracic focused assessment with sonography in trauma (T-FAST) scan is performed, if an ultrasound unit is available. This information helps guide a thoracentesis ("chest tap") with a simple butterfly catheter and large-volume syringe (see Table 3.10). If a T-FAST scan is not available, it is far better to attempt to tap air off the chest and find none than to try to perform radiographs in a patient with a pneumothorax. A repeat of the T-FAST and a more thorough auscultation are performed after the tap. A small amount of air may be introduced into the thorax in the event of negative tap; while this is clinically of little consequence, radiographs may reveal this air and the primary clinician may be misled if they are not informed about a tap.

Blood work, including a CBC, chemistry, arterial blood gas (when possible), chest/abdominal radiographs, and a full thoracic ultrasound, is performed to work up the disease in stabilized patients. A CT scan is also recommended in cases requiring surgical planning. These diagnostics indicate the type of space-occupying disease present, help rule out possible causes, and quantify the degree of severity.

When air or fluid is the cause of the space-occupying disease (e.g., pneumothorax or pyothorax), thoracocentesis or chest tube placement is performed immediately following diagnosis. Supplemental oxygen is available to the patient at all times.

1. Anesthesia concerns/common complications

- *Atelectasis*: Space occupation results in lung atelectasis and subsequent hypoxemia. Monitoring at minimum includes frequent blood gas analysis (q 30–60 min), EtCO$_2$ and SpO$_2$. IBP, Doppler, and ECG are recommended.
- *Elective procedures*: As with all respiratory diseases, elective procedures are not performed until the underlying disease is addressed and stabilized.
- *Hypoventilation*: Hypoventilation, defined by an increase in CO$_2$, results from space occupation. Respiratory acidosis is evident as well. In the stable patient prior to anesthesia with gas or fluid present in the chest, a thoracocentesis is performed prior to induction of anesthesia (see Table 3.10). Because hypoventilation results from most anesthetics, it is imperative that any gas or fluid is removed from the thoracic cavity. The anesthetist must not allow residual volume to compound anesthetic hypoventilation.
- *Hypovolemia*: Hemothorax will result in hypovolemia and a decrease in effective circulating volume as well as space occupation. In cases of hemothorax, a cross-match and/or blood type is performed and blood is available for administration.
- *Mechanical ventilation*: Defining the underlying etiology in cases of pneumothorax is necessary before MV is safely started. For example, in case of trauma, MV may rupture bullae that are currently stable. Therefore, in cases of trauma, it is best to cautiously, manually assist ventilation with a second set of hands rather than place the patient on a ventilator. In other cases of space occupation, MV is safe and often necessary. EtCO$_2$ target range is 30–35 mmHg. High positive inspiratory pressure (PIP; 20–25 cmH$_2$O) provides effective ventilation due to the space-occupying disease (i.e., increased resistance). PEEP valves may need to be used in certain cases, especially those with severe atelectasis and hypoxemia.

2. Anesthesia protocol

Intravenous catheterization is usually accomplished without sedation in compromised patients. However, premedication involving an opioid with minimal respiratory effects (i.e., methadone) in combination with a sedative (i.e., midazolam or low dose of acepromazine) is administered IM to facilitate catheterization and reduce stress when necessary, or IV after catheter placement to reduce the amount of induction drug necessary and provide preemptive analgesia. A fentanyl bolus and a subsequent fentanyl CRI are typically incorporated for these patients, and may be used as premedication. The patient is continuously monitored after premedication when respiratory disease exists. All patients are preoxygenated. When possible, prior to the administration of drugs, place monitoring equipment (i.e., ECG, Doppler, NIBP) on the patient.

A smooth, rapid-sequence induction allows quick access to the airway so assisted manual ventilation is started immediately. Drug selection will depend greatly on the degree of compromise to the patient. In severely compromised patients, the premedication IV may allow intubation. If that is not sufficient, propofol or alfaxalone are the induction agents of choice, combined with benzodiazepines to reduce the dose needed.

Maintenance with inhalant anesthetics is routine. Often CRIs are necessary in critical patients to reduce MAC of inhalant and provide other benefits (i.e., analgesia). Supporting ventilation is important in these cases. If chest tubes are not present prior to induction, the anesthetist must have all equipment needed to tap the chest (see Tables 3.9, 3.10) readily available in case suspect pneumothorax occurs. In patients with pulmonary contusions or possible bullae, conservative IPPV or manual ventilation with low PIP (10–12 cmH_2O) is recommended. Chest tubes, if placed, are left in place for recovery. Check for negative pressure with the patient in multiple positions (i.e., lateral and sternal recumbency). If negative pressure is not achieved, a chest drain system, such as a Pleur-evac®, for continual suction is necessary. The arterial line is maintained (if possible) for continued blood gas analysis and IBP.

The patient remains intubated as long as possible; the anesthetist must have the supplies on hand to reintubate, if necessary. Supplemental oxygen is provided either in an oxygen cage with 40–60% O_2 or via nasal cannulas or facemask (see Chapter 3, p.69). Try to create a quiet, calm environment during recovery. Provide adequate analgesia. Continue monitoring oxygenation using pulse oximetry.

VII. Other conditions that influence anesthesia

A. Age

Patients who are young or old have different physiology from the average adult patient.

1. Anesthesia concerns/common complications

- *Anesthetic risk*: When assessing a large number of patients, studies indicate age does not increase anesthetic risk in a patient 11 years or younger [54,55]. Breed is likely to play some role in this, as a Great Dane is unlikely to ever reach 11 years of age and a toy poodle may live well beyond that.

Chapter 5

- *Inhalant requirement*: Inhalant requirement (i.e., MAC) is highest at puberty, and steadily declines after that in humans [56]. If this is true in dogs, it is likely the geriatric patient has a low MAC requirement, whereas the patient approaching puberty may require more inhalant to prevent movement.
- *Altered drug disposition*: Reduced liver and renal function, due to organ immaturity in the very young and decrease in organ mass in the aged, will result in a reduction in the amount of drug that is metabolized and excreted. In addition to drug metabolism, the liver is responsible for many other important functions, including production of proteins. Hypoalbuminemia may be present in both the young and the elderly [57]. Because many of our anesthetic drugs are highly protein bound, hypoalbuminemia results in a higher free fraction of circulating drug, leading to a greater effect than intended. These factors combine to create the possibility of relative overdosing of a patient. Reduce drug dosage and use short-acting, reversible drugs (i.e., opioids or benzodiazepines) when possible.

a. Geriatrics

These animals are characterized by those patients which have reached 75% of their expected lifespan. As patients age, physiologic changes (as listed in Table 5.10) may affect general anesthesia; additionally, concurrent systemic diseases may manifest over time. A thorough preanesthetic exam and history (with a focus on systemic disease and current medications) is evaluated and addressed prior to anesthesia. This includes CBC, chemistry, urinalysis, and ECG. Newly made diagnoses such as chronic renal disease, Cushing disease, and neoplasia

Table 5.10 Geriatric changes.

Cardiovascular system	Decreased arterial compliance Decreased myocardial compliance Decreased maximal heart rate Decreased maximal cardiac output Blunted beta-adrenergic receptor activity
Respiratory system	Reduced gas exchange efficiency Reduced vital capacity Increased work of breathing Decreased thoracic compliance Decreased lung elasticity Increased closing volume
Nervous system	Altered sympathetic activity and outflow Downregulation of beta-adrenergic receptors Decreased parasympathetic activity Decreased central neurotransmitter activity
Renal and hepatic systems	Decreased drug clearance Decreased glomerular filtration rate Decreased capability to handle water and sodium loads
Body composition	Decreased skeletal muscle mass Increased lipid fraction Decreased perfusion and organ blood flow Decreased tissue mass

have arisen from preanesthetic BW in geriatric patients [58]. This may or may not delay the anesthetic procedure to a later time based on the findings. Thoracic radiographs and abdominal ultrasound are also considered as part of a full workup.

(1) Anesthetic goals/considerations for geriatrics:

- *Hypothermia*: As animals age and become geriatric, unless they have underlying disease (i.e., hypothyroidism), they tend to lose both fat and muscle mass. This decrease in weight often leads to difficulty thermoregulating when anesthetized. Circulating warm water blankets, forced air warming units, and fluid warmers are necessary to reduce the hypothermia these patients experience under anesthesia.
- *Patient positioning*: Osteoarthritis is an insidious disease occurring in our geriatric patients that, because of its slow progression, owners may not notice in their pet. Tension on joints and pressure points on muscles during anesthesia result in considerable pain postoperatively, so care is taken to pad the patient and position them appropriately. Gentle handling when moving patients between tables (i.e., from the prep table, to the gurney, on to the OR table) is considered good practice.
- *Physiologic reserve*: Physiological parameters are important due to geriatrics' limited functional reserve of organ systems.
  - Cardiovascular: As a patient ages, in addition to decreased organ mass, there is also stiffening of cardiac and vascular tissues, which increases afterload and may manifest as hypertension. A patient's response to catecholamines decreases as well. Age-related cardiovascular structural changes (e.g., mitral and tricuspid regurgitation) occur and progress over time.
  - Neurologic: A generalized cerebral atrophy occurs as a patient ages; this manifests as an increase in anxiety and possible cognitive dysfunction. Anesthetic drugs (e.g., sedatives) may enhance these behaviors.
  - Respiratory: As thoracic wall compliance and lung capacity decrease, a decrease in functional lung capacity occurs. These patients are at increased risk for hypoxemia and hypoventilation, especially when administered anesthetics.
  - Renal: Renal function decreases over time due to a decrease in functioning glomeruli and decreased tubular function. This is present in some patients in spite of laboratory changes (see this chapter, "Renal insufficiencies," p.170); anesthesia goals for geriatric patients include supporting BP to maintain perfusion to the kidney.

(2) Anesthetic protocol for geriatrics (Table 5.11): Premedication with an opioid, without a sedative, is suitable for many geriatric patients. If a sedative is required and the patient's temperament is appropriate, a benzodiazepine such as midazolam is included in the premedication. If additional sedation is required, low-dose acepromazine is used. While multiple induction agents are suitable in the elderly, titrating the drug to effect is appropriate, as less drug is generally required. Inclusion of a benzodiazepine, if not administered as part of the premed, is appropriate to reduce the amount of induction drug. Maintenance with inhalant anesthesia is suitable, but an opioid CRI is almost always included in an effort to reduce the amount of inhalant necessary. Local blocks are performed if appropriate to reduce inhalant requirement and provide analgesia. Maintain HR within 25% of baseline rate and manage hypotension as necessary (see Chapter 3, "Hypotension," p.61).

Table 5.11 Geriatric protocol.

Premedication (mg/kg)	Induction (mg/kg)	Maintenance	Intraoperative analgesia (mg/kg/h)	Postoperative analgesia (mg/kg)
Opioid[a] (select one) (a) Methadone 0.3 IM, 0.2 IV OR (b) Hydromorphone 0.05 IM, IV OR (c) Buprenorphine 0.01–0.03 IM, IV OR (d) Butorphanol 0.1–0.4 IM, IV Sedative (if needed) (a) Midazolam 0.1 IM OR (b) Acepromazine 0.005–0.02 IM, IV +/– (c) Alfaxalone 0.5–2 IM	(a) Alfaxalone 1–3 IV +/– midazolam 0.1–0.2 IV OR (b) Propofol 2 + ketamine 2 ("ketofol") to effect +/– midazolam 0.2 OR (c) Propofol to effect +/– midazolam 0.2 IV OR (d) Etomidate 1–2 IV +/– midazolam 0.1–0.2 IV OR (e) Fentanyl 0.005–0.01 and midazolam 0.1 (canine)	(a) Sevoflurane OR (b) Isoflurane AND Opioid CRI for reduction of inhalant requirement	(a) Opioid CRI (i) Fentanyl 0.012–0.042 OR (ii) Remifentanil 0.012–0.042 +/– (b) Lidocaine CRI 1–3 (dogs only) +/– (c) Ketamine 0.6 +/– (d) Local regional block	(a) Intermittent opioid bolus (select one): (i) Methadone 0.3 IV q 4–6 h OR (ii) Hydromorphone 0.05–0.1 IV q 4–6 h OR (iii) Buprenorphine 0.01–0.03 IM, IV q 6–12 h OR (b) Fentanyl CRI 0.002–0.005 AND (c) NSAID where not contraindicated +/– (d) Liposomal encapsulated bupivacaine infiltrative block 5.3

"AND" means that multiple choices from this column are selected, "+/–" means it is up to the anesthetist if they would like to combine multiple choices, "OR" means that the anesthetist will choose one or the other selection. For example, the postoperative analgesia column would be interpreted as including an opioid from the options (either as a CRI or intermittently given), an NSAID, and optional long0acting local anesthetic block.

[a]Opioid selection is based on anticipated degree of pain the procedure will involve. Preoxygenate patient.

CRI, constant-rate infusion; IM, intramuscular; IV, intravenous.

b. Neonatal and pediatric patients

A dog or cat is considered a neonate in the first 4 weeks of life (Figure 5.3). A pediatric patient is 5–20 weeks of life. Differences impacting neonatal and pediatric anesthesia are listed in Table 5.12. Minimal laboratory tests include PCV, total proteins (TP), and BG; care is taken to minimize the blood collected from these animals, as too much blood collected results in a decrease in effective circulating volume. Patients less than 6 weeks of age are not fasted. Patients less than 8 week or 2 kg are fasted for no longer than 1–2 hours [22]. Do not withhold water.

(1) Anesthetic goals/considerations for neonatal and pediatric patients:
- *Blood–brain barrier*: The blood–brain barrier is more permeable in young patients, and therefore drugs that cross into the CNS have a more profound effect.
- *Cardiovascular*: Cardiac output is highly dependent on HR, as SV is relatively fixed in the young (reminder: CO is equal to HR × SV). Because systemic vascular resistance (SVR) is naturally low due to the immature sympathetic system in the young, it is imperative that HR is maintained at or above resting rate. This is usually achieved by the avoidance of drugs such as alpha-2 agonists and with the use of anticholinergics.
- *Hypoglycemia*: If a patient's liver has not fully matured (usually between 4 and 6 months), glycogen storage is imperfect. Young patients may experience hypoglycemia during an anesthesia procedure. Monitoring of BG every 30–60 min and supplementing with 2.5–5% dextrose in crystalloid solution, as needed, is warranted.
- *Hypothermia*: Because these patients have a very large body surface area to body mass ratio, they often become hypothermic during a procedure. Minimizing heat loss

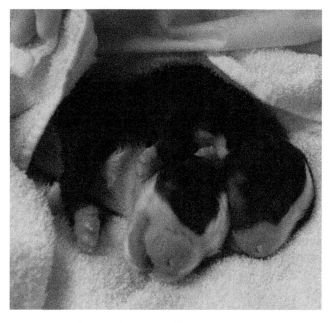

Figure 5.3   Neonate patients. *Source:* Courtesy of Anderson da Cunha.

Table 5.12   Differences impacting neonatal and pediatric anesthesia.

Cardiovascular system	Low myocardial contractility Low ventricular compliance Low cardiac reserve Cardiac output dependent on heart rate Increased cardiac index Poor vasomotor control
Respiratory system	High oxygen consumption High minute volume (higher respiratory rate) Low pulmonary reserve
Renal and hepatic system	Immature glomerular filtration rate Inability to metabolize drugs due to immature liver
Body composition	Limited thermoregulation Low body fat and muscle ratio Hypoalbuminemia Low hematocrit High total body water content Large extracellular fluid compartment Fixed and centralized circulating fluid volume
Nervous system	Increased permeability of blood–brain barrier Immature sympathetic nervous system

through the use of bubble wrap over the animal, fluid warmers, circulating warm water blankets, and forced air warming devices is warranted. Prewarming these patients is extremely important and effective at maintaining a normal body temperature. Continuous temperature checks are taken to ensure that the patient is not overheating.

- *Respiratory*: Until the bones further calcify, the thorax of these young patients remains very compliant, and at least in the first 6 weeks of life, lungs are still relatively stiff. While overall this results in normal ventilation, anesthesia disrupts this balance. Mechanical ventilation is not often warranted in these patients, but the anesthetist may need to hand ventilate the patient in periods of relatively minimal stimulation.
- *Venous access*: In small patients IV access is difficult to obtain. Interosseous (IO) catheters are useful in emergency situations. An 18 G or 20 G needle works nicely as an IO catheter but requires more advanced experience to place and may be difficult to stabilize in place.

(2) Anesthetic protocol for neonatal and pediatric patients (Table 5.13): Neonate and pediatric patients present challenges to the anesthetist due to their size. Premedication with an opioid, without a sedative, is suitable for most young patients. If a sedative is required and the patient's temperament is appropriate, a benzodiazepine such as midazolam is included in the premedication. Reversal drugs for the premed are at least calculated if not drawn up. Oxygen is administered for at least 5–10 minutes before induction occurs. Drug dose volumes are often so small that dilutions are necessary to ensure adequate dose delivery.

Table 5.13 Neonate/pediatric protocol.

Premedication (mg/kg)	Induction (mg/kg)	Maintenance	Intraoperative analgesia (mg/kg/h)	Postoperative analgesia (mg/kg)
Opioid (select one)	(a) Ketamine 5 + midazolam 0.25 IV	(a) Sevoflurane	Local blocks as necessary	(a) Intermittent opioid bolus:
(a) Methadone 0.1–0.5 IM	OR	OR		(i) Methadone 0.3 IV q 4–6 h
OR	(b) Propofol 2 + ketamine 2 ("ketofol") to effect	(b) Isoflurane		OR
(b) Hydromorphone 0.05–0.15 IM	+/– midazolam 0.2	Fluids: 10 mL/kg/h balanced crystalloid solution + 2.5–5% dextrose additive		(ii) Hydromorphone 0.05–0.1 IV q 4–6 h
OR	OR			OR
(c) Morphine 0.1–0.5 IM	(c) Alfaxalone 1–3 to effect IV			(iii) Buprenorphine 0.01–0.03 IV, IM q 6–12 h
OR	+/– midazolam 0.2			AND
(d) Buprenorphine 0.01–0.03 IM	OR			(b) NSAID where not contraindicated
OR	(d) Propofol 2–4 to effect IV			
(e) Butorphanol 0.1–0.4 IM	+/– midazolam 0.2			

Sedatives (if needed)
(a) Midazolam 0.1 IM
+/–
(b) Alfaxalone 0.5–2 IM

Glycopyrrolate is included in premedication at 0.01 mg/kg IM, or atropine at 0.02 mg/kg.
IM, intramuscular; IV, intravenous; NSAID, nonsteroidal antiinflammatory drug.

Chapter 5

Induction drugs are carefully titrated to minimize cardiopulmonary side-effects, using the smallest volume syringe suitable (e.g., 1 mL of propofol is drawn up in a 1 mL syringe, NOT a 3 mL syringe). Alfaxalone can be diluted with saline for easier titration and delivery. A ketamine and midazolam induction is also considered as ketamine may help with maintaining heart rate, causing transient tachycardia and an increase in BP. However, this may not occur with patients that have an immature nervous system. Some authors suggest that neuronal degeneration may occur when using NMDA antagonists (ketamine), although other studies show these same drugs as neuroprotective [59]. This suggests we should reserve general anesthesia only for patients where it is an absolute necessity. While use of heparinized saline for IV catheter flush is no longer routine, one should pay attention to how much flush is administered to the patient [60], especially if heparin is included. Small volumes of just several milliliters are often the patient's hourly fluid dose.

Crystalloid fluid therapy with 2.5–5% dextrose at 10 mL/kg/h due to a higher fluid requirement is recommended. Use a syringe pump or buretrol for accurate hourly delivery and monitor blood glucose every 30–60 min. With today's injectable profile of medications (i.e., alfaxalone [61]), mask induction with inhalants is rarely required but is an option when injectable options are exhausted or unavailable. The addition of an opioid is also recommended for analgesia. Eutectic mixture of lidocaine and prilocaine cream applied topically facilitates IV catheterization. Inhalant anesthesia maintenance is recommended for procedures of more than 15 min. Intubate immediately and use a nonrebreathing circuit or small pediatric circle/universal circuit system, depending on the patient's weight.

Monitoring of cardiopulmonary function is mandatory. Normal vital parameters for neonates and pediatrics can be found in Table 5.14. Shivering postoperatively increases oxygen consumption, requiring supplemental oxygen during the recovery period.

B. Body condition

An animal's body condition score is assigned as part of a routine PE. Body condition score reflects overall health and is also related to anesthetic risk. Research supports obesity being classified as a chronic inflammatory condition, which may alter other body systems including the cardiovascular, endocrine, and respiratory system [62].

1. Anesthesia concerns/common complications

- *Anesthesia risk*: In a recent study examining factors associated with increased anesthetic morbidity and mortality, it was found that underweight canine patients had an

Table 5.14   Normal vital parameters for neonates and pediatric patients.

Vital parameter	Low	High
Heart rate	140 bpm	240 bpm
Respiratory rate	24 breaths/min	40 breaths/min
Mean arterial pressure	50–60 mmHg	–
Temperature	100 °F	103 °F
Glucose	70 mg/dL	120 mg/dL

increase in anesthetic mortality compared to their normal-weight counterparts [63]. Interestingly, both under- *and* overweight felines had an increase in anesthesia-related mortality [64].

- *Drug dosage*: Because fat serves as a depot for lipid-soluble anesthetic drugs, it is appropriate to calculate a patient's anesthetic drug dosage based on ideal body weight in obese animals; emergency drugs are calculated for actual body weight.
- *Thermoregulation*: Patients at either extreme of body condition will thermoregulate differently from their normal-weight counterparts, because of changes in body surface area to mass ratios. Underweight patients will experience a worsened degree of hypothermia. Obese patients are hard to rewarm once hypothermic but are also prone to hyperthermia.

2. Anesthesia protocol

No drugs are specifically contraindicated or indicated; a protocol is selected based on the patient's temperament, signalment, comorbidities, and anticipated procedure. Temperature is diligently monitored.

3. Key points

Obesity predisposes patients to hypoventilation, which results in a respiratory acidosis and difficulty maintaining anesthetic plane due to the decreased uptake of inhalant agents. It is often necessary to mechanically ventilate obese patients.

C. Pregnancy

The heavy focus on neutering animals in veterinary medicine makes obstetric anesthesia relatively uncommon in modern practice. However, some breeds, such as the bulldog, require a cesarean section (C-section) for successful delivery. Pregnancy leads to significant physiological changes (see Chapter 4, "C-section," p.119).

1. Anesthetic goals/considerations

- *Drug disposition*: Pregnancy activates the endogenous endorphin system; in combination with the mild sedative effect of progesterone, there is a decrease in MAC requirement and an increase in pain threshold for these dogs. There is also a reduction in epidural volume. This is likely due to decreased epidural space from engorged vessels.
- *Electrolyte imbalances*: If the mother has been in labor for an extended period of time, hypocalcemia is a concern. All electrolytes, including ionized calcium, are evaluated prior to induction. Calcium is supplemented if required.
- *Fetal viability*: It is imperative the anesthetist know whether the owner prioritizes general fetus health (which may compromise the mother) or the mother's systemic health (which may compromise the fetus). While every effort is made to deliver healthy fetuses, in cases of dystocia it is difficult to prioritize both mother and neonates. If fetuses are the top priority, fetal viability is assessed before anesthesia is performed, usually by ultrasound. If the fetuses are distressed (i.e., HR is decreased), atropine will cross the placental barrier and may increase fetal HR for long enough to

Chapter 5

deliver the pups. To prevent drug-induced sedation and increase viability of the young, minimal drugs are administered to the mother; selection of drugs which are cardiovascular and respiratory friendly, reversible, and minimally metabolized is ideal. Morphine is often the opioid of choice, as it is very hydrophilic [65]. However, it is not usually given until all the fetuses have been delivered or removed from the uterus, as opioids cause respiratory depression in the puppies. Some form of analgesia must be provided for the patient experiencing an invasive abdominal procedure, such as a C-section. An epidural with lidocaine and preservative-free morphine is ideal in patients where systemic opioids are minimized initially (although they are administered after puppies are no longer present in the uterus). Liposomal encapsulated bupivacaine incorporated into the incision at closure may provide the mother with prolonged analgesia, with minimal impacts on the young.

- *Hypotension*: CO is increased during pregnancy and there is also a rise in maternal blood volume. However, inhalant anesthetics are negative inotropes and therefore still result in some degree of hypotension. This is concerning because there is no autoregulation of blood flow to the uterus, and therefore uterine BP is determined in large part by maternal BP. Maintaining BP is often challenging in that the anesthetist strives to minimize drugs administered to the patient (which ultimately go to the fetuses). Keeping the vaporizer setting low in this situation is therefore reliant on MAC decrease secondary to pregnancy. Providing analgesia to the mother therefore assists in reducing inhalant requirements, helping to maintain maternal BP and thus uterine perfusion (i.e., oxygen to the fetus). Fluid boluses and glycopyrrolate, to maintain HR, are other means of improving BP; glycopyrrolate does not cross the placental barrier. In the human medical field, ephedrine is the drug of choice for maintaining BP during pregnancy. Little work is available for the dog or cat but work in sheep suggests a beneficial effect [66]. Drugs that cause vasoconstriction are avoided (i.e., phenylephrine) as they could reduce uterine perfusion and thus oxygen to the fetus.
- *Patient positioning*: Patients in late pregnancy are not placed in dorsal recumbency if avoidable to reduce the negative impact on hypoventilation and venous return. Consider a dorsal oblique position with the cranial aspect of the mother elevated above the abdomen to assist with ventilation and venous return.
- *Physiologic changes.*
  - Cardiovascular changes include increased CO, decreased SVR, increased intravascular volume, and mild increase in HR.
  - Hepatic/renal: There is a mild and transient increase of some liver enzymes including ALP, cholesterol and LDH. Both organs positively benefit from the increase in CO secondary to pregnancy, in that blood flow increases to these organs as well.
  - RBC volume: In a possible physiologic attempt to reduce blood viscosity, there is a so-called "anemia of pregnancy." In essence, this is a dilutional anemia resulting from increasing plasma volume to a greater extent than RBC volume (although RBC volume is increased as well) [67].
  - Respiratory: Changes associated with pregnancy include increased minute ventilation, RR and V_T, and decreased functional residual capacity (FRC) from atelectasis and lung compliance. Overall, this leads to an increase in PaO_2 and a decrease

in $PaCO_2$. In spite of the increase in PaO_2, these patients, at the end of pregnancy, desaturate approximately twice as fast as nonpregnant animals, making preoxygenation critical for the mother as well as the young.

2. Anesthetic protocol

For "C-section" or dystocia procedures, see Chapter 4, p.119. Obtaining IV access is usually accomplished without sedation, as high progesterone levels present in the pregnant animal facilitate handling. If IM sedation is required to obtain IV access, opioids are preferred as they are reversible. Crystalloid fluids, ideally containing calcium (e.g., LRS), are started.

The patient is provided supplemental oxygen via oxygen mask during preoperative preparation. Preparation includes clipping the surgical area and epidural area, as well as a dirty scrub before induction (try to allow patient to remain in sternal/standing position). Induce with propofol or alfaxalone IV to effect (ideally in the OR, with the patient already on the OR table). Apgar scores were higher for the first 60 min after delivery in patients receiving alfaxalone versus propofol. However, overall survival was the same [68]. Additional work found that, in large-breed dogs, alfaxalone provided higher Apgar scores vs propofol after an elective C-section [69], so there is evidence for both drugs having utility in C-sections. If no IM sedation was used, a higher dose of induction agent (ex. propofol at 4–8 mg/kg) may be needed to intubate the patient.

It is the helpful for one anesthetist to perform the epidural while another anesthetist induces the patient, so there is a rapid transition to surgery. Inhalants are used for maintenance anesthesia. Without premedication, inhalant requirements are high. Regional anesthetic techniques will minimize inhalant requirement. Epidurals (morphine 0.1 mg/kg and bupivacaine 0.5–1 mg/kg or lidocaine 0.5 mg/kg) are administered if the anesthetist is experienced and administration is quick. If an epidural was not placed during induction or immediately following, low dose of opioids with a preference for morphine, buprenorphine or bolus of fentanyl (0.002–0.005 mg/kg) IV will provide analgesia and reduce inhalant requirement. Opioids will cross the placental barrier and may result in respiratory depression in the puppies/kittens, but these effects are reversible with naloxone. If an epidural was performed, opioids are administered once the puppies are removed from the uterus. An incisional block with bupivacaine (preferably liposomal encapsulated bupivacaine due to its 3-day duration) is also performed. Recovering the mother involves providing adequate analgesia without significant sedation; NSAIDs are often utilized.

The anesthetist focuses on the mother during anesthesia, while other people provide care for the puppies. An organized team with supplies ready will optimize neonatal outcome.

D. Shock/trauma patient

Shock refers to inadequate delivery of oxygen to tissues. There are several forms of shock: hemorrhagic, anaphylactic, cardiogenic, and septic shock, amongst others. Ultimately, shock is a life-threatening condition requiring immediate intervention, and therefore the anesthetist commonly sees the patient after stabilization. However, in some cases, such as septic shock and hemorrhagic shock, surgical intervention is necessary to address the nidus of the disease. This section will focus on these two forms of shock.

1. Anesthesia concerns/common complications

- *Decreased effective circulating volume (ECV)*: A decrease in ECV is due to either true volume loss (hemorrhagic shock) or ineffective circulating volume due to vasodilation (septic shock). In either case, improving effective circulating volume is critical. Aggressive volume resuscitation with crystalloids, colloids (hypertonic saline, hetastarch, plasma), and other blood products is indicated to improve BP and perfusion. A CRI of positive inotropic agents such as dopamine or dobutamine also improves BP and supports myocardial function. Vasopressors such as epinephrine, norepinephrine, and phenylephrine are often necessary as well (see Table 10). Norepinephrine is the vasopressor of choice for septic patients as it may help with capillary beds that may be vasodilated due to sepsis [70]. When vasopressors are used, monitoring of lactate is recommended. Physiologic doses of steroids, such as dexamethasone-SP, are also considered if other treatments have not successful in raising BP.
- *Management of underlying disease*: Shock is a symptom of a severe underlying disease, rather than a disease itself. In order to resolve, not just manage, shock, the underlying disease must be addressed.
- *Tissue hypoxemia*: Tissue hypoxemia results in lactic acidosis (see Chapter 3 "Metabolic acidosis," p.74); supplemental oxygen may not restore the delivery of oxygenation, but it will improve the concentration of oxygen available.
- *Circulatory collapse/cardiac arrest*: As multiple organ systems become starved for oxygen and appropriate perfusion, circulatory collapse and cardiac arrest become evident (see Chapter 3, p.58 and Appendix B for CPR).

2. Anesthesia protocol

Multiple large-gauge IV catheters are placed; no premedication is necessary. Preoxygenate the patient for as long as possible. IV drug administration is preferred as IM injections are compromised due to poor peripheral blood flow. Stabilization with appropriate fluid therapy is ideal before anesthesia and a normalized BP is preferred. Large volume replacement is indicated (shock doses 50–60 mL/kg in cats, 90 mL/kg in dogs). Goal-directed therapy is important with aliquots of fluids given with reevaluation of blood gases and BP. The start of norepinephrine and possibly positive inotropes is considered *before* inducing anesthesia to obtain a normal BP.

When patients require anesthesia, drugs are selected based on short duration and reversibility. This makes fentanyl, midazolam, and CRI loading doses (i.e., lidocaine in dogs) the ideal combination as a neuroleptic induction. If required, low doses of alfaxalone given very slowly to effect are useful to further facilitate intubation. Prompt placement of the ET tube (rapid-sequence induction) and inflation of the cuff are recommended to guard against aspiration. Lidocaine is used on the larynx to help smooth intubation.

Either isoflurane or sevoflurane is used to maintain anesthesia; the most important factor is using low vaporizer settings. Supplement with opioid or lidocaine CRIs to maintain a suitable depth and analgesia level; note, lidocaine CRIs are limited to the canine patient due to the cardiovascular disruption cats experience with lidocaine CRIs. The patient is kept as light as possible to optimize hemodynamic function. Monitoring is critical and preplaced to the fullest extent possible. IBP measurement and blood gas analysis are indicated, beginning preoperatively and continuing into recovery. The patient must recover where 24-h care, pressure support, and oxygen supplementation are available.

www.wiley.com/go/shelby/anesthesia2

Please go to the companion website for access to videos relating to the book

References

1. Pouchelon JL, Atkins CE, Bussadori C, et al. Cardiovascular-renal axis disorders in the domestic dog and cat: a veterinary consensus statement. J Small Anim Pract. 2015;56(9):537–52.
2. Coleman AE, Shepard MK, Schmiedt CW, Hofmeister EH, Brown SA. Effects of orally administered enalapril on blood pressure and hemodynamic response to vasopressors during isoflurane anesthesia in healthy dogs. Vet Anaesth Analg. 2016;43(5):482–94.
3. van Meel JC, Diederen W. Hemodynamic profile of the cardiotonic agent pimobendan. J Cardiovasc Pharmacol. 1989;14 Suppl 2:S1–6.
4. Boswood A, Haggstrom J, Gordon SG, et al. Effect of pimobendan in dogs with preclinical myxomatous mitral valve disease and cardiomegaly: the EPIC Study – a randomized clinical trial. J Vet Intern Med. 2016;30(6):1765–79.
5. Wagner KA, Gibbon KJ, Strom TL, Kurian JR, Trepanier LA. Adverse effects of EMLA (lidocaine/prilocaine) cream and efficacy for the placement of jugular catheters in hospitalized cats. J Feline Med Surg. 2006;8(2):141–4.
6. van Oostrom H, Knowles TG. The clinical efficacy of EMLA cream for intravenous catheter placement in client-owned dogs. Vet Anaesth Analg. 2018;45(5):604–8.
7. Crisi PE, De Santis F, Giordano MV, et al. Evaluation of eutectic lidocaine/prilocaine cream for jugular blood sampling in cats. J Feline Med Surg. 2021;23(2):185–9.
8. Muir W, Lerche P, Wiese A, Nelson L, Pasloske K, Whittem T. Cardiorespiratory and anesthetic effects of clinical and supraclinical doses of alfaxalone in dogs. Vet Anaesth Analg. 2008;35(6):451–62.
9. Pypendop BH, Barter LS, Pascoe PJ, Ranasinghe MG, Pasloske K. Hemodynamic effects of subclinical, clinical and supraclinical plasma alfaxalone concentrations in cats. Vet Anaesth Analg. 2019;46(5):597–604.
10. Rodriguez JM, Munoz-Rascon P, Navarrete-Calvo R, et al. Comparison of the cardiopulmonary parameters after induction of anaesthesia with alphaxalone or etomidate in dogs. Vet Anaesth Analg. 2012;39(4):357–65.

Chapter 5

11. Lagos-Carvajal A, Queiroz-Williams P, da Cunha A, Liu CC. Determination of midazolam dose for co-induction with alfaxalone in sedated cats. Vet Anaesth Analg. 2019;46(3):299–307.
12. Carter JE, Motsinger-Reif AA, Krug WV, Keene BW. The effect of heart disease on anesthetic complications during routine dental procedures in dogs. J Am Anim Hosp Assoc. 2017;53(4):206–13.
13. Nikolaidis LA, Trumble D, Hentosz T, et al. Catecholamines restore myocardial contractility in dilated cardiomyopathy at the expense of increased coronary blood flow and myocardial oxygen consumption (MvO2 cost of catecholamines in heart failure). Eur J Heart Fail. 2004;6(4):409–19.
14. Fox PR, Keene BW, Lamb K, et al. Long-term incidence and risk of noncardiovascular and all-cause mortality in apparently healthy cats and cats with preclinical hypertrophic cardiomyopathy. J Vet Intern Med. 2019;33(6):2572–86.
15. Wiese AJ, Barter LS, Ilkiw JE, Kittleson MD, Pypendop BH. Cardiovascular and respiratory effects of incremental doses of dopamine and phenylephrine in the management of isoflurane-induced hypotension in cats with hypertrophic cardiomyopathy. Am J Vet Res. 2012;73(6):908–16.
16. Lamont LA, Bulmer BJ, Sisson DD, Grimm KA, Tranquilli WJ. Doppler echocardiographic effects of medetomidine on dynamic left ventricular outflow tract obstruction in cats. J Am Vet Med Assoc. 2002;221(9):1276–81.
17. Davis H, Jensen T, Johnson A, et al. 2013 AAHA/AAFP fluid therapy guidelines for dogs and cats. J Am Anim Hosp Assoc. 2013;49(3):149–59.
18. Baxter AL, Ewing PH, Young GB, Ware A, Evans N, Manworren RC. EMLA application exceeding two hours improves pediatric emergency department venipuncture success. Adv Emerg Nurs J. 2013;35(1):67–75.
19. Haga HA, Bettembourg V, Lervik A. Rocuronium infusion: a higher rate is needed in diabetic than nondiabetic dogs. Vet Anaesth Analg. 2019;46(1):28–35.
20. Leece EA, Clark L. Diabetes mellitus does not affect the neuromuscular blocking action of atracurium in dogs. Vet Anaesth Analg. 2017;44(4):697–702.
21. Oliver JA, Clark L, Corletto F, Gould DJ. A comparison of anesthetic complications between diabetic and nondiabetic dogs undergoing phacoemulsification cataract surgery: a retrospective study. Vet Ophthalmol. 2010;13(4):244–50.
22. Grubb T, Sager J, Gaynor JS, et al. 2020 AAHA Anesthesia and Monitoring Guidelines for Dogs and Cats. J Am Anim Hosp Assoc. 2020;56(2):59–82.
23. Monticelli P, Dawson C, Adami C. Life-threatening hyperkalaemia in a diabetic dog undergoing anaesthesia for elective phacoemulsification. Vet Anaesth Analg. 2018;45(6):881–2.
24. Merlin T, Veres-Nyeki K. Anaesthetic management and complications of canine adrenalectomies: 41 cases (2007–2017). Acta Vet Hung. 2019;67(2):282–95.
25. Preda VA, Sen J, Karavitaki N, Grossman AB. Etomidate in the management of hypercortisolaemia in Cushing's syndrome: a review. Eur J Endocrinol. 2012;167(2):137–43.
26. Van Lanen K, Sande A. Canine hypoadrenocorticism: pathogenesis, diagnosis, and treatment. Top Compan Anim Med. 2014;29(4):88–95.
27. Stock E, Daminet S, Paepe D, et al. Evaluation of renal perfusion in hyperthyroid cats before and after radioiodine treatment. J Vet Intern Med. 2017;31(6):1658–63.
28. Robertson SA, Gogolski SM, Pascoe P, Shafford HL, Sager J, Griffenhagen GM. AAFP Feline Anesthesia Guidelines. J Feline Med Surg. 2018;20(7):602–34.
29. Wagner K, Gibbon K, Strom T, Kurian J, Trepanier L. Adverse effects of EMLA (lidocaine/prilocaine) cream and efficacy for the placement of jugular catheters in hospitalized cats. J Feline Med Surg. 2006;8(2):141–4.
30. Sturtevant F, Drill V. Tranquilizing drugs and morphine-mania in cats. Nature. 1957;179(4572):1253.
31. Brosnan R, Pypendop B, Siao K, Stanley S. Effects of remifentanil on measures of anesthetic immobility and analgesia in cats. Am J Vet Res. 2009;70(9):1065–71.

32. Yuan Z, Liu J, Liang X, Lin D. Serum biochemical indicators of hepatobiliary function in dogs following prolonged anaesthesia with sevoflurane or isoflurane. Vet Anaesth Analg. 2012;39(3):296–300.

33. Ambrisko TD, Hikasa Y. Neurohormonal and metabolic effects of medetomidine compared with xylazine in beagle dogs. Can J Vet Res. 2002;66(1):42–9.

34. Warne LN, Beths T, Whittem T, Carter JE, Bauquier SH. A review of the pharmacology and clinical application of alfaxalone in cats. Vet J. 2015;203(2):141–8.

35. Atkins JH, Smith DS. A review of perioperative glucose control in the neurosurgical population. J Diabetes Sci Technol. 2009;3(6):1352–64.

36. Ovbey DH, Wilson DV, Bednarski RM, et al. Prevalence and risk factors for canine post-anesthetic aspiration pneumonia (1999–2009): a multicenter study. Vet Anaesth Analg. 2014;41(2):127–36.

37. Levy N, Ballegeer E, Koenigshof A. Clinical and radiographic findings in cats with aspiration pneumonia: retrospective evaluation of 28 cases. J Small Anim Pract. 2019;60(6):356–60.

38. Baetge C, Cummings KJ, Deveau M. Reduced risk of pneumonia after changes in anesthetic procedures for dogs receiving repeated anesthesia for radiation treatment. Vet Radiol Ultrasound. 2019;60(2):241–5.

39. Dehuisser V, Bosmans T, Kitshoff A, Duchateau L, de Rooster H, Polis I. Cardiovascular effects, induction and recovery characteristics and alfaxalone dose assessment in alfaxalone versus alfaxalone-fentanyl total intravenous anaesthesia in dogs. Vet Anaesth Analg. 2017;44(6):1276–86.

40. Dehuisser V, Bosmans T, Devreese M, et al. Alfaxalone total intravenous anaesthesia in dogs: pharmacokinetics, cardiovascular data and recovery characteristics. Vet Anaesth Analg. 2019;46(5):605–12.

41. Trevejo RT, Lefebvre SL, Yang M, Rhoads C, Goldstein G, Lund EM. Survival analysis to evaluate associations between periodontal disease and the risk of development of chronic azotemic kidney disease in cats evaluated at primary care veterinary hospitals. J Am Vet Med Assoc. 2018;252(6):710–20.

42. Greene JP, Lefebvre SL, Wang M, Yang M, Lund EM, Polzin DJ. Risk factors associated with the development of chronic kidney disease in cats evaluated at primary care veterinary hospitals. J Am Vet Med Assoc. 2014;244(3):320–7.

43. Mathur VS, Swan SK, Lambrecht LJ, et al. The effects of fenoldopam, a selective dopamine receptor agonist, on systemic and renal hemodynamics in normotensive subjects. Crit Care Med. 1999;27(9):1832–7.

44. Halpenny M, Markos F, Snow HM, et al. Effects of prophylactic fenoldopam infusion on renal blood flow and renal tubular function during acute hypovolemia in anesthetized dogs. Crit Care Med. 2001;29(4):855–60.

45. Kyles AE, Hardie EM, Wooden BG, et al. Management and outcome of cats with ureteral calculi: 153 cases (1984–2002). J Am Vet Med Assoc. 2005;226(6):937–44.

46. Garcia de Carellan Mateo A, Brodbelt D, Kulendra N, Alibhai H. Retrospective study of the perioperative management and complications of ureteral obstruction in 37 cats. Vet Anaesth Analg. 2015;42(6):570–9.

47. Flournoy W, Wohl J, Albrecht-Schmitt T, Schwartz D. Pharmacologic identification of putative D1 dopamine receptors in feline kidneys. J Vet Pharmacol Ther. 2003;26(4):283–90.

48. Gruenheid M, Aarnes TK, McLoughlin MA, et al. Risk of anesthesia-related complications in brachycephalic dogs. J Am Vet Med Assoc. 2018;253(3):301–6.

49. Cazzola M, Page CP, Calzetta L, Matera MG. Pharmacology and therapeutics of bronchodilators. Pharmacol Rev. 2012;64(3):450–504.

50. Burburan SM, Xisto DG, Rocco PR. Anaesthetic management in asthma. Minerva Anestesiol. 2007;73(6):357–65.

Chapter 5

51. Hartland BL, Newell TJ, Damico N. Alveolar recruitment maneuvers under general anesthesia: a systematic review of the literature. Respir Care. 2015;60(4):609–20.
52. Mitchell SL, McCarthy R, Rudloff E, Pernell RT. Tracheal rupture associated with intubation in cats: 20 cases (1996–1998). J Am Vet Med Assoc. 2000;216(10):1592–5.
53. Morath U, Gendron K, Reves NV, Adami C. Perioperative and anesthetic management of complete tracheal rupture in one dog and one cat. J Am Anim Hosp Assoc. 2015;51(1):36–42.
54. Brodbelt D, Pfeiffer D, Young L, Wood J. Results of the confidential enquiry into perioperative small animal fatalities regarding risk factors for anesthetic-related death in dogs. J Am Vet Med Assoc. 2008;233(7):1096–104.
55. Brodbelt D, Pfeiffer D, Young L, Wood J. Risk factors for anaesthetic-related death in cats: results from the confidential enquiry into perioperative small animal fatalities (CEPSAF). Br J Anaesth. 2007;99(5):617–23.
56. Eger EI. Age, minimum alveolar anesthetic concentration, and minimum alveolar anesthetic concentration-awake. Anesth Analg. 2001;93(4):947–53.
57. Brock F, Bettinelli LA, Dobner T, Stobbe JC, Pomatti G, Telles CT. Prevalence of hypoalbuminemia and nutritional issues in hospitalized elders. Rev Lat Am Enfermagem. 2016;24:e2736.
58. Joubert KE. Pre-anaesthetic screening of geriatric dogs. J S Afr Vet Assoc. 2007;78(1):31–5.
59. Yan J, Jiang H. Dual effects of ketamine: neurotoxicity versus neuroprotection in anesthesia for the developing brain. J Neurosurg Anesthesiol. 2014;26(2):155–60.
60. Ueda Y, Odunayo A, Mann FA. Comparison of heparinized saline and 0.9% sodium chloride for maintaining peripheral intravenous catheter patency in dogs. J Vet Emerg Crit Care. 2013;23(5):517–22.
61. de Carellan Mateo AG, Alvarez ER, Ros C. Comparison of the efficacy of 2 sedative protocols in pediatric dogs undergoing brainstem auditory-evoked response testing. Can Vet J. 2020;61(11):1175–80.
62. Love L, Cline MG. Perioperative physiology and pharmacology in the obese small animal patient. Vet Anaesth Analg. 2015;42(2):119–32.
63. Brodbelt DC, Pfeiffer DU, Young LE, Wood JL. Results of the confidential enquiry into perioperative small animal fatalities regarding risk factors for anesthetic-related death in dogs. J Am Vet Med Assoc. 2008;233(7):1096–104.
64. Brodbelt DC, Pfeiffer DU, Young LE, Wood JL. Risk factors for anaesthetic-related death in cats: results from the confidential enquiry into perioperative small animal fatalities (CEPSAF). Br J Anaesth. 2007;99(5):617–23.
65. Vilar JM, Batista M, Perez R, et al. Comparison of 3 anesthetic protocols for the elective cesarean-section in the dog: effects on the bitch and the newborn puppies. Anim Reprod Sci. 2018;190:53–62.
66. Erkinaro T, Mäkikallio K, Acharya G, et al. Divergent effects of ephedrine and phenylephrine on cardiovascular hemodynamics of near-term fetal sheep exposed to hypoxemia and maternal hypotension. Acta Anaesthesiol Scand. 2007;51(7):922–8.
67. Nivy R, Mazaki-Tovi M, Aroch I, Tal S. Time course of serum cobalamin, folate, and total iron binding capacity concentrations in pregnant bitches and association with hematological variables and survival. J Vet Intern Med. 2019;33(4):1627–34.
68. Doebeli A, Michel E, Bettschart R, Hartnack S, Reichler IM. Apgar score after induction of anesthesia for canine cesarean section with alfaxalone versus propofol. Theriogenology. 2013;80(8):850–4.
69. Melandri M, Alonge S, Peric T, Bolis B, Veronesi MC. Effects of alfaxalone or propofol on giant-breed dog neonates viability during elective caesarean sections. Animals. 2019;9(11):962.
70. Mazzaferro E, Wagner AE. Hypotension during anesthesia in dogs and cats: recognition, causes, and treatment. Compendium 2001;23:728–37.

Chapter 5

Chapter 6

Anesthesia and analgesia in the exotic patient

Amanda M. Shelby and Carolyn M. McKune

Exotic pet owners seek veterinary care when they observe an abnormal behavior in their pets. Often, these animals are not truly domesticated, which may take up to six generations. Therefore, handling for medical procedures often requires anesthesia. The infrequency and inexperience of the veterinary staff with exotic species may contribute to the increase in morbidity and mortality seen in these species [1]. Previous chapters have outlined the preanesthetic recommendations that apply to all species in regard to anesthesia. This chapter is designed to give information regarding differences and suggestions for performing anesthesia and providing analgesia. The reader is referred to additional sources (see end of chapter) for a more extensive review on specific species.

I. Common exotic mammals

Metabolic rate scales allometrically by species; that is, the smaller the species, the greater its metabolic rate. This will influence drug metabolism. Other parameters influenced by a change in metabolic rate include body temperature and oxygen consumption (Table 6.1).

A. Ferrets

1. Characteristics

- Ferrets are often treated like cats in regard to drug dosing and intubation.
- If not descented, ferrets may spray scent glands when stressed or threatened.
- Ferrets have thick skin, requiring confidence when administering a SC injection.
- Ferrets produce copious respiratory secretions, making inclusion of an anticholinergic a suitable choice for anesthesia when not contraindicated.

2. Anesthetic considerations

- *Handling and restraint*: If required, squeeze cages might be helpful in restraining the unfriendly ferret. They have very sharp teeth and inflict severe bites. For the tame ferret,

Small Animal Anesthesia Techniques, Second Edition. Edited by Amanda M. Shelby and Carolyn M. McKune.
© 2023 John Wiley & Sons, Inc. Published 2023 by John Wiley & Sons, Inc.
Companion website: www.wiley.com/go/shelby/anesthesia2

Table 6.1 Exotic small mammal vital normal ranges

Species	Adult weights (kg)	HR[a] (bpm)	RR[a] (breaths/min)	Temperature (°F)	Fasting recommendation
Ferret	0.7–3.0	200–275	30–35	100–104	6–8 h (unless the patient has a suspected insulinoma)
Hedgehog	0.3–1.2	200–280	25–50	95–99	Not recommended
Pot-bellied pig	40–90	70–120	25–35	101–104	12–24 h
Rabbits	1–6	130–325	30–60	99–103	2–4 h for food only
Rats	0.25–0.5	250–450	70–130	99–100	Not recommended
Mice	0.02–0.04	350–800	60–200	98–100.5	Not recommended
Hamster	0.085–0.15	250–500	40–140	101–103	Not recommended
Gerbil	0.05–0.10	250–500	90–150	99–102	Not recommended
Guinea pig	0.7–1.2	230–380	50–100	101–103	2–4 h
Chinchilla	0.4–0.6	200–350	45–80	102–103	Not recommended

Sources: See Further reading.
[a]Respiratory rates and heart rates may be lower during anesthesia.
bpm, beats per minute; RR, respiratory rate.

scruffing the nape of the neck and supporting the lower half of the body with the other hand works well for restraint (Figure 6.1).

- *Premedication*: Agents that sedate and provide preemptive analgesia help to facilitate catheter placement and reduce induction and maintenance drug requirements; a variety of agents are suitable in the healthy ferret (Table 6.2). The hindlimb muscles are common locations for IM injections; sadly, for these little creatures, the patient is often sore on the limb afterwards and may limp where the injection was given, espe-

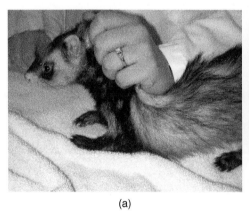
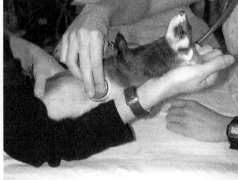

(a)   (b)

Figure 6.1 Scruff restraint technique of a ferret. *Source*: Courtesy of Jody Nugent-Deal.

Table 6.2 Anesthetic protocol for ferrets.

	ASA 1 or 2	ASA 3, 4, or 5

Premedication	1. Opioid (select most appropriate) [50]:
	  (a) Hydromorphone 0.1 mg/kg IM or SC
	  (b) Butorphanol 0.4 mg/kg IM or SC
	  (c) Buprenorphine 0.02 mg/kg IM or SC
	2. +/– Glycopyrrolate 0.01 mg/kg IM or SC
	3. Sedative option (select most appropriate):
	  (a) Acepromazine 0.01–0.03 mg/kg IM or SC or
	  (b) Dexmedetomidine 0.003–0.01 mg/kg IM or SC
		1. Opioid (select most appropriate):
		  (a) Hydromorphone 0.1 mg/kg IM or SC
		  (b) Methadone 0.1–0.5 mg/kg IM
		  (c) Buprenorphine 0.02 mg/kg IM or SC
		2. Sedative option:
		  (a) Midazolam 1 mg/kg SC or IM

Induction	Select one: (a) Alfaxalone 3–5 mg/kg IM or if IV available, 1–3 mg/kg to effect following premed (b) Propofol 4–6 mg/kg IV (c) Ketamine 10 mg/kg + midazolam 1 mg/kg IM or IV (d) Tiletamine-zolazepam 1.5–3 mg/kg IV	Select one: (a) Alfaxalone 1–3 mg/kg IV +/– midazolam 1 mg/kg IV (b) Propofol 2–4 mg/ kg +/–midazolam 1 mg/kg IV (c) Fentanyl 0.02 mg/ kg + diazepam 1–2 mg/kg IV
Maintenance, Intraoperative analgesia	Gas inhalant with continued appropriate analgesia (a) Local anesthetic block (b) Additional opioid	Gas inhalant with: (a) Local anesthetic block (b) Fentanyl CRI 0.012–0.042 mg/kg/h

Postoperative analgesic	(a) NSAID [51,52]:
	  i. Carprofen 4 mg/kg SC SID or
	  ii. Meloxicam 0.2 mg/kg SC SID
	AND
	(b) Opioid boluses
		(a) Opioid boluses

IM, intramuscular; IV, intravenous; SC, subcutaneous; SID, semel in die (once a day).

cially if large volumes are given. IV access includes the cephalic, jugular, and saphenous veins (Figure 6.2). It is helpful to nick the skin prior to attempting catheterization. Alfaxalone (5 mg/kg) has proven useful, in combination with butorphanol (0.2 mg/kg), with mild transient cardiorespiratory derangements [2].

- *Induction*: If IV access is not achieved under premedication, mask or box inductions with isoflurane or sevoflurane is the most common approach. If IV access is available, IV induction agents are administered (see Table 6.2).
- *Intubation*: Intubation is achieved with small endotracheal (ET) tubes similar to intubating a cat. The patient is placed in sternal recumbency with the head and neck hyperextended by an assistant. Some individuals suggest extending the head toward the person intubating while keeping the body straight. Lidocaine is used on the arytenoids to minimize laryngeal spasms. The tongue is pulled gently out of the mouth and a laryngeal scope is used for visualization. Small ET tubes ranging from 2.0 to 3.5 mm internal diameter (ID) (cuffed or noncuffed) are commonly used. Placement of the ET tube is verified by auscultation of lungs bilaterally for respiratory noises on inspiration or with the use of a capnograph.

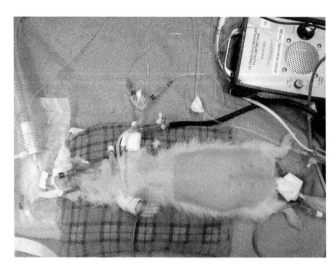

Figure 6.2   Ferret under anesthesia, intubated. Endotracheal tube secured with suture. Monitoring devices in place with intravenous catheterization and arterial catheter in place. *Source*: Courtesy of Jody Nugent-Deal.

- *Maintenance*: All the modern inhalants are commonly used. Total intravenous anesthesia (TIVA) is also used if IV access is available.
- *Monitoring during anesthesia (see Figure 6.2)*: An ECG and Doppler are recommended. Blood pressure (BP) is obtained with a cuff and sphygmomanometer. Pulse oximetry is obtained by placing a probe over a foot. Anesthetic depth is monitored similarly to the average small animal patient. Jaw tone, eye position, and palpebral reflex are indicators of depth. Additionally, changes in respiratory rate (RR) and BP may indicate changes in anesthetic depth.
- *Recovery*: Keep the patient warm in recovery and continue to monitor vital signs. Because ferrets have such a variety of endocrinologic disease requiring anesthesia and surgery, tailor each recovery to the specific patient. Additional analgesia is administered.

3. Common complications

- *Intraoperative hypothermia*: Forced air warming units, circulating hot water blankets, and/or companion animal warming units are helpful to maintain body temperature.
- *Hypoglycemia*: Hypoglycemia occurs due to high metabolic rates; 2.5% dextrose is added to the anesthetic maintenance fluids to correct this. The ferret with an insulinoma is a particular challenge in this regard, as it is a balance between providing enough dextrose without triggering release of an insulin surge.

B. Hedgehogs

1. Characteristics

- Some species of hedgehog (European) hibernate when conditions are extreme (unlikely in the household pet).

- Nocturnal (i.e., normally inactive during the day and active in the evening).
- Spines cover the dorsal aspect of body.

2. Anesthetic considerations

- *Handling and restraint*: Handling and restraint are difficult, especially if the patient rolls into a ball. Some will unroll if rump spines are stroked. Leather gloves are recommended. While these animals rarely bite, they are reclusive by nature and often resent handling, regardless of the degree of socialization.
- *Premedication*: Often patients are masked or boxed down without the use of injectable premedications. However, SC injections are given with the assistance of forceps to grasp a fold of skin between the spines over the flank of the patient. IM injections are given in the thigh. Soreness results if large volumes are administered IM (Table 6.3).
- *IV access*: Catheters are placed in the jugular or saphenous vein. Intraosseous (IO) catheters are placed in the proximal femur.
- *Induction*: Attempts at intubation are made using a 1–1.5 mm ID ET tube; however, care is taken to avoid trauma to the larynx which causes swelling, bleeding, and airway obstruction. Supraglottic airway devices designed for rabbits have shown promise in reducing trauma to the airway while providing quick access and adequate ventilation as well as delivery of inhalant anesthetics to produce maintenance anesthesia (see Table 6.3).

Table 6.3   Anesthetic protocol for hedgehog.

	ASA 1 or 2	ASA 3, 4 or 5
Premedication	1. Opioid (select most appropriate): (a) Hydromorphone 0.1 mg/kg SC (b) Butorphanol 0.4 mg/kg SC (c) Buprenorphine [53] 0.01–0.05 mg/kg SC 2. Sedative (select most appropriate): (a) Midazolam 1 mg/kg (b) Dexmedetomidine 0.03–0.05 mg/kg SC or IM 3. Injectable anesthetic [54,55]: (a) Ketamine 10–30 mg/kg SC or IM (b) Alfaxalone 2–3 mg/kg SC or IM	1. Opioid (select most appropriate): (a) Hydromorphone 0.1 mg/kg SC (b) Methadone 0.3–0.5 mg/kg SC (c) Buprenorphine 0.02–0.05 mg/kg SC 2. Sedative: (a) Midazolam 1 mg/kg SC or IM 3. Injectable anesthetic: (a) Alfaxalone 2–3 mg/kg SC or IM
Induction, Maintenance, Intraoperative analgesia	Mask/chamber with gas inhalant	Mask/chamber with gas inhalant with: (a) Fentanyl CRI 0.012–0.042 mg/kg/h if IV or IO access available
Postoperative analgesic	(a) Meloxicam 0.2 mg/kg SC SID and/or (b) Buprenorphine 0.02 mg/kg SC	(a) Buprenorphine 0.02 mg/kg SC

IM, intramuscular; IO, intraosseous; IV, intravenous; SC, subcutaneous; SID, semel in die (once a day).

- *Maintenance*: Mask induction and maintenance with an inhalant anesthetic is common clinical practice.
- *Monitoring*: A Doppler is vital for monitoring the heart rate (HR) in these animals. Pulse oximetry is useful if the probe is placed on a foot in the unrolled hedgehog. ECG provides information on HR, but most monitors are only capable of displaying up to 250 bpm. RR is monitored by watching chest excursions.
- *Recovery*: Recover hedgehogs in a quiet, nonstimulating environment. Keep the patient warm in recovery and continue to monitor vital signs. Additional analgesia is administered as warranted.

3. Common complications

Complications are typically a result of the hedgehog's high metabolic rate and the anesthetist's underestimation of the patient's requirements.

- *Hypoglycemia*: Do not fast and administer 2.5% dextrose in fluids for extended procedures.
- *Hypothermia*: Hypothermia due to small body size, use of nonrebreathing (NRB) circuits, and decreased metabolism is common. Esophageal temperature probes for continuous monitoring and forced air warming units are helpful.

C. Pot-bellied pigs (PBPs)

1. Characteristics

- PBPs have small tracheas compared to body weight; additionally, there is a sigmoid curvature to the airway and a ventral diverticulum anteroventral to the arytenoid fold preventing a straightforward intubation.
- PBPs have a high fat to muscle ratio (anatomically present as a thick layer of subcutaneous fat), making the effect of drug injections less predictable and intra-fat (rather than IM) injection more likely.
- Pigs are cannibalistic.
- Twelve- to 24-hour fasting of adult pigs is recommended.
- Difficulty accessing veins means most anesthetic plans are developed with minimal biochemical and hematologic information.

2. Anesthesia considerations

- *Handling and restraint*: Pigs are difficult to restrain due to their shape and size. Often chemical restraint is used to avoid stress. Large pigs are controlled with a board or cage door front "squeezed" against a wall while an IM injection is given, or snared just behind the canine teeth. Small pigs are manually restrained (Figure 6.3).
- *Premedication*: Behind the ear is the most common site for IM injections. In young PBPs, there is less fat in this area so the effectiveness of the drugs is more predictable. The epaxial muscles are avoided because of the large layer of back fat and the tradition of avoiding this muscle group in pigs for market. Injection in the semimembranosus and semitendinosus muscles with a 3.5 inch stylet from a catheter is a possible

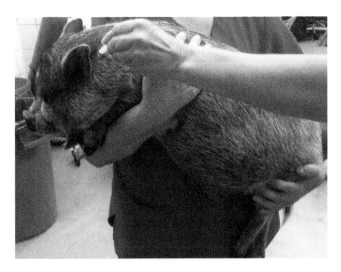

Figure 6.3   PBP restraint and IM injection behind the ear. *Source*: Courtesy of Amanda M. Shelby.

alternative. Intranasal midazolam 0.5 mg/kg may quiet the pig to a degree and facilitate limited handling. In general, pigs are less susceptible to the sedative effects of
opioids, phenothiazines, and alpha-2 agonists. Butyrophenones, such as azaperone
(2.5 mg/kg IM), are often used for sedation in noncompanion pigs and are potentially
useful in the PBP. Alfaxalone has proved useful in commercial swine, with or without
the use of an alpha-2 agonist, and may be useful in the PBP [3,4] (Table 6.4).
*   *IV access*: Veins are difficult to access. The easiest vessels for catheterization include
    the medial and lateral auricular veins (Figure 6.4) and lateral saphenous veins, which
    are typically catheterized following induction. Cephalic veins are occasionally
    attempted, but venipuncture in this area is performed blindly, as these vessels are dif-
    ficult to palpate and visualize.
*   *Induction*: If IV access is obtained following premedication, injectable agents are
    given to facilitate intubation. Otherwise, mask induction with isoflurane or sevoflu-
    rane is most common until the patient is intubated (see Table 6.4).
*   *Intubation*: Intubation in pigs is a challenge for a number of reasons. The mouth does
    not open widely, and the larynx is at an angle to the trachea. Pigs have a pharyngeal
    diverticulum, as well as a tracheal bronchus; inaccurate placement of the tube in
    either of these areas results in trauma, swelling, or bleeding. Stylets or ET tubes inad-
    vertently placed in the tracheal bronchus cause pneumomediastinum and inadequate
    ventilation. Cuffed ET tubes of various sizes (smaller than for an equivalent-sized
    canine patient) are used; for an average 60 kg PBP, an 8–9 mm ID ET tube is used.
    Place the patient in sternal recumbency. Gauze or dog leashes facilitate visualization,
    when placed behind the canine teeth and used to open the mouth. A long blade laryn-
    goscope is helpful in visualizing the larynx by placing the blade at the base of the
    tongue and pressing down to displace the epiglottis. Lidocaine is placed on the aryt-
    enoids to minimize laryngeal spasms, which readily occur. Introduce a long, thin
    stylet (crafted from small French urinary catheters connected together with tape or
    glue, approximately three times the length of the ET tube) into the trachea to assist

Table 6.4　Anesthetic and analgesic drugs for pot-bellied pig.

	ASA 1 or 2	ASA 3, 4 or 5
Premedication	Opioid (select most appropriate): (a) Hydromorphone 0.1 mg/kg IM (b) Methadone 0.1–0.5 mg/kg IM (c) Buprenorphine 0.03 mg/kg IM (d) Butorphanol 0.2–0.4 mg/kg IM Sedative (select one): (a) Dexmedetomidine 5–10 µg/kg IM (b) Midazolam 0.2–0.5 mg/kg IM, intranasal Injectable anesthetic (select one): (a) Telazol 2–3 mg/kg IM (b) Ketamine 7.5–10 mg/kg IM (c) Alfaxalone 3–5 mg/kg IM	Opioid (select most appropriate): (a) Hydromorphone 0.1 mg/kg IM (b) Methadone 0.1–0.5 mg/kg IM (c) Buprenorphine 0.03 mg/kg IM (d) Butorphanol 0.2–0.4 mg/kg IM Sedative (select one): (a) Midazolam 0.2–0.5 mg/kg IM, intranasal Injectable anesthetic: (a) Alfaxalone 3–5 mg/kg IM
Induction	Mask until intubation	Alfaxalone 1–2 mg/kg IV to effect
Maintenance	Gas inhalant	Gas inhalant
Intraoperative analgesia	(a) Local blocks where possible (b) Opioid bolus or CRI	(a) Local blocks where possible (b) Opioid bolus or CRI
Postoperative analgesia	Flunixin 0.5–1.0 mg/kg SC or IV and Opioid (select most appropriate): (a) Buprenorphine 0.01–0.05 mg/kg IV or IM q 8 h (b) Methadone 0.1–0.5 mg/kg IM q 4–6 h	Opioid (select most appropriate): (a) Fentanyl patch 50–100 µg/h (b) Buprenorphine 0.01–0.05 mg/kg IV or IM q 8 h (c) Methadone 0.1–0.5 mg/kg IM q 4–6 h

CRI, constant-rate infusion; IM, intramuscular; IV, intravenous.

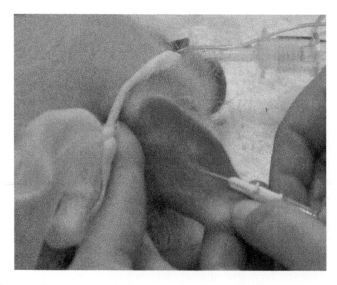

Figure 6.4　IV access in the ear of a PBP. *Source*: Courtesy of Patricia Queiroz-Williams.

intubation. If no resistance is encountered, an ET tube is passed over the stylet and gently rotated 180° once it passes beyond the larynx. Laryngeal mask airways are used with success in pigs and may reduce the potential for airway trauma. Auscultation and capnography confirm appropriate placement. If resistance is encountered, rotating the stylet gently while advancing it forward may help; however, significant resistance warrants backing out of the trachea and trying again. Intubation attempts are minimized to prevent trauma.

- *Maintenance*: Inhalant anesthetics are most commonly used following intubation. IM injectable drugs, in combination with local blocks, facilitate adequate sedation and immobilization for minor procedures like castration, hoof trim, or tusk filing.
- *Monitoring anesthetic depth*: Palpebral reflex and jaw tone will give an indication of the depth of anesthesia. PBPs have small eyes, making ocular signs of anesthetic depth difficult to obtain. Vital parameters may also indicate changes in depth. An ECG and Doppler are recommended for monitoring the HR and rhythm. Pigs have little excess skin, so using sticky pads to monitor ECG is preferable to ECG clips. The Doppler crystal, BP cuff, and a sphygmomanometer give an indication of trends. The Doppler is often placed distal to the accessory claw, with the cuff below the carpus on the forelimb, or on the hindlimb above the hock. Invasive blood pressure (IBP) is obtained from placing a catheter in the artery of the ear or dorsal pedal artery. It is also useful to monitor RR and $EtCO_2$. Pulse oximetry is obtained by placing a pulse oximeter probe on the tongue. Temperature is continuously monitored during anesthesia and into recovery.
- *Recovery*: Pigs are recovered without herd mates and only returned to the herd once completely recovered. They are placed in sternal recumbency for recovery, if possible. Pigs may obstruct post extubation due to laryngeal swelling. It is important to ensure they are capable of swallowing and adequate independent ventilation is present prior to extubation. Nonsteroidal antiinflammatory drugs (NSAIDs) are used, if not otherwise contraindicated, to minimize any airway swelling. Pigs experience postanesthetic sleep; although they appear conscious enough to extubate, once extubated, they sleep quite heavily, which contributes to the possibility of postextubation obstruction. Temperature is monitored during and following recovery. Additional analgesic drugs are administered as warranted.

3. Common complications

- Airway obstruction at extubation is possible. The anesthetist must be ready with additional induction agent (IV catheter remains in place until the patient is fully recovered) and a size smaller ET tube to intubate the patient if an obstruction occurs.
- Hypoventilation, if not from excessive anesthetic depth, is often addressed with mechanical ventilation (MV).
- Hypothermia (especially in in small pigs) occurs intraoperatively and postoperatively. Use of circulating warm water blankets and forced air warming units reduces the degree of hypothermia.
- Dysphoric or rough recoveries are possible, especially in stimulating environments and with inadequate analgesia and sedation.

Chapter 6

D. Rabbits

1. Characteristics

- Rabbits are obligate nasal breathers (require patency of the nares and nasopharynx).
- It is common for rabbits to have inconspicuous respiratory infections; as a prey species, they are remarkably good at hiding signs of illness and pain.
- Rabbits do not regurgitate or vomit.
- Some rabbits have circulating levels of atropinesterase [5], which makes the use of atropine less effective. Glycopyrrolate is a suitable alternative.
- Rabbits have extremely powerful kick strength; their kick is strong enough to fracture their own spine if they are not properly restrained.
- Because rabbits are a prey species, they are remarkably efficient at hiding signs of pain and distress. Preemptive and appropriate postoperative analgesia is administered to these animals without expecting a behavioral qualification of pain.

2. Anesthesia considerations

- *Handling and restraint (Figure 6.5)*: Rabbits are very easily stressed; it is wise to handle them in a quiet, dim environment to minimize stress until they are anesthetized.

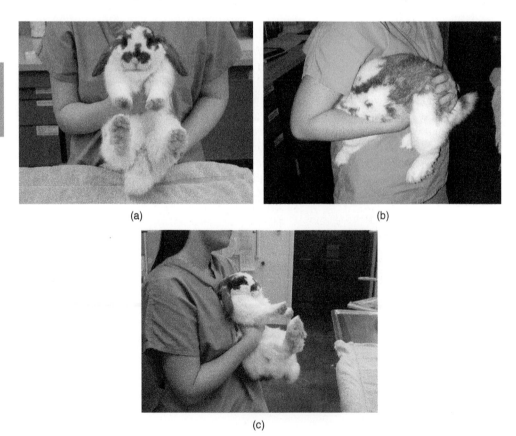

(a)

(b)

(c)

Figure 6.5   (a–c) Restraint techniques for rabbits. *Source*: Courtesy of Jody Nugent-Deal.

One method of restraint is to cradle the rabbit in one arm with the head tucked into the body of the handler. Alternatively, the handler grasps the patient by the scruff and supports the patient's hind end. Do not pick up by the ears!

- *Premedication*: SC injections are an effective technique for premedication, and preferred, if possible, to IM injections. IM injections are administered in the muscular bodies on either side of the spine or hindlimb. Squeeze boxes work nicely for IM injections in feral rabbits. Intranasal administration for soluble drugs, such as midazolam, is an alternative to a needle. While a variety of injectable agents are useful in rabbits, alfaxalone alone or in combination with an opioid and/or an alpha-2 agonist such as dexmedetomidine is useful to achieve moderate (alfaxalone alone) to deep sedation (combination) in rabbits [6–8].
- *Induction*: Because rabbits become stressed and excited, it is recommended that they are sedated prior to boxing down with a gas anesthetic when IV induction cannot be performed.
- *Intubation*: Intubation is a precarious maneuver in the rabbit (Figure 6.6). For an average size rabbit, a 2–2.5 mm uncuffed ET tube or supraglottic airway device (SGAD) such as a v-gel® is used to secure an airway [9]. A SGAD may result in a quicker and less traumatic intubation [10]; if rabbits are a significant part of one's practice, investing

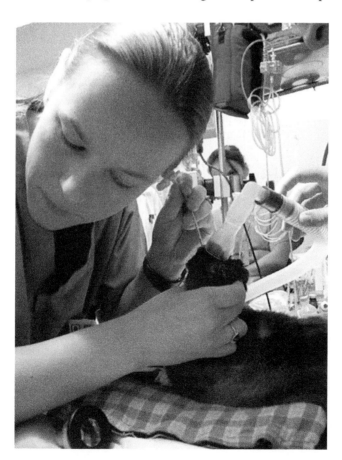

Figure 6.6   Blind technique for intubation in a rabbit. *Source*: Courtesy of Jody Nugent-Deal.

in these tubes is appropriate. Traditional intubation is only attempted a maximum of two or three times. Traumatic or repetitive intubation attempts cause laryngeal swelling and airway obstruction after extubation. See Table 6.5 for intubation techniques.

- *Vascular access*: Catheterization is performed when patient allows, often after induction. When clipping a site for catheterization, use gentle technique as the rabbit's thin skin is easily traumatized. The cephalic vein is suitable for venous access, and may reduce the possibility of damage to the ear. The lateral saphenous vein is accessible as well. IO catheters are placed in the proximal femur, tibia, or humerus. In an emergency, the auricular artery is used to provide arterial access; however, this may result in sloughing of the ear due to reduced perfusion. Therefore, routine catheterization of the auricular artery is not advised.

- *Maintenance*: The patient is typically maintained on gas inhalants, but a TIVA technique is possible if surgeon access to the airway is required and a catheter is in place (Table 6.6). Certain drug combinations, such as alfaxalone with midazolam and dexmedetomidine for premedication, may result in hypoxemia and hypoventilation; capnography and ventilatory support are advised [11].

- *Monitoring*: An ECG will display the patient's cardiac rhythm and HR; however, most monitors only read up to 250 bpm. A Doppler over the radial artery or directly over the heart works well to confirm mechanical (not just electrical) function of the heart. The forelimb is also a useful site for BP monitoring with a sphygmomanometer and Doppler crystal. Fluctuation in the volume of the Doppler may indicate changes in BP. Obtain RR by watching the chest rise and fall; if the patient is intubated, $ETCO_2$ confirms cardiac output and gives information about ventilation. Esophageal temperature probes are recommended for continuous monitoring of core body temperature.

- *Monitoring anesthetic depth*: Most reflexes are absent at a surgical plane of anesthesia but the palpebral reflex is maintained even at a deep anesthetic plane. A light plane

Table 6.5   Blind intubation technique in rabbits.

Materials: Appropriately sized endotracheal tube (2–4 mm ID)
Blind technique:
1. The patient is anesthetized adequately with a regular respiratory pattern.
2. Maintain the patient in sternal recumbency with the head and neck hyperextended. It is best if the patient is grasped from behind the head with the holder's thumb and forefinger by the ramus of the mandible. Nose is essentially directed toward the ceiling.
3. Place a lidocaine drop on the arytenoids to decrease spasms.
4. Advance the ET tube over the base of the tongue.
5. The anesthetist places their ear near the end of the ET tube and advances toward the larynx until respiratory noises are the loudest. Advance the ET tube into the trachea during the next breath; it is helpful to rotate the tube as you advance to pass between the arytenoids. Alternatively, the capnograph adaptor is placed on the end of the ET tube. When $EtCO_2$ is seen on the capnograph, advance the ET tube into the trachea during the next breath.
6. If no respiratory noise is ausculted with administration of a breath, the ET tube is likely in the esophagus and should be withdrawn.

ET, endotracheal; ID, internal diameter.

Table 6.6   Anesthetic protocol for rabbits.

	ASA 1 or 2	ASA 3, 4 or 5

Premedication	1. Opioid (select most appropriate):
	  (a) Hydromorphone 0.2 mg/kg IM
	  (b) Butorphanol 0.4 mg/kg IM
	  (c) Buprenorphine 0.03 mg/kg IM
	2. Sedative (select most appropriate):
	  (a) Midazolam 1 mg/kg IM, SC, or intranasal
	  (b) Acepromazine 0.025–0.05 mg/kg IM or SC
	  (c) Dexmedetomidine 0.1–0.2 mg/kg IM or SC
	3. Injectable anesthetic (select most appropriate):
	  (a) Alfaxalone 2.5–5 mg/kg IM
	  (b) Ketamine 5–10 mg/kg IM
		1. Opioid (select most appropriate):
		  (a) Hydromorphone 0.2 mg/kg IM
		  (b) Butorphanol 0.4 mg/kg IM
		  (c) Buprenorphine 0.03 mg/kg IM
		2. Sedative:
		  (a) Midazolam 0.5–1 mg/kg IM or SC or intranasal
		3. Injectable anesthetic (consider if desired):
		  (a) Alfaxalone 2.5–5 mg/kg IM

Induction	1. Injectable induction (choose one):
	  (a) Alfaxalone 1–3 mg/kg IV to effect
	  (b) Propofol 2–6 mg/kg IV to effect
	2. Mask/chamber with gas inhalant (author strongly opposes inhalant inductions when avoidable)
		Injectable induction (choose one):
		  (a) Alfaxalone 1–3 mg/kg IV to effect
		  (b) Propofol 2–6 mg/kg IV to effect

Maintenance	Gas inhalant	Gas inhalant
Intraoperative analgesia	(a) Local blocks where applicable (b) Opioid bolus or CRI	(a) Local blocks where applicable (b) Fentanyl CRI 0.010–0.06 mg/kg/h

Postoperative analgesia	1. NSAID (choose one):
	  (a) Flunixin 0.3–1.0 mg/kg SC or IV SID
	  (b) Meloxicam 1.0 mg/kg PO SID
	2. Opioid (choose most appropriate):
	  (a) Buprenorphine 0.05–0.3 mg/kg SC q 8 h
	  (b) Hydromorphone 0.2 mg/kg IM q 4 h
	  (c) Methadone 0.1–0.3 mg/kg IM q 4 h
		Opioid (choose most appropriate):
		  (a) Buprenorphine 0.05–0.3 mg/kg SC q 8 h
		  (b) Hydromorphone 0.2 mg/kg IM q 4 h
		  (c) Methadone 0.1–0.3 mg/kg IM q 4 h

CRI, constant-rate infusion; IM, intramuscular; I, intravenous; PO, per os (by mouth); SC, subcutaneous; SID, semel in die (once a day).

of anesthesia is identified by response to a toe pinch, ear twitch, or surgical incision. A rabbit that is at a light plane of anesthesia may shake its head in response to painful stimuli. A deep plane of anesthesia is identified by fixed dilated pupils unresponsive to light with no corneal reflex, depressed ventilation, and minimal response to surgical stimulus.

• *Recovery*: Rabbits are recovered in a quiet, dim environment to prevent startling and kicking at arousal. Additional analgesia is administered as warranted.

Chapter 6

3. Common complications

- Rabbits are very susceptible to corneal ulcers. The eyes cannot be lubricated enough; constant lubrication is recommended. Alternatively, some anesthetists tape the eyes shut.
- Fracture of the spine during improper restraint or boxing down occurs. Avoid boxing down the nonsedated rabbit.
- Hyperthermia is common during restraint and handling due to stress. Try to minimize stress during the preanesthetic and recovery phase.
- Hypothermia is common during anesthesia. The use of plastic surgical drapes, forced air warming units, and circulating warm water blankets is helpful in maintaining body temperature.
- The thoracic cavity of the rabbit is quite small compared with the large abdominal cavity, thus increasing the chance of hypoventilation. Intermittent hand ventilation is recommended.
- Gastrointestinal complications noticed by decreased stool production and stasis commonly occur in rabbits post anesthetic procedures [12].

E. Rodents (chinchillas, gerbils, guinea pigs, hamsters, mice, rats)

1. Characteristics

- Many rodents are obligate nasal breathers.
- Undetected respiratory disease is common in rodents.
- Some species, such as hamsters, are nocturnal.
- Hamsters and guinea pigs have cheek pouches, for storage of food particles, which may result in aspiration pneumonia in the sedated or anesthetized animal.
- Rodents are prone to self-mutilation. Avoid giving IM injections especially with irritating solutions or in large volumes.
- Several species of rodent are capable of shedding their tails if picked up.
- Guinea pigs have a palatal ostium, which makes traditional intubation of this species virtually impossible [13].
- Some species, such as the rat, mouse, and gerbil, do not vomit.

2. Anesthetic considerations

- *Handling and restraint*: Grasping the tail of rodents is avoided. If the rodent is tame, simply cupping it in the palm of a hand is ideal. Grasping the nape or scruff of the neck is the most acceptable means of restraint, especially when giving injections.
- *Premedication*: A variety of premedicants are suitable for rodents; in addition to the SC and IM routes, some medications are administered intraperitoneally (IP). Administration of drugs IP takes practice, so it is advisable for only experienced personnel to use this route (Table 6.7). The muscle bodies for IM administration are small, and certain drugs may irritate tissues, so SC injection is often preferable. Generally speaking, the larger rodents (i.e., guinea pig) will require the lower dose range of agents listed in Table 6.8, while small rodents (i.e., mouse) will require the higher end of the dosage range.

Table 6.7 Intraperitoneal injection in rodents.

Materials: Second person to restrain, 25 G needle, drug for administration
Technique:
1. It is helpful for an additional team member to restrain the animal. This individual inverts the rodent with the head down, to displace abdominal viscera.
2. Enter the caudal quadrant of the abdomen at a 20° angle. The right caudal quadrant is used for most small rodents. The exception is the rat, in which the left caudal quadrant is used.
3. Aspirate prior to drug administration.
4. Inject drug; maximum volume is 1–3 mL.

Table 6.8 Anesthetic protocols for rodents.[a]

	ASA 1 or 2	**ASA 3, 4 or 5**
Premedication	1. Opioid (select most appropriate): (a) Buprenorphine 0.05–0.5 mg/kg SC (b) Butorphanol 0.5–5 mg/kg SC 2. Sedative (select one): (a) Midazolam 0.5–2 mg/kg SC (b) Acepromazine 0.5–5.0 mg/kg SC 3. Anticholinergic (select one): (a) Atropine 0.05 mg/kg SC (b) Glycopyrrolate 0.01–0.02 mg/kg SC 4. Injectable anesthetic (select one): (a) Ketamine 5–10 mg/kg SC (b) Alfaxalone 2–20 mg/kg SC, IM	1. Opioid (select most appropriate): (a) Buprenorphine 0.05–0.5 mg/kg SC (b) Morphine 2–5 mg/kg SC 2. Sedative option: (a) Midazolam 0.5–1 mg/kg SC 3. Anticholinergic (select one): (a) Atropine 0.05 mg/kg SC (b) Glycopyrrolate 0.01–0.02 mg/kg SC
Induction	Mask/chamber with gas inhalants	Mask/chamber with gas inhalants
Maintenance	Gas inhalants	Gas inhalants
Postoperative analgesia	(a) Carprofen 4–10 mg/kg SC SID (b) Buprenorphine 0.05 mg/kg SC q 6–8 h	1. Opioid (select most appropriate): (a) Buprenorphine 0.05 mg/kg SC q 6–8 h (b) Morphine 2–5 mg/kg SC q 4 h

[a]great variation in dosing exists between species of rodents.
IM, intramuscular; SC, subcutaneous; SID, semel in die (once a day).

- *Induction*: Usually, rodents are masked or boxed down in a small enclosure with inhalants (Figure 6.7). The patient is removed from the box when the "righting" reflex is absent and a facemask is placed until the patient is relaxed. Alternative options include injectable anesthetic such as alfaxalone and ketamine administered by a variety of routes and in combination with opioids and sedatives to produce a balanced, effective anesthetic plan [14,15].
- *Intubation*: Larger rodents are intubated, but care is taken during the intubation process to avoid trauma, which may lead to swelling and subsequent airway obstruction. Minimal attempts are made, especially in small rodents. Rats are intubated with the

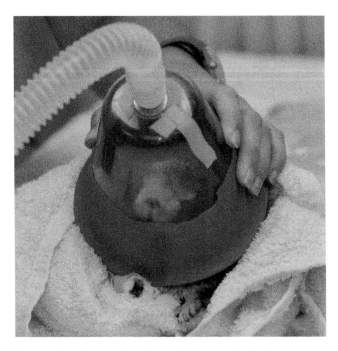

Figure 6.7 Masking a rodent. *Source*: Courtesy of Anderson da Cunha.

assistance of a modified #2 otoscope ear speculum to allow visualization of the larynx. Lidocaine on the arytenoids will help minimize laryngeal spasms. Catheters (16–20 G) work well in place of ET tubes.

- *IV access*: Catheterization in large rodents is accomplished in the cephalic, the tail (in rats), or saphenous veins. IO catheters, if used, are commonly placed in the proximal femur, tibia, or humerus.
- *Maintenance*: Typically, gas inhalants are used to maintain anesthesia in nonlaboratory settings.
- *Monitoring during anesthesia.*
  - Vitals: HR is monitored with a Doppler over an artery or directly over the heart. ECG may be of limited use, as most monitors only read up to 250 bpm. In small rodents, a wire suture is placed in the skin of the animal to clip ECG leads to. Capnography is often inaccurate in small rodents but may assist with confirmation for placement of the ET tube. Instead, monitor chest wall excursions visually to obtain RR.
  - Anesthetic depth: Trends in HR and RR assist with assessment of depth of anesthesia. Responses to toe pinch, tail pinch, or skin incision all suggest too light a plane of anesthesia for surgery. A guinea pig may shake its head in response to surgical stimulus.
  - Recovery: Continued thermal support is important in the recovery phase, as is oxygen supplementation and additional analgesic drugs as warranted.

3. Common complications

- Hypoxemia may result because an airway is difficult to secure in several rodent species. Oxygenation by mask is a reasonable part of the plan.
- Hypoglycemia occurs in small rodent species that are used to free choice availability of food. Unfortunately, lack of venous access for administration of 2.5–5% dextrose complicates this. Therefore, preemptive steps, such as access to food before and immediately after anesthesia, are crucial to preventing hypoglycemia.
- Hypothermia occurs due to large surface area to body mass ratio, use of NRB circuits, and depressed metabolism. External heat support is necessary.
- Respiratory obstruction results from traumatic intubation; in some cases, it is preferable to use a mask as opposed to attempting intubation. Copious respiratory secretions may also obstruct the ET tube; look for increased respiratory effort, which may indicate the ET tube is obstructed.

II. Avians

1. Characteristics

- Birds have a highly efficient respiratory system compared to mammals. Birds have higher V_T, lower RR, and larger minute ventilation. Inspiration and expiration are both active phases in the bird; that is, respiratory movements are accomplished by cervical, thoracic, and abdominal muscle contractions (there is no diaphragm to contribute to the active phase). Two complete respiratory cycles exchange inhaled gases via cross-current gas exchange.
- The trachea is longer and has an increased diameter compared to mammals, resulting in more dead space. Unlike mammals, the tracheal rings are complete. For this reason, the anesthetist utilizes uncuffed ET tubes. It is wise to review the specific species with regard to variations in respiratory anatomy; for example, some penguins have a double trachea and emus have a tracheal diverticulum.
- The epiglottis is absent.
- Birds have high metabolic rates which require higher substrate levels (blood glucose [BG] is greater than 200 mg/dL) and higher fluid rates (10–30 mL/kg/h).
- Cardiovascular differences include larger stroke volume (SV), increased cardiac output (CO), and higher mean arterial pressure (MAP). HR varies considerably depending on the size of the patient.
- Circulation influences the effect of various drugs. Birds possess a renal portal system. This network of vessels around the kidney, which selectively channels blood through or past it, results in a potential first-pass effect of drugs administered in the caudal half of the body, altering the drug's intended effect. When a drug is given in the lower half of the body, it is metabolized by the renal portal system before reaching the central nervous system, the target site for effect.
- Fasting is highly variable depending on the size of the bird; in general, fasting is usually less than 3 hours, but may not be performed at all for very small birds.

2. Anesthetic considerations

- *Handling and restraint*: It is important to minimize stress while restraining birds. Ideally, a bird is allowed to acclimatize to the hospital environment before handling. In an emergency situation, acclimatization is not possible. Covering the eyes of the patient with a hood or towel helps to reduce stress. For smaller birds, utilize the hand technique: place the head gently between the thumb and forefinger with the body supported in the palm.
- *Preanesthetic assessment*: The physical examination (PE) begins before the bird is removed from its housing. Visually assess RR and effort prior to handling. Look at the bird's posture and whether the feathers are "fluffed." When the bird is removed from its surroundings, a hands-on examination of the bird commences. This includes ausculting air sacs ventrally, lungs dorsally, and over the trachea for abnormal airway sounds. The heart is ausculted as well. Obtaining an accurate body weight is key to drug dosages and fluid rates; palpation of the keel gives an indication of body condition of the bird to know whether this weight is appropriate for the patient. Color of the urate is helpful in suggesting liver dysfunction when preoperative bloodwork (BW) is unavailable. Hydration status is assessed by moistness of the cloaca, ocular mucous membranes, and elasticity of skin. Sunken eyes and cold extremities suggest dehydration and/or shock.
- *Premedication*: Anticholinergics are controversial for use in the bird; while an increase in HR is desirable, increased thickness of respiratory secretions increases the chance of ET tube occlusion. Additionally, some herbivorous birds may possess atropinesterases. Injectable premedication with sedatives, analgesics, and anesthetics will minimize stress during induction (Table 6.9). The pectoral muscles are utilized for IM injections (Figure 6.8), although consideration is given to a captive bird that may be released, as soreness may result in limited flight activity. However, when

Table 6.9   Common anesthetic and analgesic protocols in birds.

	ASA 1 or 2	**ASA 3, 4 or 5**
Premedication	1. Butorphanol 1.0–2.5 mg/kg IM [56,57] (chickens, parrots) OR 2. Methadone 6 mg/kg IM [58] (chickens) OR 3. Concentrated buprenorphine 0.3 mg/kg, SC (raptors) [59] +/– 4. Midazolam 1–2 mg/kg IM +/– 5. Ketamine 10–20 mg/kg IM OR 6. Alfaxalone 10–20 mg/kg IM	1. Butorphanol 1.0–2.0 mg/kg IM [57] (chickens, parrots) OR 2. Fentanyl 20–30 μg/ kg [60] (raptors) +/– 3. Midazolam 1 mg/kg IM +/– 4. Alfaxalone 10 mg/kg IM
Induction	Mask with gas inhalant	Mask with gas inhalant OR If IV access present, alfaxalone 2 mg/kg IV to effect

	ASA 1 or 2	**ASA 3, 4 or 5**
Maintenance	Gas inhalant Alfaxalone for short procedures	Gas inhalant
Intraoperative analgesia	1. Local blocks where appropriate AND 2. Butorphanol boluses (chickens, parrots) OR 3. Methadone boluses 6 mg/kg IM [58] (chickens)	1. Local blocks where appropriate AND 2. Butorphanol CRI 0.1–0.4 mg/kg/h following loading dose premedication (chickens, parrots) OR 3. Fentanyl CRI 30 µg/kg/h following loading dose [61,62] (raptors) OR 4. Methadone 6 mg/kg IM [58] (chickens)
Postoperative analgesia	1. Butorphanol 1.0 mg/kg IV or IM (chickens, parrots) OR 2. Concentrated buprenorphine 0.3 mg/kg, SC (raptors) [59] AND 3. Carprofen 1 mg/kg IM SID OR 4. Meloxicam 1.0 mg/kg PO SID	1. Butorphanol 1.0 mg/kg IV or IM (chickens, parrots) OR 2. Concentrated buprenorphine 0.3 mg/kg, SC (raptors) [59]

CRI, constant-rate infusion; IM, intramuscular; IV, intravenous; SC, subcutaneous; SID, semel in die (once a day).

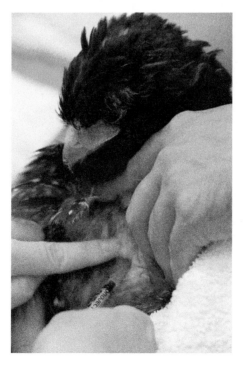

Figure 6.8   IM injection in the pectoral muscle of a bird. *Source*: Courtesy of Anderson da Cunha.

Chapter 6

administered into the lower half of the body, the drugs pass through the portal venous system, which may result in altered drug metabolism.

- *Induction*: Preoxygenate if possible. The most common means of induction is masking the patient down with an inhalant (Figure 6.9). In the small avian, the mask is made with a syringe casing so the whole head of the patient fits in the "mask." An examination glove with a hole cut in the end is used as a diaphragm to create a sealed fit. The patient's HR and RR are monitored closely during induction because there is a tendency to achieve an excessive depth resulting in hypoventilation and bradycardia. Injectable agents are used if an IV catheter is available. Vessels suitable for catheterization include the cutaneous ulnar or basillic vein, medial metatarsal, or jugular vein (Figure 6.10). Preference is given to the upper half of the body due to the circulatory pattern and its influence on drug metabolism. IO catheters are placed in the proximal ulna or cranial tibiotarsus; other bones are pneumatic.

  Alfaxalone and its favorable IM route is gaining attention for avian anesthesia. Several species, including parrots, lovebirds and budgerigars, exhibit sedation after an IM injection with alfaxalone [16–19] and, indeed, alfaxalone may prove a suitable alternative to other sedatives or isoflurane for minimally noxious procedures [20,21]. If only alfaxalone is used for induction, muscle tremors and hyperexcitation may occur during induction, Premedication with midazolam may help alleviate that [18]. Dosage of alfaxalone for effect varies considerably by the breed of bird, so the reader is referred to species-specific dosing when possible.

- *Intubation*: The glottis is readily visible for intubation (Figure 6.11). Uncuffed ET tubes are used.
- *Maintenance*: Inhalants in oxygen or TIVA are the most common techniques.

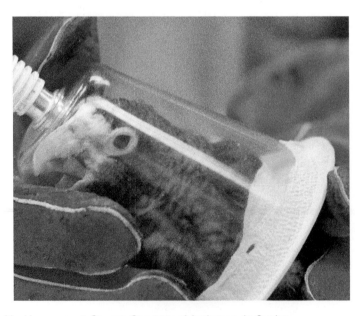

Figure 6.9   Masking a parrot. *Source*: Courtesy of Anderson da Cunha.

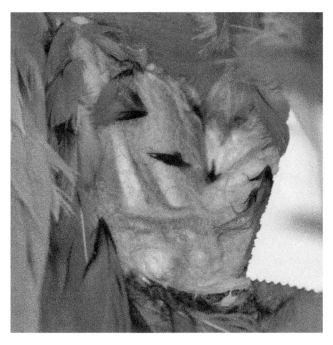

Figure 6.10   Cutaneous ulnar or basillic vein for IV catheterization in a bird. *Source*: Courtesy of Anderson da Cunha.

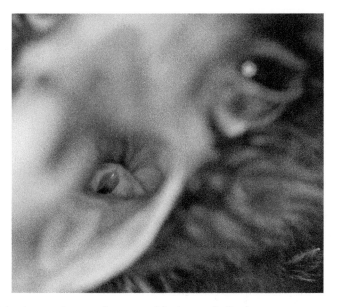

Figure 6.11   Avian larynx. *Source*: Courtesy of Anderson da Cunha.

- *Analgesia*: Local techniques are used when possible. Toxic doses vary among species and between local anesthetics [22]. Eutectic mixture of local anesthetic (EMLA) cream is used but is limited to small areas. In some species of birds, there is a prevalence of kappa receptors, making kappa agonists such as butorphanol or nalbuphine suitable analgesics in birds. However, there is conflicting information about pure mu agonists, such as hydromorphone or tramadol, altering a bird's response to nociception [23–26]. The reader will note that a variety of opioids are listed in Table 6.9. Some newer data suggest that some raptorial species of birds may have more mu receptors compared to kappa receptors [27] and thus a partial or full mu opioid may be more appropriate for these species [28]. Most studies in parrots and chickens show that full mu opioids are likely not as effective for analgesia [26,29], but may work for sedation [30] or maintenance agent reduction [31–34]. With a huge number of species to evaluate, it is not possible to create a blanket statement on which opioid is most appropriate for all avian species, and the reader is encouraged to look for studies that pertain to the species of bird they most often encounter.

- *Monitoring suggestions*: A Doppler is considered essential monitoring for assessing HR; while an ECG is useful, many ECG units only count up to 250 bpm. Additionally, the thin skin of the bird makes ECG clips unsuitable for use, so a small wire suture or needle is placed in the skin as an alternative site for clips. An esophageal stethoscope is a suitable means of HR monitoring as well. Use of a Doppler and sphygmomanometer, with a BP cuff, allows the anesthetist to obtain BP trends. Additionally, in large birds, arterial access is possible. The brachial or carotid arteries are accessible; the use of EMLA cream may facilitate arterial line placement. Respiration is monitored. Ideally, there are minimal respiratory noises in the intubated patient, although the intubated bird, unlike mammals, has the ability to vocalize due to the caudal location of the syrinx. Apnea for a period greater than 10–20 seconds warrants a manual breath; most birds benefit from MV under anesthesia. Capnography is helpful in assessing quality of ventilation and confirming that perfusion of the lungs is occurring; however, birds are one of the few animals where the $EtCO_2$ is possibly greater than $PaCO_2$. The benefits are considered in light of the possible increase in dead space or oversampling of a capnograph adapter. Pulse oximeters are not accurate in birds, due to the difference in avian hemoglobin. A cloacal or esophageal temperature is monitored to guide thermoregulatory management.

- *Monitoring anesthetic depth*: Reaction to toe pinch, cere pinch, cloacal pinch, or feather plucking, and increased jaw tone are all indications of a light plane of anesthesia. Muscle tone, such as neck or wing tone, may give an indication of depth as well. Slight palpebral and corneal reflexes are typical in the surgical plane of anesthesia. Decreases in HR, BP, RR, and apnea are indications of a deep plane of anesthesia.

- *Recovery*: Indications of recovery include wing and leg movement. Jaw tone returns as anesthetic depth decreases and the patient is extubated when this occurs. Continued oxygen supplementation is administered after extubation. Additional analgesics are administered as warranted.

3. Common complications

- Hypothermia occurs due to large surface area to body mass ratio, use of NRB circuits, and depressed metabolism. External heat support is provided.

Chapter 6

- ET tube occlusions secondary to mucus plugs are extraordinarily common in birds; any resistance to administering a breath or difficulty ventilating a patient warrants an exchange of ET tube due to the possibility of occlusion.
- Hypoventilation which is prevalent in this species often necessitates MV.

III. Reptiles

1. Characteristics

- The heart has three chambers (two atria, one ventricle). This allows for mixing of oxygenated and deoxygenated blood with changes in vascular resistance under anesthesia. This "shunting" significantly worsens perfusion of vital tissues.
- Reptiles are ectothermic; therefore, body temperature influences drug metabolism and clearance, as well as physiologic parameters.
- Prior to anesthetizing a reptile, the reader is advised to review the individual species variations in regard to respiratory anatomy and physiology, as this is beyond the scope of this chapter. For example, many reptiles do not possess a diaphragm. Instead, abdominal, pectoral, and pelvic muscles control ventilation. However, crocodilians have a nonmuscular tissue which functions as a rudimentary diaphragm. Most snakes possess a single elongated right lung, although boas possess the left lung lobe in addition to the right. Most reptiles have simplified sacs with folds allowing for respiratory gas exchange, but there is a whole spectrum of complexity. The trachea in a turtle is short and bifurcates early compared with most reptiles. Some reptiles, such as turtles, possess complete tracheal rings.
- A renal portal system is present in reptiles as it is in birds. This network of vessels around the kidney, which selectively channels blood through or past it, results in a potential first-pass effect of drugs administered in the caudal half of the body, altering the drug's intended effects.
- Although fasting is often not required, timing of last large meal (especially for snakes) is important to know. A recent large meal affects the patient's ability to adequately ventilate.

2. Anesthesia considerations

- *Restraint and handling*: This varies greatly by species restrained. All reptiles are capable of biting; many have claws and tails that are used in defense. Leather gloves are useful in preventing trauma to the handler for large reptile species. Nonpoisonous snakes are grasped at the base of the head with one hand while the other hand supports the body. Lizards are similarly handled, although the body is often tucked under the arm of the handler or restrained in the other hand (Figure 6.12). Turtles and tortoises are held at the shell; the length of the neck determines how far caudal on the carapace the animal is restrained. Some species of turtles have extremely long necks and can deliver a powerful bite to an unsuspecting restrainer.
- *Preanesthetic assessment*: In nonpoisonous and tame species, perform a PE prior to anesthesia to obtain a baseline HR, RR, body temperature, and accurate body weight.

Chapter 6

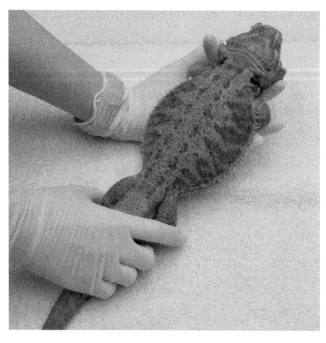

Figure 6.12   Restraint of a bearded dragon. *Source*: Courtesy of Amanda M. Shelby.

Physical parameters such as HR are greatly influenced by body temperature, environmental stress, and presence of noxious stimuli. Due to the large variation in reptilian species, normal physical parameters are based on species-specific reference material and the patient's examination.

- *Premedication*: Benefits of a premedication in animals include reduced dosages of induction drugs, analgesia, and sedation. However, clearance is prolonged in reptiles compared to mammals. Therefore, reversible drugs are chosen when possible. Some reptiles have mu opioid receptors, making mu opioids such as morphine an effective analgesic option, although respiratory depression may result [35,36]. Other opioids may be effective at providing analgesia but differences between species are notable [37,38]. Other alternative analgesic drugs, including alpha-2 agonists such as dexmedetomidine and medetomidine, may provide analgesia in some retiles [39–41]. Any injectable premedication is administered in the cranial portion of the animal if possible [42]; more effective sedation with injectable drugs such as alfaxalone was evident when the drug was administered cranially [43]. However, safety of the handler is prioritized over concern regarding the renal portal system. There is also evidence that intracelomic administration of alfaxalone is a viable route in snakes [44,45]. Indeed, with its favorable routes of administration, alfaxalone is a versatile drug for use in many reptile species [46,47].
- *Induction*: When premedication is insufficient, reptiles can be induced with inhalants via mask or chamber (Figure 6.13). Inhalants are administered to the patient until it is relaxed and intubation is accomplished (Table 6.10). Turtles and tortoises may be induced with IV induction agents by IV access or injection through

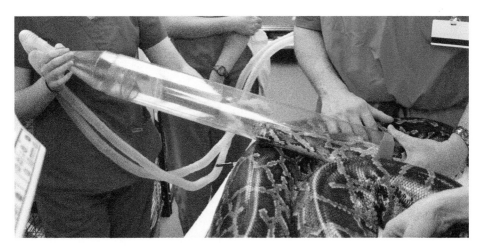

Figure 6.13   Masking a snake. *Source*: Courtesy of Anderson da Cunha.

Table 6.10   Anesthetic protocol for reptiles.

	Snake	Lizard	Turtle/tortoise
Premedication (*Note*: No premedication in aggressive or poisonous species)	Opioid premedication: Butorphanol 20 mg/kg IM Sedative agent (select one): (a) Midazolam 0.5–1.0 mg/kg IM (b) Dexmedeto-midine 0.05–0.1 mg/kg IM/SC Injectable anesthetic (select one): (a) Ketamine 5–10 mg/kg IM (b) Alfaxalone 5–20 mg/kg IM or 10–30 mg/kg intracolemic (c) Propofol 15 mg/kg IV	1. Morphine 0.4–1.5 mg/kg 2. Midazolam 1.0–2.0 mg/kg IM 3. Dexmedetomidine 0.1–0.2 mg/kg IM 4. Injectable anesthetic (select one): (a) Ketamine 5–10 mg/kg IM (b) Alfaxalone 5–15 mg/kg IM or 10–20 mg/kg SC [63]	1. Opioid (select one): (a) Hydromorphone 0.5 mg/kg IM (b) Morphine 0.4–1.5 mg/kg IM 2. Sedative (select one): (a) Midazolam 1.0–2.0 mg/kg IM (b) Medetomidine 0.05 mg/kg IM 3. Injectable anesthetic (select one): (a) Ketamine 5–10 mg/kg IM (b) Alfaxalone 10 mg/kg IM
Induction	1. Proper premedication dosing can facilitate intubation 2. Mask/chamber with gas inhalants; due to breath holding, this can take several minutes and exposes staff to waste anesthetic gas	1. Proper premedica-tion dosing can facilitate intubation 2. Mask/chamber with gas inhalants	1. Mask/chamber with gas inhalants OR 2. Propofol via frontal sinus or IV 2–4 mg/kg to effect OR 3. Alfaxalone via frontal sinus or IV 3–10 mg/kg to effect (Note: assisted ventilation is necessary if the high end of the dose range is used) [64]

(Continued)

Chapter 6

Table 6.10 (Continued)

	Snake	Lizard	Turtle/tortoise
Maintenance	Gas inhalants	Gas inhalants OR Alfaxalone in some lizard species [65]	Gas inhalants
Intraoperative analgesia	Local blocks where applicable	Local blocks where applicable (Note: Neuroaxial anesthesia with lidocaine or bupivacaine is feasible in the bearded dragon [66,67])	Local blocks where applicable
Postoperative analgesia	1. Butorphanol 20 mg/kg IM 2. Carprofen 1–4 mg/kg IM SID	1. Morphine 0.4–1.5 mg/kg IM 2. NSAID (select one): (a) Carprofen 1–4 mg/kg IM SID (b) Meloxicam 0.2 mg/kg PO or IV	1. Tramadol 5–10 mg/kg PO 2. Carprofen 1–4 mg/kg IM SID

IM, intramuscular; IV, intravenous; NSAID, nonsteroidal antiinflammatory drug; PO, per os (by mouth); SC, subcutaneous; SID, semel in die (once a day).

the subcarapacial sinus under their shells (Figure 6.14). Intubation of snakes and lizards is straightforward, as the position of the glottis is rostral (Figure 6.15). Noncuffed ET tubes, Cole tubes, or 16–19 G catheters are used for smaller reptiles. Typically, the best method of securing the ET tube is taping it to the patient's lower jaw. In turtles (Figure 6.16), the glottis is located at the base of the tongue. They have short tracheas so care is taken to ensure ET tubes are not advanced too far, causing an endobronchial intubation. In reptiles, IV access is infrequently achieved. In turtles and tortoises, catheterized vessels include the jugular or coccygeal veins; alternatively, IO catheters are commonly placed (Figure 6.17).

- *Maintenance*: General anesthesia is maintained primarily with inhalant anesthetics. Alfaxalone has potential for a surgical plane of anesthesia in some lizard species [48]. Because these animals are ectothermic, external heat support is necessary throughout the anesthetic period to keep them in their optimal thermoregulatory range.
- *Monitoring vitals*: A Doppler is useful for monitoring HR (Figure 6.18); a pencil probe is ideal for the anesthetist to obtain HR via the ocular artery by placing this probe (well lubed) onto the eye. An esophageal stethoscope is also useful for obtaining HR. RR is visually observed. Assisted ventilation of 1–4 breaths per minute is recommended due to the long periods of apnea; MV is indicated for most reptiles. Capnography is not an adequate representation of ventilation due to intrapulmonary shunting (i.e., $EtCO_2$ is increased compared to true $PaCO_2$), but does provide some

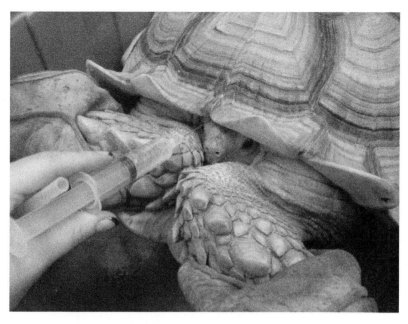

Figure 6.14   Subcarapacial sinus injection in a tortoise. *Source*: Courtesy of Anderson da Cunha.

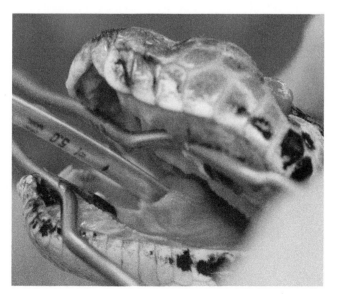

Figure 6.15   Intubation of a snake. *Source*: Courtesy of Anderson da Cunha.

evidence for the presence of CO_2. Pulse oximetry is not accurate in reptiles due to their alternative form of hemoglobin and difficulty placing the probe.

- *Monitoring anesthetic depth*: Muscle tone will decrease in the reptile as it becomes anesthetized. In the snake, relaxation occurs initially at the head, then through the

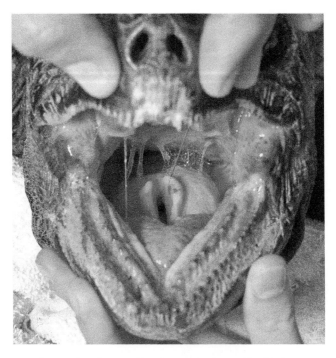

Figure 6.16   Larynx of a tortoise. *Source*: Courtesy of Anderson da Cunha.

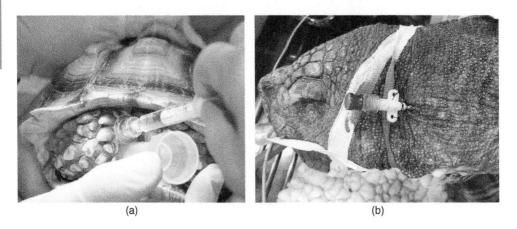

(a)   (b)

Figure 6.17   (a) IO catheter in a tortoise. *Source*: Courtesy of Anderson da Cunha. (b) Jugular catheter in a tortoise. *Source*: Courtesy of Jody Nugent-Deal.

torso, and proceeds caudally, lastly affecting the tail; recovery occurs in the opposite order. In snakes, the tongue retraction reflex will only subside in a deep plane of anesthesia. Palpebral reflexes may give an indication of anesthetic depth. Corneal reflexes are also lost in a deep plane. Toe or tail pinch is absent during the surgical plane of anesthesia. Jaw tone is also monitored in species where this is safe to assess.

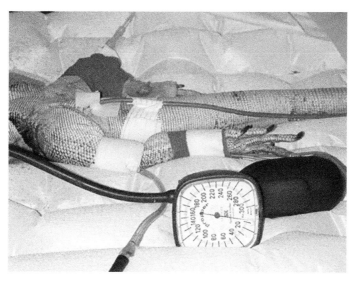

Figure 6.18 Doppler and blood pressure monitoring of a reptile. *Source*: Courtesy of Jody Nugent-Deal.

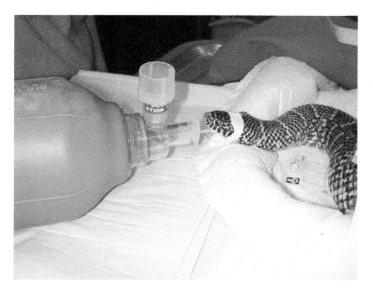

Figure 6.19 Snake placed on Ambu-bag on room air for recovery. *Source*: Courtesy of Jody Nugent-Deal.

- *Recovery*: Snakes typically take longer than lizards to recover; turtles, especially those that are capable of holding their breath, take an extraordinarily long time to recover. There is evidence that administration of epinephrine may expedite recovery from inhalant in sea turtles [49]. Maintaining optimal body temperature is critical to recovery. All reptiles are placed on room air to recover due to the downregulation of

Chapter 6

a reptile's respiratory system secondary to increased FiO_2. Continuing assisted ventilation is often necessary on room air (Figure 6.19). Extubation occurs once the patient is capable of spontaneous ventilation and pharyngeal reflexes have returned. Additional analgesia is administered as warranted.

3. Common complications

- *Hypothermia*: Hypothermia is reduced by using circulating hot water blankets and forced air warming units.
- *Hypoventilation*: Hypoventilation secondary to apnea and respiratory depression is common in most reptiles, requiring assisted ventilation.

www.wiley.com/go/shelby/anesthesia2

Please go to the companion website for access to videos relating to the book

References

1. Brodbelt D, Blissitt K, Hammond R, et al. The risk of death: the confidential enquiry into perioperative small animal fatalities. Vet Anaesth Analg. 2008;35(5):365–73.
2. Milloway MC, Posner LP, Balko JA. Sedative and cardiorespiratory effects of intramuscular alfaxalone and butorphanol at two dosages in ferrets (Mustela Putorius Furo). J Zoo Wildlife Med. 2021;51(4):841–7.
3. Bigby SE, Carter JE, Bauquier S, Beths T. The use of alfaxalone for premedication, induction and maintenance of anaesthesia in pigs: a pilot study. Vet Anaesth Analg. 2017;44(4):905–9.
4. Santos M, Bertran de Lis BT, Tendillo FJ. Effects of intramuscular dexmedetomidine in combination with ketamine or alfaxalone in swine. Vet Anaesth Analg. 2016;43(1):81–5.
5. Tucker FS, Beattie RJ. Qualitative microtest for atropine esterase. Lab Anim Sci. 1983;33(3):268–9.
6. Marin P, Belda E, Laredo FG, Torres CA, Hernandis V, Escudero E. Pharmacokinetics and sedative effects of alfaxalone with or without dexmedetomidine in rabbits. Res Vet Sci. 2020;129:6–12.
7. Ishikawa Y, Sakata H, Tachibana Y, et al. Sedative and physiological effects of low-dose intramuscular alfaxalone in rabbits. J Vet Med Sci. 2019;81(6):851–6.
8. Bradley MP, Doerning CM, Nowland MH, Lester PA. Intramuscular administration of alfaxalone alone and in combination for sedation and anesthesia of rabbits (Oryctolagus cuniculus). J Am Assoc Lab Anim Sci. 2019;58(2):216–22.
9. Fusco A, Douglas H, Barba A, et al. V-Gel® guided endotracheal intubation in rabbits. Front Vet Sci. 2021;8:684624.

10. Engbers S, Larkin A, Rousset N, et al. Comparison of a supraglottic airway device (v-gel®) with blind orotracheal intubation in rabbits. Front Vet Sci. 2017;4:49.

11. Rousseau-Blass F, Pang DS. Hypoventilation following oxygen administration associated with alfaxalone-dexmedetomidine-midazolam anesthesia in New Zealand White rabbits. Vet Anaesth Analg. 2020;47(5):637–46.

12. Lee HW, Machin H, Adami C. Peri-anaesthetic mortality and nonfatal gastrointestinal complications in pet rabbits: a retrospective study on 210 cases. Vet Anaesth Analg. 2018;45(4):520–8.

13. Timm KI, Jahn SE, Sedgwick CJ. The palatal ostium of the guinea pig. Lab Anim Sci. 1987;37(6):801–2.

14. Arenillas M, Gomez de Segura IA. Anaesthetic effects of alfaxalone administered intraperitoneally alone or combined with dexmedetomidine and fentanyl in the rat. Lab Anim. 2018;52(6):588–98.

15. Parkinson L, Mans C. Anesthetic and postanesthetic effects of alfaxalone-butorphanol compared with dexmedetomidine-ketamine in chinchillas (Chinchilla lanigera). J Am Assoc Lab Anim Sci. 2017;56:290–5.

16. Romano J, Hasse K, Johnston M. Sedative, cardiorespiratory, and thermoregulatory effects of alfaxalone on budgerigars (Melopsittacus Undulatus). J Zoo Wildlife Med. 2020;51(1):96–101.

17. Kruse TN, Messenger KM, Bowman AS, Aarnes TK, Wittum TE, Flint M. Pharmacokinetics and pharmacodynamics of alfaxalone after a single intramuscular or intravascular injection in mallard ducks (Anas platyrhynchos). J Vet Pharmacol Ther. 2019;42(6):713–21.

18. Whitehead MC, Hoppes SM, Musser JMB, Perkins JL, Lepiz ML. The use of alfaxalone in Quaker parrots (Myiopsitta monachus). J Avian Med Surg. 2019;33(4):340–8.

19. Greunz EM, Limon D, Bertelsen MF. Alfaxalone sedation in black-cheeked lovebirds (Agapornis nigrigenis) for non-invasive procedures. J Avian Med Surg. 2021;35(2):161–6.

20. Balko JA, Lindemann DM, Allender MC, Chinnadurai SK. Evaluation of the anesthetic and cardiorespiratory effects of intramuscular alfaxalone administration and isoflurane in budgerigars (Melopsittacus undulatus) and comparison with manual restraint. J Am Vet Med Assoc. 2019;254(12):1427–35.

21. Escalante GC, Balko JA, Chinnadurai SK. Comparison of the sedative effects of alfaxalone and butorphanol-midazolam administered intramuscularly in budgerigars (Melopsittacus undulatus). J Avian Med Surg. 2018;32(4):279–85.

22. DiGeronimo PM, da Cunha AF, Pypendop B, et al. Cardiovascular tolerance of intravenous bupivacaine in broiler chickens (Gallus gallus domesticus) anesthetized with isoflurane. Vet Anaesth Analg. 2017;44(2):287–94.

23. Geelen S, Sanchez-Migallon Guzman D, Souza MJ, Cox S, Keuler NS, Paul-Murphy JR. Antinociceptive effects of tramadol hydrochloride after intravenous administration to Hispaniolan Amazon parrots (Amazona ventralis). Am J Vet Res. 2013;74(2):201–6.

24. Guzman DS, Drazenovich TL, Olsen GH, Willits NH, Paul-Murphy JR. Evaluation of thermal antinociceptive effects after intramuscular administration of hydromorphone hydrochloride to American kestrels (Falco sparverius). Am J Vet Res. 2013;74(6):817–22.

25. Sanchez-Migallon Guzman D, Douglas JM, Beaufrere H, Paul-Murphy JR. Evaluation of the thermal antinociceptive effects of hydromorphone hydrochloride after intramuscular administration to orange-winged Amazon parrots (Amazona amazonica). Am J Vet Res. 2020;81(10):775–82.

26. Houck EL, Guzman DS, Beaufrere H, Knych HK, Paul-Murphy JR. Evaluation of the thermal antinociceptive effects and pharmacokinetics of hydromorphone hydrochloride after intramuscular administration to cockatiels (Nymphicus hollandicus). Am J Vet Res. 2018;79(8):820–7.

27. Guzman DS, Drazenovich TL, KuKanich B, Olsen GH, Willits NH, Paul-Murphy JR. Evaluation of thermal antinociceptive effects and pharmacokinetics after intramuscular administration of butorphanol tartrate to American kestrels (Falco sparverius). Am J Vet Res. 2014;75(1):11–18.

28. Gleeson MD, Guzman DS, Knych HK, Kass PH, Drazenovich TL, Hawkins MG. Pharmacokinetics of a concentrated buprenorphine formulation in red-tailed hawks (Buteo jamaicensis). Am J Vet Res. 2018;79(1):13–20.

29. Guzman DS, Houck EL, Knych HKD, Beaufrere H, Paul-Murphy JR. Evaluation of the thermal antinociceptive effects and pharmacokinetics after intramuscular administration of buprenorphine hydrochloride to cockatiels (Nymphicus hollandicus). Am J Vet Res. 2018;79(12):1239–45.

30. Singh PM, Johnson CB, Gartrell B, Mitchinson S, Jacob A, Chambers P. Analgesic effects of morphine and butorphanol in broiler chickens. Vet Anaesth Analg. 2017;44(3):538–45.

31. Pavez JC, Hawkins MG, Pascoe PJ, Knych HK, Kass PH. Effect of fentanyl target-controlled infusions on isoflurane minimum anaesthetic concentration and cardiovascular function in red-tailed hawks (Buteo jamaicensis). Vet Anaesth Analg. 2011;38(4):344–51.

32. Hawkins MG, Pascoe PJ, DiMaio Knych HK, Drazenovich TL, Kass PH, Sanchez-Migallon Guzman D. Effects of three fentanyl plasma concentrations on the minimum alveolar concentration of isoflurane in Hispaniolan Amazon parrots (Amazona ventralis). Am J Vet Res. 2018;79(6):600–5.

33. Santos EA, Monteiro ER, Herrera JR, et al. Total intravenous anesthesia in domestic chicken (Gallus gallus domesticus) with propofol alone or in combination with methadone, nalbuphine or fentanyl for ulna osteotomy. Vet Anaesth Analg. 2020;47(3):347–55.

34. Escobar A, da Rocha RW, Pypendop BH, Zangirolami Filho D, Sousa SS, Valadao CA. Effects of methadone on the minimum anesthetic concentration of isoflurane, and its effects on heart rate, blood pressure and ventilation during isoflurane anesthesia in hens (Gallus gallus domesticus). PLoS One. 2016;11(3):e0152546.

35. Sladky KK, Miletic V, Paul-Murphy J, Kinney ME, Dallwig RK, Johnson SM. Analgesic efficacy and respiratory effects of butorphanol and morphine in turtles. J Am Vet Med Assoc. 2007;230(9):1356–62.

36. Leal WP, Carregaro AB, Bressan TF, Bisetto SP, Melo CF, Sladky KK. Antinociceptive efficacy of intramuscular administration of morphine sulfate and butorphanol tartrate in tegus (Salvator merianae). Am J Vet Res. 2017;78(9):1019–24.

37. Hawkins SJ, Cox S, Yaw TJ, Sladky K. Pharmacokinetics of subcutaneously administered hydromorphone in bearded dragons (Pogona vitticeps) and red-eared slider turtles (Trachemys scripta elegans). Vet Anaesth Analg. 2019;46(3):352–9.

38. Kharbush RJ, Gutwillig A, Hartzler KE, et al. Antinociceptive and respiratory effects following application of transdermal fentanyl patches and assessment of brain mu-opioid receptor mRNA expression in ball pythons. Am J Vet Res. 2017;78(7):785–95.

39. Bunke LG, Sladky KK, Johnson SM. Antinociceptive efficacy and respiratory effects of dexmedetomidine in ball pythons (Python regius). Am J Vet Res. 2018;79(7):718–26.

40. Karklus AA, Sladky KK, Johnson SM. Respiratory and antinociceptive effects of dexmedetomidine and doxapram in ball pythons (Python regius). Am J Vet Res. 2021;82(1):11–21.

41. Bisetto SP, Melo CF, Carregaro AB. Evaluation of sedative and antinociceptive effects of dexmedetomidine, midazolam and dexmedetomidine-midazolam in tegus (Salvator merianae). Vet Anaesth Analg. 2018;45(3):320–8.

42. Yaw TJ, Mans C, Johnson SM, Doss GA, Sladky KK. Effect of injection site on alfaxalone-induced sedation in ball pythons (Python regius). J Small Anim Pract. 2018;59(12):747–51.

43. James LE, Williams CJ, Bertelsen MF, Wang T. Anaesthetic induction with alfaxalone in the ball python (Python regius): dose response and effect of injection site. Vet Anaesth Analg. 2018;45(3):329–37.

44. Strahl-Heldreth DE, Clark-Price SC, Keating SCJ, et al. Effect of intracoelomic administration of alfaxalone on the righting reflex and tactile stimulus response of common garter snakes (Thamnophis sirtalis). Am J Vet Res. 2019;80(2):144–51.

Chapter 6

45. Chen K, Keating S, Strahl-Heldreth D, Clark-Price S. Effects of intracoelomic alfaxalone-dexmedetomidine on righting reflex in common garter snakes (Thamnophis sirtalis): preliminary data. Vet Anaesth Analg. 2020;47(6):793–6.

46. Kleinschmidt LM, Hanley CS, Sahrmann JM, Padilla LR. Randomized controlled trial comparing the effects of alfaxalone and ketamine hydrochloride in the Haitian Giant Galliwasp (Celestus warreni). J Zoo Wildlife Med. 2018;49(2):283–90.

47. Bertelsen MF, Buchanan R, Jensen HM, Leite CAC, Abe AS, Wang T. Pharmacodynamics of propofol and alfaxalone in rattlesnakes (Crotalus durissus). Comp Biochem Physiol A Mol Integr Physiol. 2021;256:110935.

48. Rasys AM, Divers SJ, Lauderdale JD, Menke DB. A systematic study of injectable anesthetic agents in the brown anole lizard (Anolis sagrei). Lab Anim. 2020;54(3):281–94.

49. Balko JA, Gatson BJ, Cohen EB, Griffith EH, Harms CA, Bailey KM. Inhalant anesthetic recovery following intramuscular epinephrine in the loggerhead sea turtle (Caretta caretta). J Zoo Wildlife Med. 2018;49(3):680–8.

50. Katzenbach JE, Wittenburg L, Allweiler S, et al. Buprenorphine, butorphanol and hydromorphone in the domestic ferret (Mustela putorius furo). J Exotic Pet Med 2018;27(2):95–102.

51. Hawkins MG. Advances in exotic mammal clinical therapeutics. Vet Clin North Am Exot Anim Pract. 2015;18(2):323–37.

52. Chinnadurai SK, Messenger KM, Papich MG, Harms CA. Meloxicam pharmacokinetics using non-linear mixed-effects modeling in ferrets after single subcutaneous administration. J Vet Pharmacol Ther. 2014;37(4):382–7.

53. Doss GA, Mans C. Antinociceptive efficacy and safety of subcutaneous buprenorphine hydrochloride administration in African pygmy hedgehogs (Atelerix albiventris). J Am Vet Med Assoc. 2020;257(6):618–23.

54. Hawkins SJ, Doss GA, Mans C. Evaluation of subcutaneous administration of alfaxalone-midazolam and ketamine-midazolam as sedation protocols in African pygmy hedgehogs (Atelerix albiventris). J Am Vet Med Assoc. 2020;257(8):820–5.

55. Bellini L, Pagani G, Mollo A, Contiero B, Loretti E, Gelli D. Evaluation of alfaxalone and dexmedetomidine for intramuscular restraint in European hedgehogs (Erinaceus europaeus). Vet Rec. 2019;185(5):145.

56. Guzman DS, Flammer K, Paul-Murphy JR, Barker SA, Tully TN Jr. Pharmacokinetics of butorphanol after intravenous, intramuscular, and oral administration in Hispaniolan Amazon parrots (Amazona ventralis). J Avian Med Surg. 2011;25(3):185–91.

57. Singh PM, Johnson CB, Gartrell B, Mitchinson S, Jacob A, Chambers P. Analgesic effects of morphine and butorphanol in broiler chickens. Vet Anaesth Analg. 2017;44(3):538–45.

58. Escobar A, da Rocha RW, Pypendop BH, Zangirolami Filho D, Sousa SS, Valadao CA. Effects of methadone on the minimum anesthetic concentration of isoflurane, and its effects on heart rate, blood pressure and ventilation during isoflurane anesthesia in hens (Gallus gallus domesticus). PLoS One. 2016;11(3):e0152546.

59. Gleeson MD, Guzman DS, Knych HK, Kass PH, Drazenovich TL, Hawkins MG. Pharmacokinetics of a concentrated buprenorphine formulation in red-tailed hawks (Buteo jamaicensis). Am J Vet Res. 2018;79(1):13–20.

60. Hawkins MG, Pascoe PJ, DiMaio Knych HK, Drazenovich TL, Kass PH, Sanchez-Migallon Guzman D. Effects of three fentanyl plasma concentrations on the minimum alveolar concentration of isoflurane in Hispaniolan Amazon parrots (Amazona ventralis). Am J Vet Res. 2018;79(6):600–5.

61. Santos EA, Monteiro ER, Herrera JR, et al. Total intravenous anesthesia in domestic chicken (Gallus gallus domesticus) with propofol alone or in combination with methadone, nalbuphine or fentanyl for ulna osteotomy. Vet Anaesth Analg. 2020;47(3):347–55.

Chapter 6

62. Pavez JC, Hawkins MG, Pascoe PJ, Knych HK, Kass PH. Effect of fentanyl target-controlled infusions on isoflurane minimum anaesthetic concentration and cardiovascular function in red-tailed hawks (Buteo jamaicensis). Vet Anaesth Analg. 2011;38(4):344–51.
63. Ratliff C, Parkinson LAB, Mans C. Effects of the fraction of inspired oxygen on alfaxalone-sedated inland bearded dragons (Pogona vitticeps). Am J Vet Res. 2019;80(2):129–34.
64. Phillips BE, Posner LP, Lewbart GA, Christiansen EF, Harms CA. Effects of alfaxalone administered intravenously to healthy yearling loggerhead sea turtles (Caretta caretta) at three different doses. J Am Vet Med Assoc. 2017;250(8):909–17.
65. Rasys AM, Divers SJ, Lauderdale JD, Menke DB. A systematic study of injectable anesthetic agents in the brown anole lizard (Anolis sagrei). Lab Anim. 2020;54(3):281–94.
66. Ferreira TH, Mans C. Evaluation of neuraxial anesthesia in bearded dragons (Pogona vitticeps). Vet Anaesth Analg. 2019;46(1):126–34.
67. Ferreira TH, Fink DM, Mans C. Evaluation of neuraxial administration of bupivacaine in bearded dragons (Pogona vitticeps). Vet Anaesth Analg. 2021;48(5):798–803.

Further reading

Balko JA, Chinnadurai SK. Advancements in evidence-based anesthesia of exotic animals. Vet Clin North Am Exot Anim Pract. 2017;20(3):917–28.

Ballard, BM, Cheek R (eds) *Exotic Animal Medicine for the Veterinary Technician*, 3rd edn. Hoboken, NJ: Wiley and Sons, 2017.

Bryant S. *Anesthesia for Veterinary Technicians*. New York: Wiley-Blackwell, 2010.

Carpenter JW, Marion C. *Exotic Animal Formulary*, 5th edn. St Louis, MO: Elsevier, 2016.

Divers SJ, Stahl SJ. *Mader's Reptile and Amphibian Medicine and Surgery*, 3rd edn. St Louis, MO: Elsevier, 2019.

Longley LA. *Anaesthesia of Exotic Pets*. St Louis, MO: Saunders, 2008.

Quesenberry K, Carpenter JW. *Ferrets, Rabbits, and Rodents: Clinical Medicine and Surgery*, 3rd edn. Philadelphia, PA: Elsevier Saunders, 2012.

Chapter 7

Nonopioid analgesia alternatives and locoregional blocks

Vaidehi Paranjape and Stephen Cital

Opioids form an integral part of an anesthesia regime to provide perioperative analgesia, sedation, and anesthetic-sparing effects in small animals. However, their significant side-effects and restricted availability due to the ongoing abuse crisis in humans warrant their limited use. Hence, opioid alternative techniques are increasingly being used to enhance the anesthetic and postanesthetic experience in animals. These include nonopioid analgesic infusions, oral gabapentanoids, psychotropic drugs, cannabinoids, antiinflammatories, nonpharmacologic pain modalities and robust use of local-regional anesthetic techniques, which are briefly reviewed in this chapter.

I. Nonopioid analgesic constant-rate infusions

Ketamine (N-methyl-D-aspartate receptor antagonist), dexmedetomidine (alpha-2 adrenoreceptor agonist), and lidocaine (sodium channel blocker) are routinely used as constant-rate infusions (CRIs) to provide analgesia in the perioperative period. With basic understanding of the major pain pathways, these drugs are used as either primary analgesics or adjunctive analgesics to provide multimodal analgesia.

A. Ketamine

The NMDA receptor is a ligand-gated, voltage-dependent ion channel, widely distributed in the CNS and primary sensory neurons. It serves as a binding site for glutamate, which is released with noxious peripheral stimuli.

1. Clinical uses

It serves as a noncompetitive antagonist at the NMDA receptor and is used at subanesthetic doses of 0.12–1.2 mg/kg/h as an adjunctive to other analgesics. These doses are less likely to produce dissociative and cardiostimulatory effects. Activation of NMDA receptor leads to the development of cancer, chronic, neuropathic and wind-up pain, central sensitization and hyperalgesia [1]. It may be more effective for somatic pain than visceral pain [2].

Small Animal Anesthesia Techniques, Second Edition. Edited by Amanda M. Shelby and Carolyn M. McKune.
© 2023 John Wiley & Sons, Inc. Published 2023 by John Wiley & Sons, Inc.
Companion website: www.wiley.com/go/shelby/anesthesia2

Additionally, it exhibits opioid-sparing effects and counteracts opioid-induced hyperalgesia. Authors recommend its cautious use in cats with progressive renal disease and hypertrophic cardiomyopathy.

B. Dexmedetomidine

1. Pharmacology

Alpha-2 adrenoceptors are a class of G protein-coupled receptors that serve as a primary site for norepinephrine and epinephrine. They are found peripherally and at spinal and supraspinal sites within the CNS. They induce antinociception by:

- stimulation of spinal alpha-2 receptors and direct inhibition of spinal cord neurons
- presynaptic inhibition of neurotransmitter release from the primary afferents in the dorsal horn
- neuronal hyperpolarization and inhibition of substance P release via postsynaptic actions
- inhibitory neuronal action at higher supraspinal structures [3].

2. Clinical uses

Dexmedetomidine is the most selective drug for alpha-2 adrenoreceptors, with a binding affinity for alpha-2:alpha-1 receptors reported as 1620:1. It is a pure S-enantiomer of the racemic medetomidine and is twice as potent as medetomidine. Micro-bolus doses of 0.0005–0.002 mg/kg can be given intraoperatively as needed, or 0.0005–0.002 mg/kg/h administered as a CRI for sedation, anxiolytic effect, anesthetic adjunct, inhalant-sparing effect, supplemental somatic and visceral analgesia, and muscle relaxation [4]. Cardiorespiratory monitoring is essential when it is used postoperatively. If excessive sedation or significant cardiovascular effects are extended into the recovery period, reversal with atipamezole IM is considered. Side-effects requiring possible intervention include bradycardia, atrioventricular blocks, respiratory depression, nausea, vomiting, and ileus. This drug should be avoided in patients with moderate-severe cardiac disease, cardiac arrhythmias, preexisting hypertension, and hypovolemia.

C. Lidocaine

1. Pharmacology

The systemic analgesic action is thought to be due to lidocaine's interaction with Na+, Ca2+, and K+ channels and the NMDA receptor [5].

2. Clinical uses

It is the only local anesthetic that is administered intravenously to provide analgesia and inhalant-sparing effects. It possesses antiinflammatory effects and free radical scavenging properties that contribute to management of inflammatory pain. In dogs, IV loading dose of

1–2 mg/kg followed by infusion rates of 3–6 mg/kg/h are commonly used for intraoperative analgesia. Lower infusion rates of 0.6–1.5 mg/kg/h are used postoperatively. In cats, studies show that the doses required to achieve inhalant-sparing effects can cause greater cardiovascular depression compared to an equipotent dose of isoflurane alone [6].

II. Oral gabapentinoids

Gabapentin was traditionally used as an anticonvulsant, but its benefits include anxiolysis, analgesia, antiallodynia, and antihyperalgesia. Pregabalin is structurally similar to gabapentin but has higher oral bioavailability and a longer half-life. However, at the time of writing, it is expensive. This makes gabapentin a more popular gabapentanoid for use during chronic pain; the authors encourage the reader to evaluate the prices from your distributors.

1. Pharmacology

Gabapentin is a structural analogue of gamma-aminobutyric acid (GABA) but does not interact with GABA receptors to produce analgesia. It binds to the α2δ subunit on the voltage-dependent calcium channels located in neurons of the peripheral and CNS. This reduces calcium influx into neurons and inhibits release of excitatory neurotransmitters like glutamate, substance P and norepinephrine that are actively involved in pain pathways.

2. Clinical uses

- *Dogs*: The therapeutic dose of gabapentin is 10–20 mg/kg PO 2–3 times daily. Sedation is a common side-effect. When included in the analgesic regime, it successfully controls pain associated with Chiari malformation and syringomyelia [7], neuropathies, mastectomy [8], and intervertebral disc surgery [9]. When 20 mg/kg PO is given 2 h prior to anesthetic induction, isoflurane requirement is reduced by 20 ± 14% with no effect on hemodynamic variables or vital parameters [10].
- *Cats*: Pharmacokinetic data suggest a dosing regimen of 5–10 mg/kg PO every 8–12 h for chronic musculoskeletal pain [11], hyperesthesia syndrome [12], and osteoarthritis [13]. It is often recommended orally to decrease the stress associated with transportation and veterinary examinations [14]. Sedation, ataxia, hypersalivation, and vomiting are reported side-effects, which tend to resolve 8 h after oral administration. Interestingly, IV gabapentin does not have a detectable effect on isoflurane requirement in cats [15].

III. Psychotropic drugs

Neuropathic pain is a result of a lesion or disease affecting the somatosensory system and is generally chronic and challenging to treat. With prolonged use, psychotropic drugs possibly relieve neuropathic pain by (1) recruitment of noradrenergic descending pathways, (2) peripheral recruitment of noradrenaline from sympathetic fibers sprouting into dorsal root ganglia, and (3) action via adrenergic receptors. Tricyclic antidepressants (TCAs, e.g., amitriptyline), selective serotonin reuptake inhibitors (SSRIs, e.g., fluoxetine), NMDA antagonists (e.g. amantadine), and atypical antidepressants (e.g., trazodone) are often used as adjunctive therapy for managing chronic pain states [16–18].

- *Amitriptyline*: Predominantly inhibits serotonin reuptake, whereas its metabolite nortriptyline specifically inhibits norepinephrine reuptake. Analgesic action is attributed to the blockade of voltage-gated sodium channels and NMDA receptors, as well as inhibition of norepinephrine reuptake. Antagonistic effects are also seen on alpha-1, cholinergic, and histamine receptors.
- *Fluoxetine*: Exclusively inhibits serotonin reuptake with eventual downregulation of postsynaptic serotonergic receptors.
- *Amantadine*: Antagonizes NMDA receptors in the CNS which helps prevent central sensitization, wind-up, allodynia, and opioid tolerance.
- *Trazodone*: Inhibits both serotonin transporter and serotonin type 2 receptors. It inhibits serotonin reuptake and blocks the histamine and alpha-1-adrenergic receptors [19].

1. Clinical uses

Psychotropic drugs are useful in clinical scenarios manifesting neuropathic pain such as Chiari-like malformation/syringomyelia, radiculopathy caused by chronic cervical or lumbosacral disc disease, diabetic or other polyneuropathies, spinal cord injury caused by intervertebral disc extrusion, chronic osteoarthritis, and musculoskeletal pain. Drug interactions can occur when different serotonin-enhancing agents are administered together (e.g., fluoxetine with tramadol or fluoxetine with selegiline) leading to "serotonin syndrome" (see Chapter 5, p. 154) [20]. It is vital that these interactions are well known to the prescribing clinician and owners. Other common adverse effects of psychotropic drugs include lethargy, sedation, vomiting, diarrhea, panting, hyperactivity, ataxia, increased anxiety, increased appetite, shaking, restlessness, and/or agitation. Arrhythmias, tachycardia, and orthostatic hypotension can be seen with high doses of TCAs.

2. Dosage

- Amitriptyline: 2–4 mg/kg PO q12h (dogs); 0.5–1 mg/kg PO q24h (cats).
- Fluoxetine: 1–2 mg/kg PO q24h (dogs); 0.5–1 mg/kg PO q24h (cats).
- Amantadine: 3–5 mg/kg PO q24 in dogs and cats.
- Trazodone: 5–7 mg/kg PO q24 (dogs); 50–100 mg total dose PO q24 (cats).

IV. Cannabinoids

1. Endocannabinoid system (ECS) and pain

The ECS is the largest G-protein-coupled receptor system with neuromodulatory functions. It is now known as one of the key endogenous systems regulating pain sensation, with modulatory actions at all stages of pain-processing pathways. Its effects are mediated by the interaction of cannabinoid receptors (CB1, CB2), endogenous ligands, and synthesizing and hydrolyzing enzymes [21,22]. CB1 receptors are mainly present in the brain and spinal cord and are responsible for centrally mediated analgesia as well as adverse central effects. They inhibit acetylcholine, L-glutamate, GABA, norepinephrine, dopamine, and serotonin. CB2 receptors are found in the hematopoietic and immune cells, including microglial cells. These are possibly involved in immune regulation and antiinflammatory effects [23].

Phytocannabinoids are molecules produced by the *Cannabis sativa* plant which can act on the ECS receptors. Hemp and marijuana are both varieties of the *Cannabis* genus. Hemp is a variety of cannabis that produces large amounts of cannabidiolic acid compared to the amount of tetrahydrocannabinolic acid produced. The inverse is true for marijuana. After harvesting and drying of the plant material, particularly the flowering tops of female plants, the acidic forms of these two prominent phytocannabinoids become decarboxylated into their mainstream personalities – cannabidiol (CBD) and tetrahydrocannabinol (THC). Tetrahydrocannabinol is a major intoxicating compound, associated with unpleasant clinical presentation in animals that consume this molecule. Animals may experience increased anxiety with mild-moderate doses of THC. Tolerance can be built up to THC as it is the only phytocannabinoid to sit in the orthosteric binding site on the CB1 receptor. The stronger affinity of THC compared to endogenous ligands when dosed chronically can downregulate endocannabinoid production which may have adverse physiologic consequences. Also, because of the risk and particular sensitivity of THC in companion animals, it may be best to avoid THC-dominant products and utilize products derived from hemp.

In addition, newer research has shown that THC alone is not a good analgesic for chronic [24] pain states. On the other hand, CBD may possess analgesic effects, best described in chronic or neuropathic pain states. Both of these phytochemical compounds, among the hundreds of other phytocannabinoids, have predominantly allosteric binding to ECS receptors and affinity/dimerizing effects on several receptors systems related to pain signaling which include the transient receptor potential vanilloid (TRPV), NMDA, glycine, G-protein-coupled (GPR55), GABA, and serotonin (5-HT) receptors [25].

2. Clinical uses

Well-controlled studies in companion animals on the efficacy of these compounds are increasing. Three pharmacokinetic studies in dogs found that doses of 2 mg/kg create adequate serum concentrations, related to therapeutic benefits extrapolated from other lab animals and human subjects. Three long-term studies (12, 39, and 56 weeks) have been performed in dogs with doses from 2 mg/kg up to 100 mg/kg. Mild-moderate elevations of liver enzymes were noted in the higher dose long-term studies [26,27]. In cats, only two studies have been published, elucidating that a 2 mg/kg dose may need to be given more than twice a day to maintain suspected therapeutic serum concentrations [28,29].

Efficacy of hemp CBD products has also been evaluated for management of osteoarthritic pain in dogs [30–32]. These studies had successful outcomes, particularly for pets on traditional pharmaceuticals such as NSAIDs and gabapentin. Owners were also able to eliminate the traditional pharmaceuticals out of the analgesia regime. Acute pain studies are still under way in companion animals; currently, only anecdote abounds [33].

Chapter 7

Dosing of CBD-dominant products will depend on the other phytocannabinoids and terpenes present. Terpenes are aromatic molecules also produced by the *Cannabis* plant that have their own set of therapeutic potentials. Doses from the two canine studies found oral doses of a full/complete spectrum cannabinoid product of 2 mg/kg twice a day to be safe and effective. The authors would suggest a dosing range of 0.5–2 mg/kg, or higher, depending on clinical response.

Clinicians prescribing cannabinoid products must be fully aware of the primary source (hemp vs marijuana), the concentration and the phytocannabinoid/terpene profile of the product verified by a certificate of analysis (COA). There are a few different types of phytocannabinoid products on the market being sold as animal supplements [34]. Clinicians may notice increased lethargy in patients that are on concurrent oral narcotics or gabapentanoids. Doses of the cannabinoid product or pharmaceutical are adjusted to minimize this effect. Other notable drug interactions occur with benzodiazepines, where patients may seem uncoordinated or ataxic.

V. Antiinflammatories

Long-term pharmacological management of pain in small animals includes use of nonsteroidal antiinflammatory drugs (NSAIDs) or corticosteroids. Nonsteroidal drugs possess antipyretic, antiinflammatory, and analgesic effects. Significant analgesic and antiinflammatory clinical effects are due to the inhibition of the COX enzyme isoforms and central pain transmission. They are widely used to control mild-moderate pain during the perioperative period as well as for chronic pain states. On the other hand, corticosteroids inhibit the production of arachidonic acid, which can stop the inflammation and stop the production of prostaglandins, similar to NSAIDs. They do not have a direct effect on nociception and are not primary analgesics. However, they are beneficial in controlling pain mediated via inflammatory processes as seen in musculoskeletal and joint disorders. More information on this class of drugs is available in the drug formulary (Section II).

VI. Nonpharmacological pain therapy

Acupuncture and physical rehabilitation are fundamental in the multimodal management of pain, especially of a chronic nature. These aid in balancing analgesic regimes, strengthening human–pet relationships, and increasing the quality of patient care and comfort.

A. Acupuncture

Acupuncture involves placement of percutaneous needles in specific anatomic locations on the body, like nerve bifurcations or neurovascular structures in tissues, in order to stimulate an endogenous response facilitating analgesia, healing, and immunomodulation. It also improves blood flow, inhibits inflammation, reduces muscle tension, resets proprioceptive mechanisms and posture, and affects autonomic nervous system. Stimulation of A-β, A-δ and C nociceptive fibers prevents pain transmission via local spinal inhibition of nociception, spinal release of endogenous opioids, and activation of inhibitory interneurons and descending inhibitory pain pathways. The bioactive acupuncture points lie along "meridians" that serve as an energetic distribution network following specific peripheral nerve pathways targeted for preventing nociception. Stimulation of acupuncture points in animals is manifested by a response to needle placement followed by sudden relaxation.

Acupuncture is a complex intervention requiring additional training. Clinical scenarios for its use include spinal cord injury/disease [35], wounds, chronic pain, osteoarthritis [36], visceral pain, and myofascial trigger point pain [37].

B. Physical rehabilitation

Physical rehabilitation involves objective assessment, diagnosis, and treatment of musculo-skeletal and neurologic impairments during acute, subacute, and chronic pain states. The assessment utilizes careful evaluation of posture, gait, function, strength, muscle extensibility, passive range of motion, and joints to create a problem list and develop an assessment from which targeted treatment modalities are developed. These modalities provide pain relief, promote soft tissue healing, improve muscle extensibility, and facilitate muscle strengthening. Some of the commonly used physical therapy modalities are described below.

1. Superficial thermotherapy

Application of heat to tissues increases nerve conduction velocity and blood flow, facilitating healing, muscle relaxation, and resolution of local ischemia. Heat activates cutaneous thermal receptors that inhibit pain transmission. Heat can be applied with hot packs or warm baths for 15–20 min at a time. It is avoided in acute stages of tissue injury.

2. Cryotherapy

Cooling results in vasoconstriction and a reduction in tissue metabolism and oxygen requirement, sensory and motor nerve conduction velocity, edema, and muscle spasm [37]. It is used in the acute inflammatory state. Ice packs should not be placed directly over the skin and their application should not exceed 10 min at a time. Portable machines, based on active compression and cold exchange loop technology, facilitate icing of limbs with tailored protocols, and may be quite useful to practices which extensively treat orthopedic pain [39,40].

3. Laser

Low-level laser therapy is light energy used to stimulate healing, provide pain relief, and facilitate the reorganization of injured tissues. The range of therapeutic window for this therapy is 600–1000 nm. It aims at imparting analgesia within the target tissue, and causes cartilage stimulation, fibroblast production, enhancement of immune cells to combat pathogens, acceleration of collagen synthesis, and increasing vascularity of the healing tissue [41]. It is used to reduce inflammation and treat musculoskeletal, neuropathic, and osteoarthritic pain [42–45]. Studies are conflicting regarding the benefits of this therapy.

4. Transcutaneous electrical nerve stimulation (TENS)

Electrotherapy targets sensory and motor nerve fibers, causing nerve cell excitation and changes in cell membrane permeability. This enables skeletal muscle and smooth muscle contraction, enhancing muscle-pumping action and improving joint mobility and circulatory and lymphatic drainage [46]. TENS decreases pain and inflammation by providing a low-level electrical current which disrupts the normal pain perception pathways. The pulse rate and width are adjusted to deliver the desired effect [47].

5. Extracorporeal shockwave therapy

This is production of high-pressure sound waves emitted at high velocity by a generator that converts electrical energy into mechanical energy. The acoustic waves are delivered either in a focused manner, with greater penetration into the deeper tissues, or in a radial manner, affecting a wider area. Its benefits include angiogenesis, increase in collagen synthesis, increase in bone remodeling, and decrease in inflammatory mediators. It is incorporated in analgesic protocols for various musculoskeletal and joint disorders [48–50].

6. Massage, therapeutic exercises

These therapeutic novelties increase connective tissue extensibility, vascular supply, and lymphatic drainage, and improve joint range of motion. Active and passive exercises are recommended for treatment of chronic pain associated with osteoarthritis. Reduced activity and deconditioning cause decreased muscle mass and strength, loss of endurance, increased joint stiffness, and loss of cardiovascular fitness. Reduction of pain and disability is achieved through improvement of muscle strength, stability of joints, and range of motion (ROM). Passive ROM exercises are used to enhance analgesia in inflamed joints and assist tissue stretching. Active ROM exercises are required to prevent muscle atrophy, increase strength and endurance, and enhance circulation [51].

7. Glucosamine-chondroitin, hyaluronic acid (HA) and platelet-rich plasma (PRP)

Glucosamine hydrochloride and chondroitin sulfate are commonly recommended natural health products for treating osteoarthritis in small animals. Glucosamine regulates the synthesis of collagen in cartilage and possesses mild antiinflammatory effects. Chondroitin sulfate inhibits destructive enzymes in joint fluid and cartilage [52]. Other novel therapies include PRP and HA, which are gaining momentum for their beneficial effects in canine osteoarthritis, as evidenced both clinically and histologically [53,54]. Both therapies are accessible and cost-effective for veterinary practitioners using commercially available products and kits [55].

8. Other nonpharmacologic techniques

Other nonpharmacologic techniques used in adjunctive management of acute and chronic pain include pulsating electromagnetic fields (PEMF), therapeutic ultrasound, neuromuscular electrical stimulation (NMES), myofascial release and trigger point therapy, nutraceuticals, and palliative radiotherapy.

Chapter 7

VII. Local-regional anesthetic techniques

A. Local anesthetics (LAs)

1. Pharmacology

Local anesthetics consist of a lipophilic benzene ring (confers liposolubility) and a hydrophilic amine group (confers hydrosolubility). These two structures are linked together with an ester or amide linkage. Drugs with ester linkage include cocaine, procaine, tetracaine, and benzocaine that undergo hydrolysis by pseudocholinesterase in the blood and require minimal liver metabolism. Drugs with amide linkage include lidocaine, mepivacaine, bupivacaine, and ropivacaine which undergo extensive oxidative metabolism in the liver via cytochrome P450. Hepatic blood flow and hepatic function determine the clearance of these drugs. Hence, they are used cautiously in patients with liver disease. More information regarding the most commonly used LAs is provided in Table 7.1.

Table 7.1 Commonly used local anesthetics and their toxic doses.

Drug name	Onset of action	Duration of action	Comments
Lidocaine	1–3 min	1–2 h	Dose 4–6 mg/kg (dogs); 2–4 mg/kg (cats) Toxic IV dose for CNS toxicity: 20–mg/kg (dogs); 12–mg/kg (cats) Toxic IV dose for cardiovascular collapse: 80–mg/kg (dogs); 47 mg/kg (cats) Authors suggest do not exceed 6 mg/kg in dogs and 3 mg/kg in cats by any route
Mepivacaine	3–5 min	2–3 h	Dose 4–6 mg/kg (dogs); 2–3 mg/kg (cats) Toxic IV dose for CNS toxicity: 29–mg/kg (dogs) Toxic IV dose for cardiovascular collapse: 80–mg/kg (dogs); unknown in cats Authors suggest do not exceed 6 mg/kg in dogs and 3 mg/kg in cats
Ropivacaine	5–10 min	5–8 h	Dose 1–3 mg/kg (dogs); 1–2 mg/kg (cats) Toxic IV dose for CNS toxicity: 4.8 mg/kg (dogs); unknown in cats Toxic IV dose for cardiovascular collapse: 42 mg/kg (dogs); unknown in cats Authors suggest do not exceed 3 mg/kg in dogs and 2 mg/kg in cats
Bupivacaine	2–20 min	4–8 h	Dose 1–2 mg/kg (dogs); 1 mg/kg (cats) Toxic IV dose for CNS toxicity: 4–8 mg/kg (dogs); 4 mg/kg (cats) Toxic IV dose for cardiovascular collapse: 20 mg/kg (dogs); 18 mg/kg (cats) Authors suggest do not exceed 3 mg/kg in dogs and 2 mg/kg in cats

Note: It is important to bear in mind the sliding scale of toxicity of these agents. In humans, the first known side-effect of accumulating local anesthetic is tinnitus, or ringing in the ears. As this would be difficult to identify in companion animal species, veterinarians often see nausea and vomiting, which can progress to seizures (CNS toxicity) and then cardiovascular collapse. Suggested doses are given with the intent to reduce all complications, although this may vary by patient. CNS, central nervous system; IV, intravenous. *Source*: Adapted from [56].

Chapter 7

2. Analgesic action

Local anesthetics bind to sodium channels present in the peripheral neurons during their inactive state. This prevents subsequent channel activation and inhibition of sodium permeability that occurs with membrane depolarization. As the threshold level for the action potential is not attained, suppression of nerve signal transmission occurs between neurons.

3. Clinical considerations

Local anesthetics with larger molecular weights, greater lipid solubility, and higher protein binding (e.g., bupivacaine) have a longer duration of action. The onset of action is related to the lipid solubility of the drug. The rate at which a LA diffuses into a nerve is determined by its concentration. The higher the concentration, the more rapid the onset of the block. Because of the lack of evidence showing a consistent advantage of mixing LAs, the authors prefer to simply select a single agent based on its desired and predictable characteristics [57].

4. Adjuncts used with LAs

Epinephrine may be used with LAs to cause vasoconstriction and therefore prolong the duration of action of LAs and intensity of the blockade. It also reduces the systemic absorption of LAs and decreases the probability of systemic toxicity. However, caution is advised if LA with epinephrine is used on extremities, as ischemia of the tissue may result. Preservative-free buprenorphine (0.004 mg/kg) with bupivacaine injected into the epidural space provided up to 24 h analgesia in dogs undergoing stifle arthroplasty [56]. It is also used for perineural injections in order to extend the analgesic duration of LAs.

Alpha-2 agonists like dexmedetomidine when added to LAs enhance analgesia via hyperpolarization of C fibers during neuraxial anesthesia and peripheral nerve blocks. These drugs can produce analgesia through supraspinal and spinal mechanisms (via adrenergic receptors) and have inhibitory effects on conduction of nerve impulses. A dose of 0.1 µg/kg added to LA in femoral nerve blocks effectively prolongs analgesia for 24 h [56]. The same dose is also used for perineural injections.

Ketamine produces localized hypoalgesia due to its LA-like effects, which may be through its ability to inhibit neuronal sodium channels. Apart from causing NMDA blockade-mediated analgesia in the CNS and spinal cord receptors, ketamine also interacts with opioid and monoaminergic receptors. Thoracic epidural administration of lidocaine with ketamine provides longer duration of analgesia of the thorax and forelimbs bilaterally in dogs [58].

5. Local anesthetic toxicity

Administration of an incorrect dose and inadvertent IV administration are likely the most common causes of systemic toxicity. Cats are most susceptible to developing methemoglobinemia after topical exposure to products containing benzocaine, which should be avoided in these species [59]. Toxicity of local anesthetics is additive by nature and may be due to multiple routes of exposure (topical and regional), mixtures of local anesthetics, or recurrent dosing. Post IV overdose, initial clinical signs include salivation, vomiting, and hypothermia. There is an immediate progression to pronounced CNS signs like nystagmus, muscle twitching, convulsions, tremors/seizures, and generalized CNS depression. These are then followed by cardiovascular effects like hypotension, bradycardia, and arrhythmias. Muscle tremors and seizures are managed with benzodiazepines (0.2–0.4 mg/kg IV) or propofol (2–4 mg/kg IV).

Hypotension is treated with IV crystalloids and a vasopressor (phenylephrine 0.1–3 µg/kg/min). 20% lipid emulsion is recommended at 4 mL/kg initial bolus over 2 min followed by an infusion 0.25 mL/kg/min for 20–30 min. This extracts the LA from the aqueous plasma into a "lipid sink," making it unavailable to the tissues [60].

Other supportive therapy includes airway management, treating arrhythmias, and cardiopulmonary resuscitation if cardiac arrest ensues.

B. Equipment used for local-regional anesthesia

1. Needles

Small-gauge needles (25–27 G) minimize the risk of nerve injury and are generally used for infiltration anesthesia and superficial blocks (e.g., dental blocks). Large-gauge needles of a longer length (19–22 G, 1.5–3.5 inch) are used for deeper blocks (e.g., brachial plexus, epidural). Spinal needles with removable stylets are sharp, specially designed for penetrating the dura mater. Tuohy needles are blunt-ended, curved at the distal tip, and used for epidural injections or placement of indwelling epidural catheters. Insulated nerve block needles, which are also blunt-ended, are coated with a thin layer of nonconducting material over the entire length of the needle except for a small area at the distal tip. When the needle is connected to a peripheral nerve stimulator, low-intensity currents (0.2–0.5 mA) can stimulate motor fibers, allowing successful identification of the target nerves.

2. Peripheral nerve stimulator (PNS)

This device generates a square-wave electrical current to locate target nerves, when used with an insulated needle (Figure 7.1). At sufficiently low currents (0.4–1 mA), if the stimulating needle elicits contractions of the muscle group of the target nerve, it indicates that the needle-to-nerve proximity is ideal for an injection of LA to cause a sensory block. If current is still conducted at 0.4 mA or less, it is likely that the needle is intraneuronal; it is advised to back the needle out prior to injection to avoid perineural injections, which may damage the nerve.

3. Ultrasound machine

Ultrasound allows for real-time visualization of the stimulating needle, as well as identification of peripheral nerves and other anatomic structures such as vessels, muscles, and fasciae. Ultrasound guidance and electrolocation are often used together while performing nerve blocks, to increase the accuracy of nerve location and efficacy of the blockade. High-frequency linear transducers (10–15 MHz) are suitable for performing most peripheral nerve blocks, and imaging superficial nerves that are less than 5 cm in depth. It is crucial that the anesthetist has: (1) a thorough understanding of the operative functions and basic principles of the ultrasound

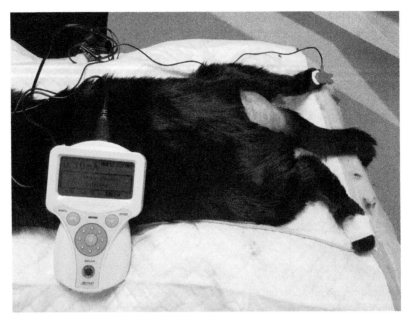

Figure 7.1   A peripheral nerve stimulator in use for the placement of a sacrococcygeal epidural injection.

machine; (2) knowledge of anatomy and landmarks surrounding the target nerves; and (3) training to identify the echogenicity of the peripheral nerves, muscles, bones, fasciae, and blood vessels.

C. Local-regional anesthesia

Injection of LA around a particular nerve or nerve roots produces loss of sensation (sensory block) with or without paralysis (motor block) in that region, depending on the drug and its concentration. Different techniques for delivering LAs include topical anesthesia, infiltration anesthesia, neuraxial anesthesia, and peripheral nerve blocks. Some of the most common techniques are briefly reviewed below but fully described in the digital addendum. Additional resources for regional anesthesia strategies in small animals are listed at the end of this chapter.

1. Topical anesthesia

Topical lidocaine spray (2%, 4% or 10% solution) is available for laryngeal desensitization before tracheal intubation. A eutectic mixture of local anesthetics (EMLA) cream or patches (2.5% lidocaine and 2.5% prilocaine) prevent pain associated with peripheral catheter placement [61,62], superficial skin closure and blood sampling [63]. The cream is applied to the skin and covered with a dressing to enable absorption of the LAs. Time to achieve local effect is 45–60 min and it lasts up to 2 h after the dressing is removed. Transdermal self-adhesive lidocaine patches (Lidoderm®, 5%, Teikoku Pharma) are used for surgical, incisional or trauma wounds. The manufacturer recommends placing the patch about 1 cm from the incision edge, covering the entire length of the incision to produce prolonged dynamic pain control and reduce requirement of systemic opioids postoperatively. However, some investigators found no adverse effects when the patch was placed directly over the incision [64]. This patch is cut to the desired length and shape. Plasma peak lidocaine concentrations are reached in 12–60 h in dogs and cats, with duration of analgesic effect lasting for 3–5 days [65,66]. Lidoderm and EMLA cream provide dermal anesthesia and minimal systemic absorption of the LA occurs via these methods.

2. Infiltration anesthesia

Incisional, intraperitoneal, and tissue infiltration of LAs is used for a variety of surgeries, wound care, multimodal analgesia, and in sterilization programs carried out in countries with limited drug availability [67]. Splash blocks are performed prior to closure of an incisional site to provide local analgesia [68] (Table 7.2). Wound infiltration using a multifenestrated catheter inserted into the surgical wound at the end of the procedure is a novel method of permitting repeated or continuous infusion of LAs for a prolonged period of time for postoperative analgesia [69] (Figure 7.2). The nerve endings in the tissues or in the area of infiltration are desensitized, thus preventing nociception. Infiltration technique should be avoided in infected tissues/wounds, as pH changes render LAs ineffective, and for masses where malignant cells may be spread beyond margins by the needle used. Care must be taken not to exceed the toxic dose for LAs (see Table 7.1).

A liposome-encapsulated injectable suspension of bupivacaine (Nocita®, Elanco) is the newest FDA-approved formulation for providing postoperative analgesia using a single injection technique at the time of incision closure for stifle surgery in dogs [70,71], and for regional analgesia following onychectomy in cats. It is also used for tissue infiltration during wound/incision closure (off-label) and nerve blocks not at incisional sites (off-label except for blockade of the radius/ulnar/musculocutaneous nerves). It consists of a unique liposomal delivery technology that encapsulates the bupivacaine with liposomal chambers.

Table 7.2   Infiltrative or splash blocks.

Materials: 20–22 G needle, appropriately sized labeled syringe with local anesthetic solution, aseptic preparation, disposable or sterile gloves
Drugs: 0.5–0.75% bupivacaine 1–2 mg/kg for dogs and 1 mg/kg for cats; 2% lidocaine 3 mg/kg in dogs and 2 mg/kg in cats. Dilution can be achieved by 0.9% normal saline
Infiltrative technique: An infiltrative block involves distribution of local anesthetic into tissue, usually subcutaneous, around a mass or area of incision. Area is clipped and aseptically prepped prior to block
Splash technique: Splash block involves the "splashing" of local anesthetic over an incision after closure of the muscle layer, but prior to closure of the skin. The solution is given sterilely to the surgeon for administration or splashed sterilely into incision

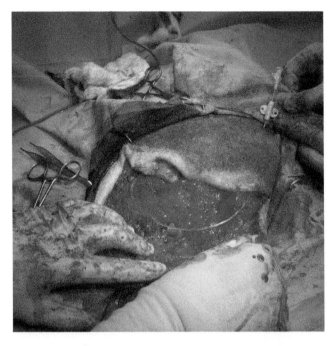

Figure 7.2 A soaker catheter placed by the surgical team for wound infiltration.

Post administration, these chambers break down, gradually releasing the bupivacaine over an extended period (72 h). Injection at closure prevents liposome disruption during surgical tissue manipulation. Slow bupivacaine release results in lower systemic exposure and decreased incidence of adverse effects. It is essential to use a 22 G or larger bore needle for the injection as smaller-bore needles can disrupt the liposomes [72]. This liposomal bupivacaine may not be as effective when used for a splash block.

Dosage for liposome-encapsulated injectable suspension of bupivacaine is as follow.

- *Dogs*: 5.3 mg/kg (0.4 mL/kg) total dose for local infiltration injection. The label indication allows for an equivalent amount of saline added to the drug to cover a larger surface area.
- *Cats*: 5.3 mg/kg per forelimb (0.4 mL/kg per forelimb) prior to onychectomy; total dose 10.6 mg/kg.

3. Neuraxial anesthesia

Epidural anesthesia is the administration of LA (or other drugs, e.g., opioids) into the epidural space (outside the dura) (Figure 7.3). If the drug is injected in the subarachnoid space, it is called spinal/intrathecal anesthesia. Epidural blocks are typically performed in anesthetized or heavily sedated patients, to relieve acute and chronic pain associated with a variety of surgeries and medical conditions. Analgesia occurs due to the bathing of the spinal nerve roots with the LAs. The extent of spinal nerve blockade following an epidural injection depends on the site of injection and the volume injected. Greater volumes cause cranial spread of the injected

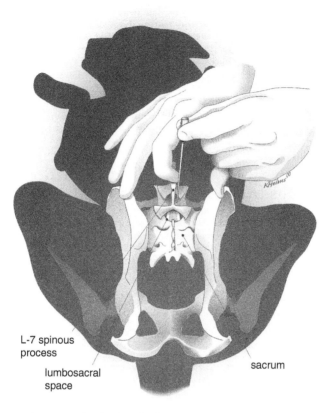

L-7 spinous
process

lumbosacral
space

sacrum

Figure 7.3   Diagram demonstrating landmarks for epidural placement. *Source:* Courtesy of
Teton NewMedia.

Chapter 7

solution, increasing the area of desensitization. Also, higher concentrations of LAs are associated with more profound and prolonged blockade.

a. Lumbosacral (LS) epidural anesthesia (Table 7.3)
- *Area and nerves blocked*: Pelvic plexus nerves, pelvic limbs, perineum, and tail. If total injectate volume is 0.2–0.3 mL/kg, desensitization can extend up to T13.
- *Landmarks*: Dorsal midline between L7 and S1.
- *Indications*: To provide analgesia for procedures involving the perineal/urogenital region, middle and caudal abdomen, pelvic limbs, and tail.
- *Complications*: (1) Excess injectate volume can cause cranial migration, leading to blockade of the diaphragm, impairing ventilation; (2) urinary retention if preservative-free morphine is used; (3) spinal injection can cause hypotension, cardiovascular collapse, and apnea; (4) LA toxicity can occur with high doses; (5) spinal cord and nerve root damage; (6) intravascular injection in the internal venous plexus.
- *Contraindications*: Skin infection over lumbosacral region, abnormal pelvic anatomy, patients with bleeding disorders, uncorrected hypovolemia or hypotension, neoplasia at the site of injection, sepsis.

Table 7.3   Lumbosacral (LS) epidural placement (Figures 7.4–7.7).

Materials: Aseptic skin preparation supplies, sterile gloves, spinal needle/Tuohy needle of appropriate diameter and length, drugs in appropriately labeled syringes, +/– glass syringe, +/– nerve stimulator and appropriate insulated needle, +/– sterile 0.9% normal saline

Drugs: Preservative-free (PF) morphine 0.1 mg/kg +/– bupivacaine PF 0.5–1.0 mg/kg or lidocaine PF 0.5 mg/kg not to exceed calculated total volume[a]

Technique:

1. Once patient is heavily sedated or anesthetized, place animal in lateral or sternal recumbency and pull hindlimbs ventral (forward).

2. Clip a 10 × 10 cm square area over the LS space; aseptically prepare site.

3. Open gloves and sterilely place necessary materials on glove cover paper; glove carefully, avoiding contaminating materials.

4. Palpate the iliac wings with thumb and middle finger. Use index finger to palpate the LS junction (usually just caudal to a line drawn between the two iliac wings).

5. In the canine, on midline, insert the needle perpendicular to the skin, approximately halfway between the spinous process of L7 and the sacrum (S1). In the feline, the junction is slightly more caudal.

6. Remove stylet from the spinal needle, once through the skin, and place a few drops of sterile 0.9% normal saline in the needle hub. On further advancement of the needle, feel for two "pops" (resistance which dissipates abruptly). The first minor pop is passage through muscle fascia. The next, more prominent pop signifies passing through the ligamentum flavum. If bone is encountered while advancing the needle, withdraw the needle to just below the surface of the skin, reassess location, and redirect the needle if no blood is present in the needle hub. At this point, the saline is pulled into the epidural space ("sucked") from the hub of the needle. Positive "hanging drop" test signifies aspiration of fluid in the hub of the needle as the epidural space is entered.

7. The other confirmatory tests are loss of resistance (LOR) and nerve stimulation.
    LOR: Place 1–2 mL of air in a glass syringe or loss of resistance syringe and secure to the spinal needle. Test for loss of resistance by injecting air to see if the plunger of the syringe advances smoothly. If there is no resistance, the needle is in the epidural space.
    Nerve stimulation: When using a nerve stimulator, a nerve stimulation test (0.7 mA, 1 Hz, 0.1 ms) will elicit muscle contraction of the pelvic limbs and tail. However, it does not differentiate if the needle tip is in the epidural or subarachnoid space.

8. If cerebrospinal fluid (CSF) is present in the needle hub, reduce the dose of drugs by 50%. CSF is more likely to be encountered in cats because the spinal cord ends (L7–S1) more caudally than in dogs. If blood is present in the needle hub, remove needle completely. Another fresh attempt can be made or adopt an alternative analgesic technique.

9. A 1 mL air bubble placed in the drug syringe helps to confirm that the needle remained in the epidural space (during injection of drugs, the air bubble will not collapse). Some anesthesiologists recommend aspirating prior to drug injection for blood or CSF. Inject drugs slowly over 90–120 seconds; injections should be smooth (no resistance).

10. The authors advocate putting the affected limb down to encourage epidural spread to that region, especially if local anesthetics were used.

[a]Total volume calculation options: 1 mL/10 kg for perianal, 1 mL/7 kg for hindlimb procedures, 1 mL/5 kg for thoracic/abdominal procedure. Avoid total volumes over 6 mL. Sterile 0.9% normal saline is used to add volume if desired.

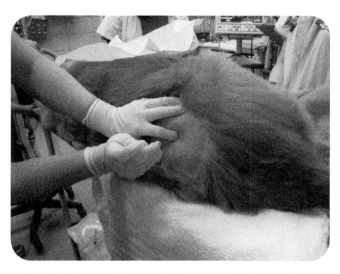

Figure 7.4   L7–S1 epidural placement in a canine patient in lateral recumbency.

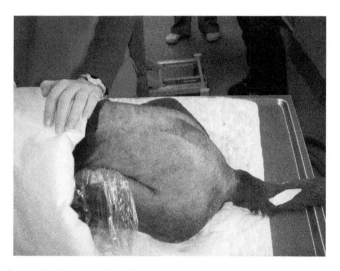

Figure 7.5   Canine patient in sternal positioning during an epidural technique.

- *Practical points*: (1) Epidural catheters are an option in larger dogs and maintained for several days to allow continuous or intermittent delivery of analgesic drugs; (2) in cats, there is a risk of spinal cord damage with traumatic injection as their spinal cord ends at L7, as opposed to the canine patient whose spinal cord ends at L5–6; (3) epidural anesthesia may provide long duration (12–24 h) of analgesia, and reduce inhalant requirements; (4) preservative-free drugs are recommended; (4) postoperative expression of urinary bladder must be performed (more so if morphine is used), and the patient is observed to ensure normal urination for 24 h post epidural.

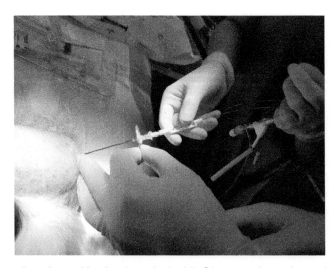

Figure 7.6   Threading of an epidural catheter in the L7–S1 space of a canine patient.

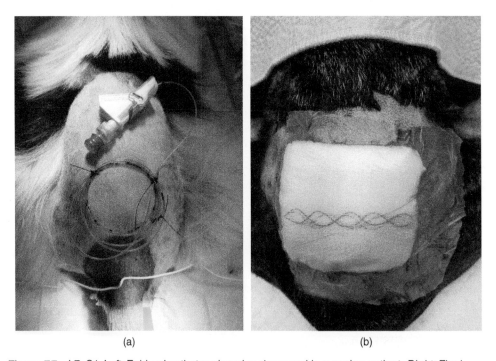

(a)   (b)

Figure 7.7   L7–S1. *Left*: Epidural catheter placed and secured in a canine patient. *Right*: Final fixation of the epidural catheter with an adhesive plaster.

b. Sacrococcygeal (SC) or intercoccygeal (IC) epidural anesthesia (Table 7.4)
   • *Area and nerves blocked*: Pudendal, pelvic, and caudal nerves supplying soft tissue structures of the sacrum, perineum, and tail region.
   • *Landmarks*: SC space or IC articulation between first and second coccygeal vertebrae.

Table 7.4 Sacrococcygeal (SC) or intercoccygeal (IC) epidural anesthesia placement.

Materials: Aseptic skin preparation supplies, sterile gloves, spinal needle or hypodermic needle of appropriate diameter and length, drugs in appropriately labeled syringes, +/− nerve stimulator and appropriate insulated needle, +/− sterile 0.9% normal saline

Drugs: Preservative-free (PF) morphine 0.1 mg/kg +/− 0.5% bupivacaine PF 0.5 mg/kg or 2% lidocaine PF 0.5 mg/kg not to exceed calculated total volume[a]

Technique:

1. Once patient is heavily sedated/anesthetized, place animal in sternal recumbency.
2. Clip a 10 × 10 cm square area over the SC or IC space; aseptically prepare site.
3. Open gloves and sterilely place necessary materials on glove cover paper; glove carefully, avoiding contaminating materials.
4. Palpate the most mobile joint caudal to the sacrum with the nondominant index finger (sacrococcygeal or 1st intercoccygeal space). It is identified by up-and-down movement ("pumping") of the tail. An attendant mobilizes the tail to avoid breaking sterility.
5. The dominant hand is used to insert a hypodermic or spinal needle at a 30–45° angle through the skin on the dorsal midline. Remove stylet from the spinal needle, once through the skin. If the needle hits the vertebral bone, it is repositioned by making slight changes in the angle of entry until it pierces through the ligamentum flavum, generating a palpable "pop".
6. Confirmation of accurate needle tip placement: (1) palpable "pop" may be encountered as the needle penetrates the ligamentum flavum (sharpness of hypodermic needles can cause lack of "pop" response in spite of being in the correct location); (2) loss of resistance while injecting; (3) relaxation of the rectum and tail muscles; (4) nerve stimulation test (0.7 mA, 0.1 ms, 1 Hz) will elicit muscle contraction of the middle and distal third of the tail (SC approach).
7. If blood is present in the needle hub, remove needle completely. Another fresh attempt can be made or adopt an alternative analgesic technique.
8. A 1 mL air bubble placed in the drug syringe helps to confirm that the needle remained in the epidural space (during injection of drugs, the air bubble will not collapse). Inject drugs slowly over 90–120 seconds; injections should be smooth (no resistance).
9. If tail/anus relaxation does not occur within 5 min (within 8–10 min with bupivacaine), the injection may have been made subcutaneously.

[a]Total volume calculation options: 1. To block pelvic limb motor function, use total volume of 0.2 mL/kg; 2. for tail and perineal surgeries use total volume of 0.1 mL/kg. Avoid total volumes over 6 mL. Sterile 0.9% NaCl is used to add volume if desired.

- *Indications*: To provide analgesia for tail amputation, anal sacculectomy, perineal urethrostomy, perineal mass removal, deobstipation, assisted vaginal delivery of puppies or kittens, correction of urinary obstruction.
- *Complications*: (1) Excess injectate volume can cause cranial migration, leading to motor nerve blockade of the pelvic region; (2) urinary retention if morphine is used (see Practical points); and (3) LA toxicity can occur with high doses.
- *Contraindications*: Patients with bleeding disorders, uncorrected hypovolemia and hypotension, infections, and neoplasia at the site of injection and sepsis.
- *Practical points*: (1) Chances of spinal cord damage or intrathecal injection with SC and IC approach are eliminated; (2) in scenarios where these approaches cannot be performed, lumbosacral injection is considered; (3) preservative-free drugs are recommended; (4) expression of urinary bladder must be performed (more so if morphine is used), and the patient is observed to ensure normal urination for 24 h post epidural.

D. Peripheral nerve blocks

1. Head

a. Infraorbital nerve block

- *Area and nerves blocked*: Infraorbital nerves supplying the caudal, medial, and rostral superior alveolar nerves, multiple nerve branches innervating the upper lip, buccal and nasal areas (Figures 7.8. and 7.9).
- *Landmarks*: Infraorbital foramen and zygomatic arch.

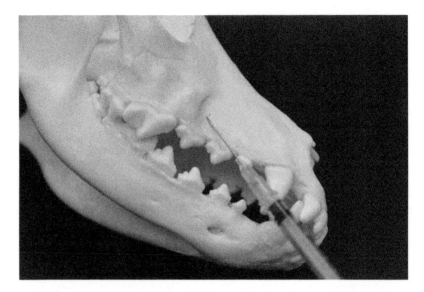

Figure 7.8   Infraorbital nerve block in canine skeleton. *Source:* Courtesy of Anderson da Cunha.

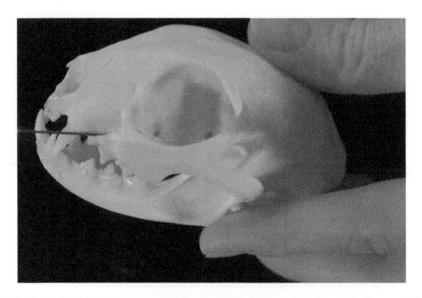

Figure 7.9   Infraorbital nerve block in the feline skeleton. *Source:* Courtesy of Anderson da Cunha.

Table 7.5 Infraorbital nerve block.

Materials: Disposable or sterile gloves, hypodermic needles (23–25 G) or 24 G catheter, drug solution labeled in 1 mL syringe
Drugs: 0.5% bupivacaine or 2% mepivacaine or 2% lidocaine 1–1.5 mg/kg. Generally, the dose per site is dependent on the patient size and weight and is 0.1–1 mL/site (dog) and 0.1–0.3 mL/site (cat)
Technique:
1. Place the heavily sedated or anesthetized patient in lateral or sternal recumbency. Palpate the infraorbital foramen (on the buccal side of the maxilla, usually above the 3rd premolar in dogs and 2nd premolar in cats).
2. Place the index finger over the foramen to guide needle and insert a 23–25 G needle or 24 G catheter (sliding catheter into the foramen into the canal) into the opening of the foramen. Inserting a needle deeper into foramen increases the chance of injecting into the nerve. A shorter needle engages into the foramen.
3. Aspirate; if no blood is present, inject local anesthetic solution over 30 seconds around opening of and slightly within the foramen. Little to no resistance to injection is felt when the needle is correctly placed.

- *Indications*: Analgesia for maxillary canine, molar, and premolar extractions, surgeries on hard and soft tissues of ipsilateral maxilla, nose, and upper lip, rhinotomy, rhinoscopy, and palatal surgery.
- *Complications*: (1) Nerve, vessel, or soft tissue injury from the needle; (2) injury to the ocular globe (especially in cats due to a short infraorbital canal).
- *Contraindications*: Infection, inflammation, or neoplasia at the site of injection.
- *Practical points*: (1) Required drug volumes are low due to small size of foramen; (2) foramen size in dogs is 1–2-cm long (shorter in brachycephalic breeds) and 4 mm long in cats, which warrants use of short needles or a 24 G catheter (Table 7.5).

b. Maxillary nerve block
- *Area and nerves blocked*: All maxillary teeth and associated soft structures, skin of the nose, cheek, upper lip and possibly ipsilateral hard and soft palate.
- *Indications*: Analgesia for performing procedures on any tooth or soft and hard tissues of the ipsilateral maxilla.
- *Landmarks*: Maxillary tuberosity, maxillary molar teeth, zygomatic arch, pterygopalatine fossa (Figures 7.10 and 7.11).
- *Complications*: Nerve, vessel or soft tissue injury from the needle; puncture or laceration of the maxillary artery.
- *Contraindications*: Infection, inflammation, or neoplasia at the site of injection.
- *Practical points*: Required drug volumes are low due to small size of foramen. This warrants short needles (Table 7.6).

c. Caudal inferior alveolar (mandibular) nerve block
- *Area and nerves blocked*: Mandibular tooth, rostral lower lip, rostral intermandibular region, lower dental arch and soft tissue and periosteum of the lingual side of the mandible (Figures 7.12–7.14).

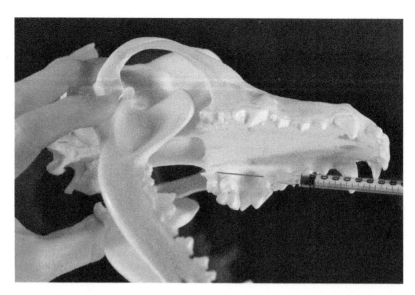

Figure 7.10   Maxillary nerve block via internal approach in the skeleton of a dog. *Source:* Courtesy of Anderson da Cunha.

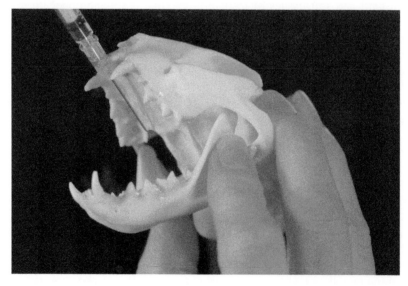

Figure 7.11   Maxillary nerve block via internal approach in the skeleton of a cat. *Source:* Courtesy of Anderson da Cunha

- *Indications*: Extraction of mandibular tooth, procedures involving lower lip and inter-mandibular region.
- *Landmarks*: Mandibular foramen, angular process of mandible, last molar tooth.
- *Complications*: Nerve, vessel or soft tissue injury from the needle
- *Contraindications*: Infection, inflammation, or neoplasia at the site of injection.
- *Practical points*: Required drug volumes are low due to small size of foramen. This warrants short needles (Table 7.7).

Table 7.6   Maxillary nerve block.

Materials: Disposable or sterile gloves, hypodermic needles (23–25 G), drug solution labeled in 1 mL syringe

Drugs: 0.5% bupivacaine or 2% mepivacaine or 2% lidocaine up to 1–1.5 mg/kg. Generally, the dose per site is dependent on the patient size and weight and is 0.1–1 mL/site (dog) and 0.1–0.3 mL/site (cat).

Technique (inside mouth approach):

1. Place the heavily sedated or anesthetized patient in lateral or dorsal recumbency. Open the mouth wide and retract lips at the lateral commissure. Laterally from the caudal nasal spine of the palatine lies the pterygopalatine fossa and pterygoid process (the maxillary nerve passes through the pterygoid fossa).

2. Insert a 23–25 G needle into the area near the pterygoid fossa, dorsally immediately caudal to the maxillary second and third molars, in a perpendicular angle to the maxilla.

3. Aspirate to rule out blood, and then inject the drug solution over 30 seconds. Little to no resistance to injection is felt when the needle is correctly placed.

Technique (from outside mouth):

1. A 23–25 G needle is inserted perpendicular to the skin just ventral to the zygomatic arch and 0.5 cm caudal to the lateral canthus of the eye. Direct the needle perpendicular to the arch.

2. Insert the needle to the level of the pterygopalatine fossa and maxillary nerve.

3. Aspirate to rule out blood, and then inject the drug solution over 30 seconds. Little to no resistance to injection is felt when the needle is correctly placed.

---

d. Mental nerve block

- *Area and nerves blocked*: Middle mental nerve, rostral alveolar branch of inferior alveolar nerve, lower incisors and canine tooth, rostral intermandibular region and lower lip (Figures 7.15 and 7.16).
- *Indications*: Analgesia for mandibular canine, molar and premolar extractions, rostral intermandibular region, and lower lip mass removal.
- *Landmarks*: Middle mental foramen, mandibular canine tooth.
- *Complications*: Nerve, vessel or soft tissue injury from the needle.
- *Contraindications*: Infection, inflammation, or neoplasia at the site of injection.
- *Practical points*: Required drug volumes are low due to small size of foramen. This warrants short needles (Table 7.8).

e. Retrobulbar nerve block

- *Area and nerves blocked*: Oculomotor, trochlear, trigeminal, and abducens nerves, ciliary ganglion, conjunctiva, cornea, and uvea [73].
- *Indications*: Analgesia for enucleation, evisceration with intrascleral prosthesis and necessity for central rotation of the globe.
- *Landmarks*: Lateral canthus, middle of lower eyelid and bony rim of the lower orbit (Figure 7.17).

Chapter 7

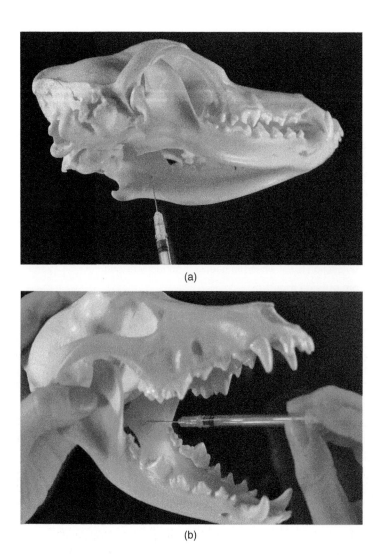

(a)

(b)

Figure 7.12 Approaches for a caudal inferior alveolar (mandibular) nerve block in a canine skull. *Source:* Courtesy of Anderson da Cunha.

- *Complications*: (1) Globe penetration; (2) nerve or vessel injury; (3) inadvertent injection of local anesthetic in the perineural optic nerve sheath; (4) retrobulbar hemorrhage and proptosis of the eye (seen with higher volumes in brachycephalic breeds); (5) intrathecal injection.
- *Contraindications*: Infection, inflammation, or neoplasia at the site of injection.
- *Practical points*: There are several approaches with different complications depending on the experience of the individual performing the block (Table 7.9).

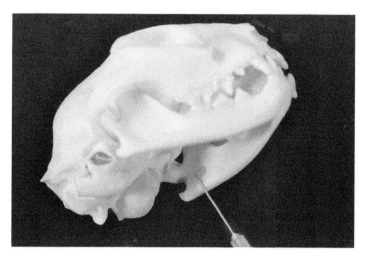

Figure 7.13 Caudal inferior alveolar (mandibular) nerve block in a feline skull. *Source:* Courtesy of Anderson da Cunha.

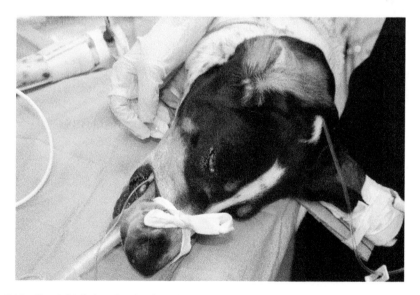

Figure 7.14 Caudal inferior alveolar (mandibular) nerve block in canine patient. *Source:* Courtesy of Anderson da Cunha.

f. Auriculotemporal nerve block and greater auricular nerve block

- *Area and nerves blocked*: Auriculotemporal nerve, great auricular nerve, external acoustic meatus, base of the auricle or pinna [74] (Figures 7.18 and 7.19).
- *Indications*: Analgesia for procedures of the external acoustic meatus, tympanic bulla, and pinna, acute and chronic auricular pain management.

Table 7.7   Caudal inferior alveolar (mandibular) nerve block.

Materials: Disposable or sterile gloves, hypodermic needles (23–25 G), drug solution labeled in 1 mLsyringe.

Drugs: 0.5% bupivacaine or 2% mepivacaine or 2% lidocaine up to 1–1.5 mg/kg. Generally, the dose per site is dependent on the patient size and weight and is 0.1–1 mL/site (dog) and 0.1–0.3 mL/site (cat).

Technique:

1. Place the heavily sedated or anesthetized patient in a lateral or dorsal recumbency. Palpate the mandibular foramen on the caudal, medial (lingual) surface of the ramus (curve of the mandible) behind the last molar. The foramen is palpable both internally on the lingual side of the ramus, or externally.

2. Use index finger of the opposite hand to guide the 23–25 G needle and a 1 mL syringe of local anesthetic near the foramen, between the mucosa and bone. If the approach is through the skin, the skin is first aseptically prepared.

3. Aspirate syringe. If no blood is present, inject local anesthetic around the mandibular foramen. Little to no resistance to injection is felt when the needle is correctly placed.

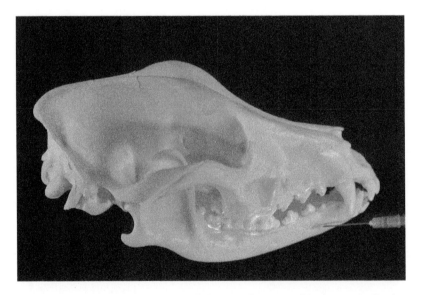

Figure 7.15   Mental nerve block in canine skull. *Source:* Courtesy of Anderson da Cunha.

- *Landmarks*: Zygomatic arch, auriculotemporal joint, auricular cartilage, and the wing of atlas [75].
- *Complications*: (1) Nerve or vessel injury; (2) parotid gland laceration; (3) lingual nerve blockade leading to desensitization of the tongue and subsequent self-mutilation lesions.
- *Contraindications*: Infection, inflammation, or neoplasia at the site of injection.
- *Practical points*: (1) In brachycephalic breeds, the location of the auriculotemporal nerve may be more ventral, towards the temporomandibular joint. (2) Due to the close proximity between auriculotemporal nerve, facial nerve and auriculopalpebral nerve,

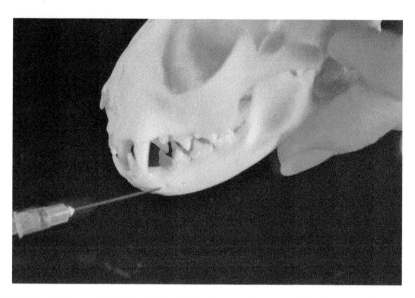

Figure 7.16   Mental nerve block in a feline skull. *Source:* Courtesy of Anderson da Cunha.

Table 7.8   Mental nerve block.

Materials: Disposable or sterile gloves, hypodermic needles (23–25 G), drug solution labeled in 1 mL syringe.

Drugs: 0.5% bupivacaine or 2% mepivacaine or 2% lidocaine up to 1–1.5 mg/kg. Generally, the dose per site is dependent on the patient size and weight and is 0.1–1 mL/site (dog) and 0.1–0.3 mL/site (cat).

Technique:

1. Place the heavily sedated or anesthetized patient in a lateral or sternal recumbency. The mandibular labial frenulum is retracted ventrally. Palpate the middle mental foramen on the buccal side of the mandible, ventral to the rostral aspect of second premolar. In cats, it is at the apex of mandibular canine.

2. Insert 23–25 G needle in front of the mental foramen.

3. Aspirate to rule out blood, and then inject the drug solution over 30 seconds. The needle can be introduced a couple of millimeters into the foramen or, in very small patients, the local anesthetic can be infiltrated on the area just outside the foramen. Little to no resistance to injection is felt when the needle is correctly placed.

desensitization of motor branches of the facial nerve can occur. Hence, evaluation of palpebral reflex and use of eye lubricants are necessary to protect the corneal surface during the duration of the nerve blockade (Table 7.10).

2. Thorax and cranial abdomen

a. Intercostal nerve block

- *Area and nerves blocked*: Intercostal nerve caudal to the associated rib, lateral chest wall and associated bony and soft tissue structures distal to the injection.

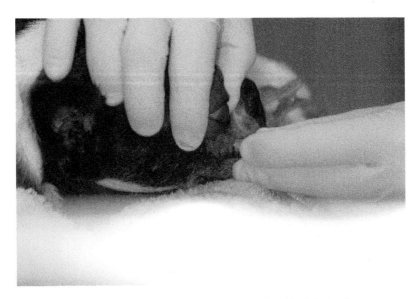

Figure 7.17   Retrobulbar nerve block. *Source:* Courtesy of Filipe Espinheira Gomes.

Table 7.9   Retrobulbar nerve block: inferior temporal palpebral technique.

Materials: 22 G spinal needle (length is dependent on size of patient but is typically 3–5 cm), drug solution labeled in a 3 mL syringe, aseptic preparation, sterile gloves

Drugs: 2% lidocaine or 0.5% bupivacaine up to 1 mg/kg; maximum volume of injection is 1–3 mL in dogs and 0.3–0.5 mL in cats. Dilution is achieved with sterile 0.9% normal saline

Technique:

1. Once animal is adequately anesthetized, aseptically prepare the injection site for the procedure.

2. Bend the needle tip to approximately 20° angle to conform to the orbit.

3. Insert the needle at the 7 o'clock position, below the eyelid. When placing the needle, preferentially allow the needle to traverse along the bony orbit to avoid puncturing the globe and/or blood vessels. The needle is directed along the floor of the orbit and then redirected dorsally and towards the nose to reach the apex of the orbit. A slight popping sensation may be detected on piercing of the orbital fascia. The needle is then redirected slightly dorsally and nasally toward the orbital apex.

4. The globe will rotate caudally until the conjunctival sac is breached, then the globe will rotate back to a standard position.

5. If any resistance is felt, immediately stop and withdraw the needle slightly.

6. Aspirate for blood, fluid, or resistance. If none is present, inject a test dosage (0.5 mL or less) of local anesthetic. If there is no resistance, and patient remains stable, continue with the rest of the injection over 30 seconds.

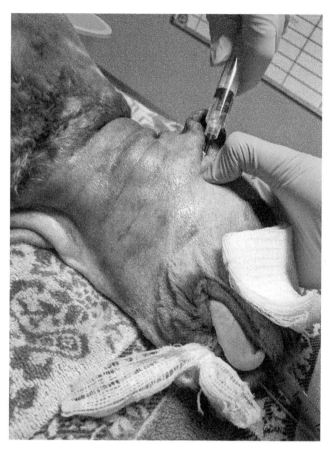

Figure 7.18 Auriculotemporal nerve block.

- *Indications*: Analgesia for lateral thoracotomies, thoracic wounds, thoracic wall tumor removal, placement and removal of thoracic drain, rib fractures, thoracic wall injury.
- *Landmarks*: Intercostal space, ribs (dependent on the affected/surgical site) (Figures 7.20 and 7.21).
- *Complications*: (1) Accidental puncture of the thoracic cavity may result in pneumothorax; (2) accidental injection into nerve, artery, or vein.
- *Contraindications*: Active infection over the site of injection, coagulopathy.
- *Practical points*: (1) Intercostal nerve blocks provide a reliable unilateral dermatomal band of analgesia for the vertebral level at which they are performed; (2) care is taken to perform this block under sterile technique to avoid infection; (2) history of coagulopathy or anticoagulation is taken into consideration to reduce the risk of bleeding; (3) systemic absorption with this block may be significant, hence always stay below the local anesthetic toxic dose range (Table 7.11).

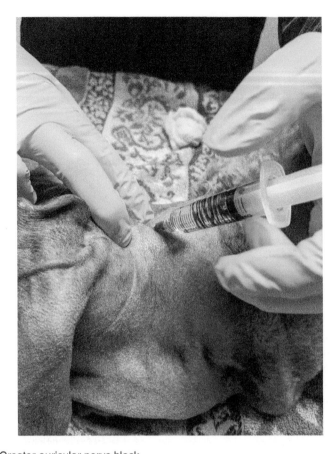

Figure 7.19   Greater auricular nerve block.

Table 7.10   Auriculotemporal nerve block and greater auricular nerve block.

Materials: 22–25 G hypodermic needle, 1 or 3 mL syringe, sterile gloves, aseptic preparation

Drugs: 0.5% bupivacaine or 2% lidocaine up to 1 mg/kg; maximum volume limited to 0.5–3 mL / site (dogs) and 0.2–0.5 mL (cats). Dilution can be achieved by sterile 0.9% normal saline.

Technique:

1. Place the heavily sedated or anesthetized patient in lateral recumbency with the affected side up. Clip and aseptically prepare the skin of the parotid region and the lateral area of the neck.

2. For auriculotemporal nerve block, the needle is inserted in the skin between the rostral aspect of the ear canal and the dorsal aspect of the most caudal part of the zygomatic arch. Once the needle is advanced half of the distance between the skin and the bone, the solution is deposited at that site.

3. For the greater auricular nerve block, the needle is inserted in the skin ventral to the wing of the atlas and caudal to the ear canal. The needle is advanced into the subcutaneous tissue, and the solution is deposited at the site caudal to the vertical ear canal.

4. Aspirate to ensure there is no air or blood. Continue to inject as the needle is withdrawn out of the skin during the greater auricular nerve block. This will maximize the success of the blockade of both the greater auricular nerve and the auricular branches of the facial nerve. If blood or air is aspirated, withdraw, reposition the needle, and then aspirate again.

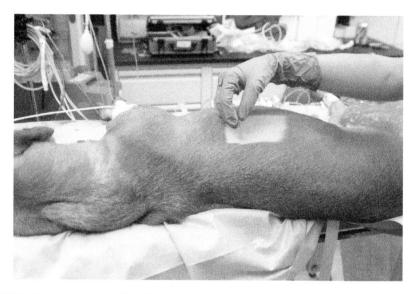

Figure 7.20 Intercostal nerve block in canine patient.

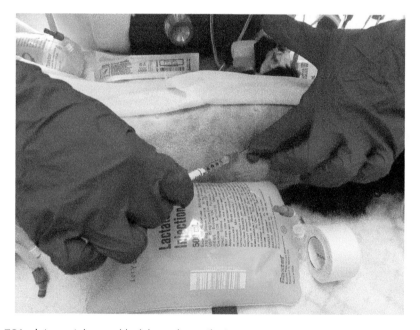

Figure 7.21 Intercostal nerve block in canine patient.

b. Transversus abdominis plane block

- *Area and nerves blocked*: Sensory blockade of abdominal wall and the parietal peritoneum. The transverse abdominal plane contains ventral branches of the last 3–4 inter-
  coastal nerves and the first 2–3 lumbar vertebrae [76,77]. If the block is performed
  bilaterally, complete desensitization of the abdominal ventral midline is achieved.

Table 7.11 Intercostal nerve block.

Materials: 22–25 G hypodermic needle, 3 mL syringe, sterile gloves, aseptic preparation

Drugs: 0.5% bupivacaine or 2% lidocaine up to 2 mg/kg; maximum volume limited to 0.5–2 mL / site (dogs) and 0.5–1 mL (cats). Dilution can be achieved by sterile 0.9% normal saline.

Technique:

1. Place the heavily sedated or anesthetized patient in lateral recumbency with the affected side up. Clip and aseptically prepare two cranial spaces, target space, and two caudal rib spaces for the block.

2. Palpate between the intervertebral foramen and the caudal border of each of the five rib spaces (two spaces cranial to the location of interest, the location of interest, and two spaces caudal to the location of interest).

3. Place needle through the skin, just below the intervertebral foramen, caudal to rib. For appropriate depth, the needle must penetrate just below the intercostal muscles. Direct the needle dorsally and medially, and "walk" the needle off the caudal border of each rib. This will help reduce the likelihood of causing pneumothorax.

4. Aspirate to ensure there is no air or blood. Inject at this point and continue to inject as the needle is withdrawn out of the muscle layers and skin. If blood or air is aspirated, withdraw and reposition the needle, and then aspirate again.

- *Indications*: Analgesia for abdominal surgeries [78,79], mastectomy [80], pancreatitis, and abdominal wall wound repairs.
- *Landmarks*: Abdominal ventral midline, interfacial plane formed by the transversus abdominis muscle and the internal oblique abdominal muscle
- *Complications*: (1) Intraperitoneal injection; (2) abdominal organ/vessel puncture.
- *Contraindications*: Soft tissue infection of the abdominal wall and skin.
- *Practical points*: Addition of dexmedetomidine to the local anesthetic solution can aid in prolonging duration of the blockade and analgesia [81] (Table 7.12).

Table 7.12 Transversus abdominis plane block.

Materials: Clippers, aseptic skin preparation solutions, disposable or sterile gloves, 20–22 G 2.5 m (cats, dogs <5 kg) and 5–6 cm (dogs) hypodermic or spinal needles, +/– extension set, drug solution in appropriately labeled syringe, ultrasound guidance using high-frequency linear transducer (7.5–15 MHz)

Drugs: 0.5% bupivacaine (preferred due to longer duration of action) 1 mg/kg or 2% lidocaine up to 2 mg/kg; maximum volume limited to 1 mL/kg/injection site. Dilution can be achieved by sterile 0.9% normal saline

Technique:

1. Clip hair at the level of lateral and ventral abdominal wall and aseptically prepare the skin for the block. This block can be approached with the anesthetized patient in either lateral or dorsal recumbency.

2. Place a high-frequency (7.5–15 MHz) linear array transducer connected to an ultrasound system in a longitudinal orientation (with the marker cranially) in the area between the posterior margin of the last rib and the anterior margin of the iliac crest at the level of the axilla (3–4 cm from the abdominal midline). Clear imaging of the three abdominal muscle layers (external abdominal oblique, internal abdominal oblique, transversus abdominis) is obtained (Figures 7.22 and 7.23).

---

3. Attach the needle (+/– extension set) to the labeled syringe with drug solution. Insert the needle tip cranial to the transducer. An "in-plane" technique is used to obtain continuous real-time visualization of the needle, advancing through the external and internal oblique abdominal muscles until the fascial plane overlying the transversus abdominis muscle is reached.

4. Aspirate to ensure there is no blood. A small test dose (0.5 mL) can be injected into the observed space to confirm the correct positioning of the needle in the transversus abdominis plane. Once space is confirmed, inject the remaining volume of the drug solution.

5. Two approaches that can be made for this block are: (1) paracostal approach: caudal to the caudal border of the last rib and dorsal to the midaxillary line; 2) umbilical approach: cranial to the iliac crest at the level of the umbilicus and dorsal to the midaxillary line. Some anesthesiologists will use both sites to provide more extensive coverage.

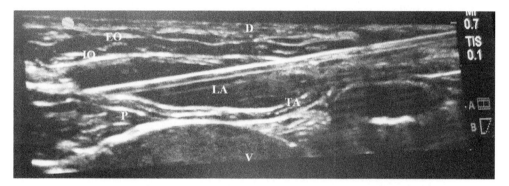

Figure 7.22   Local anesthetic solution injected in the transverse abdominis plane using an ultrasound system with linear array transducer. D, dorsal; V, ventral; EO, external oblique abdominal muscles; IO, internal oblique abdominal muscle; P, peritoneum; TA, transversus abdominis muscle.

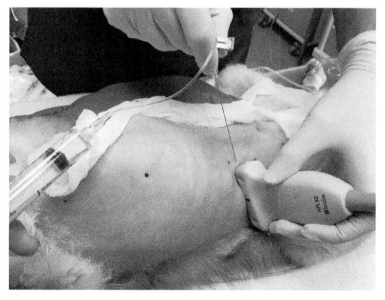

Figure 7.23   Spinal needle (attached to the syringe with the local anesthetic solution) insertion cranial to the linear array transducer (13-6 MHz) for placement of the transverse abdominis plane block.

3. Thoracic and pelvic limb

a. Brachial plexus block

- *Area and nerves blocked*: Soft tissues from the mid to distal humerus, extending to the tip of the digits supplied by the musculocutaneous, supra- and subscapular, axillary, radial, median, and ulnar nerves. Consistent desensitization of the elbow does not occur.
- *Indications*: Analgesia for procedures involving mid to distal humerus, extending to the tip of digits (e.g., amputation, fracture repair, wound explore, arthroscopy).
- *Landmarks*: Scapulohumeral joint, acromion process, greater tubercle, trachea, jugular vein, first rib.
- *Complications*: (1) Nerve trauma or hematoma compressing the nerve can cause neurologic deficits; (2) puncture of the thoracic cavity; (3) perforation of brachial artery; (4) ventricular fibrillation was reported after a stimulating needle was unintentionally introduced into the thorax [82]; (5) possible blockade of phrenic nerve.
- *Contraindications*: (1) Skin infection in area of injection; (2) blocking of both front limbs (as patient may lose motor function and therefore ability to ambulate).
- *Practical points*: The technique may be difficult to perform in obese patients. Addition of dexmedetomidine to the local anesthetic solution can enhance the duration of sensory and motor block, as well as duration of analgesia [83] (Table 7.13).

Table 7.13　Brachial plexus block (Figures 7.24–7.27).

Materials: 20 22 G 2.5–5 cm spinal needle (patient size dependent), aseptic preparation, sterile gloves, labeled syringe containing drug solution, +/− nerve stimulator with appropriately sized insulated needle

Drugs: 2% lidocaine or 0.5% bupivacaine up to 2 mg/kg; maximum volume limited to 0.2–0.3 mL/kg. Dilution can be achieved by sterile 0.9% normal saline

Technique:

1. The anesthetized patient lies in lateral recumbency with the limb to be blocked uppermost. Locate the point of the shoulder (scapulohumeral joint).

2. Clip a 5 ×5 cm area with the point of the shoulder in the center; prepare aseptically.

3. Insert the spinal needle at the point of the shoulder, through the skin.

4. The needle is placed lateral to the chest wall/medial to the scapula, and parallels the transverse processes of the cervical vertebrae, directed towards the scapula to avoid entering the thorax. The needle tip is slowly advanced caudal to the second rib.

5. With the blind technique, once the needle is inserted, attach the drug syringe, then aspirate and if no blood or air is present, approximately one-third of the drug volume is injected. The needle is withdrawn 1–2 cm, aspirate and another third of the drug volume is administered. This continues until all drug is administered.

6. With the nerve stimulator and insulated locator needle technique, once needle tip is near the musculocutaneous nerve, contractions of the biceps brachii muscle will cause flexion and supination of the elbow. Extension of the elbow indicates radial nerve response. Pronation of the extremity and flexed carpus indicates median/ulnar nerve response. Initially, locate a strong twitch with current amperage of 1.0 mA. Then follow with a reduced current amperage of 0.5 mA; decision to inject the drug solution is made when correct muscular response is still observed at <0.5 mA.

7. Aspirate to ensure there is no blood. Inject the drug solution over 30–60 seconds. No resistance should be noted during injection. To ensure effectiveness, some anesthesiologists advocate depositing local anesthetic as the needle is slowly removed.

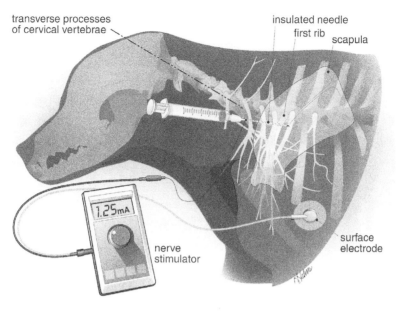

transverse processes
of cervical vertebrae

insulated needle

first rib

scapula

7.25mA

nerve
stimulator

surface
electrode

Figure 7.24   Diagram demonstrating brachial plexus block with a nerve locator and insulated needle. *Source:* Courtesy of Teton NewMedia.

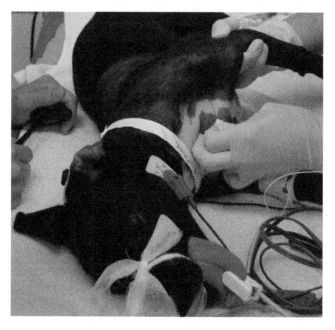

Figure 7.25   Brachial plexus block in canine patient using a peripheral nerve stimulator. *Source:* Courtesy of Patricia Queiroz-Williams.

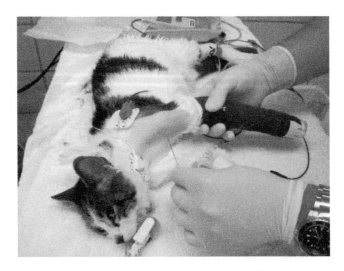

Figure 7.26   Brachial plexus block in feline patient using a nerve stimulator.

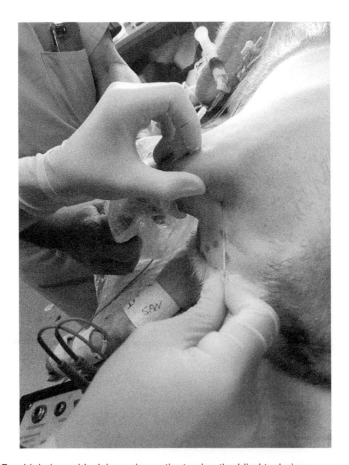

Figure 7.27   Brachial plexus block in canine patient using the blind technique.

b. Metacarpal/metatarsal ring block

- *Area and nerves blocked*: (1) Forelimb: superficial branches of the radial nerve, dorsal and palmar branches of the ulnar nerve, palmar median nerve at the level of the carpus; (2) hindlimb: superficial and deep peroneal nerve, tibial nerve, and/or lateral and plantar nerves (Figure 7.28).
- *Indications*: Analgesia for digit amputations, interdigital tumor removal and digit wounds.
- *Landmarks*: (1) Forelimb: proximal region to the carpus; (2) hindlimb: dorsal and plantar surfaces, at the level of the tarsometatarsal joint.
- *Complications*: Injection into a nerve, artery, or vein.
- *Contraindications*: (1) Skin infection in area of injection; (2) inflammation in the area of injection.
- *Practical points*: (1) Do not use epinephrine because of the potential for ischemia in extremities; (2) stay below local anesthetic toxic dose range; (3) individual digits may also be blocked by injecting the local anesthetic solution subcutaneously in a circumferential ring pattern proximal to the affected digit (Table 7.14).

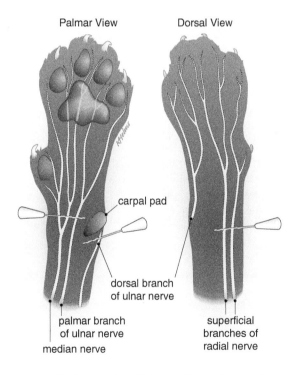

Figure 7.28 Diagram for radial, ulnar, and medial nerve block. *Source:* Courtesy of Teton NewMedia.

Table 7.14   Metacarpal/metatarsal ring block.

Materials: 22–25 G hypodermic needle, 1–3 mL syringe, local anesthetic solution, aseptic skin preparation, disposable, or sterile gloves

Drugs: 0.5% bupivacaine 1–2 mg/kg for dogs and 1 mg/kg for cats; 2% lidocaine up to 3 mg/kg in dogs and 2 mg/kg in cats. Divide this between limbs if procedure involves multiple limbs. Maximum total volume is limited to 0.1–0.3 mL/kg. This total volume is divided equally per site, depending on the total number of sites of injection. Dilution can be achieved by sterile 0.9% normal saline.

Technique:

1. Place the heavily sedated or anesthetized patient in lateral or dorsal recumbency.

2. The affected limb is aseptically prepared for block. (Remember to avoid alcohol for preparation if laser declaw method is used.)

3. For forelimb: insert the 22–25 G hypodermic needle attached to the labeled syringe with drug solution subcutaneously in three sites: (1) lateral and proximal to the accessory carpal pad, (2) medial to the accessory carpal pad, and (3) at the dorsal-medial aspect of the proximal carpus. Always aspirate to check for no blood before injecting at each site. There should be no resistance while injecting.

4. For hindlimb: insert the 22–25 G hypodermic needle attached to the labeled syringe with drug solution subcutaneously on the dorsal and plantar surfaces, at the level of the tarsometatarsal joint. Then, a simple circumferential ring block is performed at this location. Always aspirate to check for no blood before injecting at each site. There should be no resistance while injecting.

---

c. Femoral (FNB) and sciatic nerve block (SNB)

- *Area and nerves blocked*: (1) FNB: mid-diaphysis to distal end of the femur, femoroti-bial joint, femorotibial intraarticular structures, skin of dorsomedial tarsus and first digit; (2) SNB: stifle, tibia, tarsus, metatarsus, and digits (except 1st digit and proximal aspect of 2nd digit).
- *Indications*: Analgesia for stifle surgery, procedures involving mid-diaphysis to distal end of the femur, tarsus, metatarsus, and digits of pelvic limb (e.g., fracture repair, wound explore, arthroscopy).
- *Landmarks*: The femoral nerve arises from L4–L6 vertebrae, and the sciatic nerve arises from L6–S2 vertebrae. In general, the femoral nerve provides innervation to the medial aspect of the hindlimb distally to just below the stifle. The sciatic nerve, along with its branches, provides innervation to the remainder of the hindlimb. For FNB, palpate the femoral artery and femoral triangle (cranial sartorius muscle, caudal pectineus muscle, proximal iliopsoas). For SNB, palpate the greater trochanter of femur, ischiatic tuberosity, and semitendinosus muscle [84].
- *Complications*: Injection into a nerve, artery, or vein.
- *Contraindications*: (1) Skin infection in the area of injection; (2) inflammation in the area of injection.
- *Practical points*: (1) Accuracy of this nerve block is significantly increased with ultrasound guidance and/or peripheral nerve stimulation; (2) addition of dexmedeto-midine to the local anesthetic solution can aid in prolonging duration of the blockade and analgesia [85,86] (Table 7.15).

Table 7.15   Femoral (FNB) and sciatic nerve block (SNB) (Figures 7.29–7.31).

Materials: 20–22 G insulated needle (length depends on size of patient), peripheral nerve stimulator, labeled syringe with drug solution, aseptic skin preparation, sterile gloves

Drugs: Up to 2 mg/kg of 0.5% bupivacaine (preferred due to longer duration of action) or 2% lidocaine. Total injection volume is 0.1 mL /kg for each FNB and SNB [84,87].

Technique:

1. Aseptically prepare the site once the patient is heavily sedated or anesthetized. The initial setting of the nerve stimulator is set at 0.5–1.0 mA, 2 Hz, 0.10 ms.

2. FNB: The patient is placed in lateral recumbency, with the limb for blockade uppermost. The limb is abducted 90° and extended caudally with access to the medial side of the thigh. Palpate for the femoral artery in the femoral triangle. Cranial to the femoral artery, and caudal to the rectus femoris, lies the femoral nerve. A 20–22 G insulated needle is introduced through the quadriceps femoris targeting the location of the femoral nerve. Nerve stimulator-elicited muscle contraction includes contraction of the quadriceps muscle or extension of the stifle. This response is persistent even at a lower amperage of 0.4 mA. Aspirate to rule out blood and then deposit the local anesthetic solution. There should be no resistance during injection.

3. SNB: The patient is placed in lateral recumbency, with the limb for blockade uppermost. Palpate the ischiatic tuberosity and insert the 20–22 G insulated needle perpendicular to the skin through the semitendinosus muscle. Nerve stimulator-elicited muscular response includes either dorsiflexion or plantar extension of the foot. This response is persistent even at a lower amperage of 0.4–mA. Aspirate to rule out blood and then deposit the local anesthetic solution. There should be no resistance during injection.

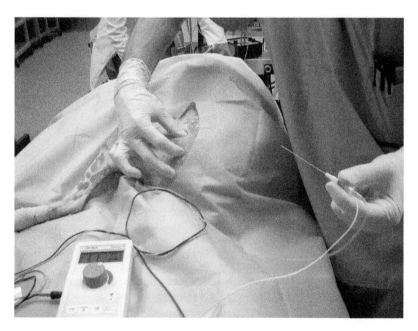

Figure 7.29   Palpation of landmarks for a sciatic nerve block with the assistance of a nerve locator and insulated needle.

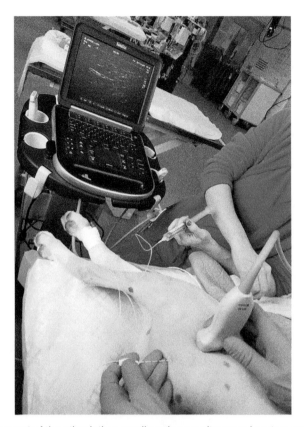

Figure 7.30   Placement of the stimulating needle using an ultrasound system and a linear array transducer (13-6 MHz) while performing a sciatic nerve block.

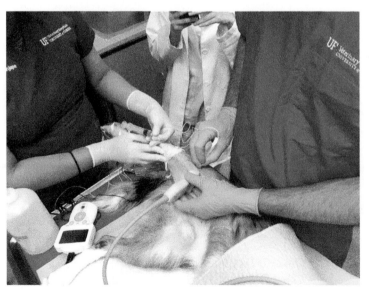

Figure 7.31   Placement of the stimulating needle using a peripheral nerve stimulator, an ultrasound system and a linear array transducer (13-6 MHz) while performing a femoral nerve block.

VIII. Conclusion

To summarize, in both acute and chronic pain settings, opioids are a mainstay in providing analgesia. However, they are associated with possible detrimental effects, as well as being subject to shortages caused by things like natural disasters or pandemics. Nonopioid analgesia alternatives include an assortment of pharmacologic and nonpharmacologic interventions. Also, development of novel regional anesthesia techniques for small animals has grown tremendously in recent times. Veterinary clinicians and technicians should be aware of these potential options and consider them when developing a multimodal approach to pain management.

www.wiley.com/go/shelby/anesthesia2

Please go to the companion website for access to videos relating to the book

References

1. Abdollahpour A, Saffarieh E, Zoroufchi BH. A review on the recent application of ketamine in management of anesthesia, pain, and health care. J Family Med Prim Care. 2020;9(3):1317–24.
2. Bredlau AL, Thakur R, Korones DN, Dworkin RH. Ketamine for pain in adults and children with cancer: a systematic review and synthesis of the literature. Pain Med. 2013;14(10):1505–17.
3. Tang C, Xia Z. Dexmedetomidine in perioperative acute pain management: a non-opioid adjuvant analgesic. J Pain Res. 2017;10:1899–904.
4. Moran-Munoz R, Valverde A, Ibancovichi JA, et al. Cardiovascular effects of constant rate infusions of lidocaine, lidocaine and dexmedetomidine, and dexmedetomidine in dogs anesthetized at equipotent doses of sevoflurane. Can Vet J. 2017;58(7):729–34.
5. Garcia ER. Local anesthetics. In: Kurt A, Grimm LAL, Tranquilli W, Greene S, Robertson S (eds) *Lumb and JonesVeterinary Anesthesia and Analgesia*, 5th edn. Ames, IA: John Wiley & Sons, 2015, pp.332–54.
6. Pypendop BH, Ilkiw JE. Assessment of the hemodynamic effects of lidocaine administered IV in isoflurane-anesthetized cats. Am J Vet Res. 2005;66(4):661–8.
7. Plessas IN, Volk HA, Rusbridge C, Vanhaesebrouck AE, Jeffery ND. Comparison of gabapentin versus topiramate on clinically affected dogs with Chiari-like malformation and syringomyelia. Vet Rec. 2015;177(11):288.
8. Crociolli GC, Cassu RN, Barbero RC, Rocha TL, Gomes DR, Nicacio GM. Gabapentin as an adjuvant for postoperative pain management in dogs undergoing mastectomy. J Vet Med Sci. 2015;77(8):1011–15.

Chapter 7

9. Aghighi SA, Tipold A, Piechotta M, Lewczuk P, Kästner SB. Assessment of the effects of adjunctive gabapentin on postoperative pain after intervertebral disc surgery in dogs. Vet Anaesth Analg. 2012;39(6):636–46.

10. Johnson BA, Aarnes TK, Wanstrath AW, et al. Effect of oral administration of gabapentin on the minimum alveolar concentration of isoflurane in dogs. Am J Vet Res. 2019;80(11):1007–9.

11. Adrian DE, Rishniw M, Scherk M, Lascelles BDX. Prescribing practices of veterinarians in the treatment of chronic musculoskeletal pain in cats. J Feline Med Surg. 2019;21(6):495–506.

12. Amengual Batle P, Rusbridge C, Nuttall T, Heath S, Marioni-Henry K. Feline hyperaesthesia syndrome with self-trauma to the tail: retrospective study of seven cases and proposal for an integrated multidisciplinary diagnostic approach. J Feline Med Surg. 2019;21(2):178–85.

13. Guedes AGP, Meadows JM, Pypendop BH, Johnson EG, Zaffarano B. Assessment of the effects of gabapentin on activity levels and owner-perceived mobility impairment and quality of life in osteoarthritic geriatric cats. J Am Vet Med Assoc. 2018;253(5):579–85.

14. van Haaften KA, Forsythe LRE, Stelow EA, Bain MJ. Effects of a single preappointment dose of gabapentin on signs of stress in cats during transportation and veterinary examination. J Am Vet Med Assoc. 2017;251(10):1175–81.

15. Reid P, Pypendop BH, Ilkiw JE. The effects of intravenous gabapentin administration on the minimum alveolar concentration of isoflurane in cats. Anesth Analg. 2010;111(3):633–7.

16. Kaye AD, Kline RJ, Thompson ER, et al. Perioperative implications of common and newer psychotropic medications used in clinical practice. Best Pract Res Clin Anaesthesiol. 2018;32(2):187–202.

17. Obata H. Analgesic mechanisms of antidepressants for neuropathic pain. Int J Mol Sci. 2017;18(11):2483.

18. Fornasari D. Pharmacotherapy for neuropathic pain: a review. Pain Ther. 2017;6(Suppl 1):25–33.

19. Stahl SM. Mechanism of action of trazodone: a multifunctional drug. CNS Spectr. 2009;14(10):536–46.

20. Crowell-Davis SL, Poggiagliolmi S. Understanding behavior: serotonin syndrome. Compend Contin Educ Vet. 2008;30(9):490–3.

21. Lu HC, Mackie K. An introduction to the endogenous cannabinoid system. Biol Psychiatry. 2016;79(7):516–25.

22. Schurman LD, Lu D, Kendall DA, Howlett AC, Lichtman AH. Molecular mechanism and cannabinoid pharmacology. Handb Exp Pharmacol. 2020;258:323–53.

23. Davis MP. Cannabinoids in pain management: CB1, CB2 and non-classic receptor ligands. Expert Opin Invest Drugs. 2014;23(8):1123–40.

24. Mucke M, Phillips T, Radbruch L, Petzke F, Hauser W. Cannabis-based medicines for chronic neuropathic pain in adults. Cochrane Database Syst Rev. 2018;3:CD012182.

25. Koppel BS, Brust JC, Fife T, et al. Systematic review: efficacy and safety of medical marijuana in selected neurologic disorders: report of the Guideline Development Subcommittee of the American Academy of Neurology. Neurology. 2014;82(17):1556–63.

26. Whalley BJ, Lin H, Bell L, et al. Species-specific susceptibility to cannabis-induced convulsions. Br J Pharmacol. 2019;176(10):1506–23.

27. Center for Drug Evaluation and Research. Non-clinical review(s). www.accessdata.fda.gov/drugsatfda_docs/nda/2018/210365Orig1s000PharmR.pdf

28. Deabold KA, Schwark WS, Wolf L, Wakshlag JJ. Single-dose pharmacokinetics and preliminary safety assessment with use of CBD-rich hemp nutraceutical in healthy dogs and cats. Animals. 2019;9(10):832.

29. Kulpa JE, Paulionis LJ, Eglit GM, Vaughn DM. Safety and tolerability of escalating cannabinoid doses in healthy cats. J Feline Med Surg. 2021;23(12):1162–75.

30. Gamble LJ, Boesch JM, Frye CW, et al. Pharmacokinetics, safety, and clinical efficacy of cannabidiol treatment in osteoarthritic dogs. Front Vet Sci. 2018;5:165.

31. Kogan LH, P. Downing, R. The use of cannabidiol-rich hemp oil extract to treat canine osteoarthritis-related pain: a pilot study. AHVMA. 2020;58(Spring):35–45.

32. Mejia S, Duerr FM, Griffenhagen G, McGrath S. Evaluation of the effect of cannabidiol on naturally occurring osteoarthritis-associated pain: a pilot study in dogs. J Am Anim Hosp Assoc. 2021;57(2):81–90.

33. Santisteban RR, Muñoz LC, Libreros P, Cristancho D. Preoperative administration of cannabidiol (CBD) in healthy dogs undergoing elective surgery in Colombia: 16 cases. 2021 ACVIM poster presentation.

34. Sarma ND, Waye A, ElSohly MA, et al. Cannabis inflorescence for medical purposes: USP considerations for quality attributes. J Nat Prod. 2020;83(4):1334–51.

35. Roynard P, Frank L, Xie H, Fowler M. Acupuncture for small animal neurologic disorders. Vet Clin North Am Small Anim Pract. 2018;48(1):201–19.

36. Teixeira LR, Luna SP, Matsubara LM, et al. Owner assessment of chronic pain intensity and results of gait analysis of dogs with hip dysplasia treated with acupuncture. J Am Vet Med Assoc. 2016;249(9):1031–9.

37. Fry LM, Neary SM, Sharrock J, Rychel JK. Acupuncture for analgesia in veterinary medicine. Top Compan Anim Med. 2014;29(2):35–42.

38. Kieves NR, Bergh MS, Zellner E, Wang C. Pilot study measuring the effects of bandaging and cold compression therapy following tibial plateau levelling osteotomy. J Small Anim Pract. 2016;57(10):543–7.

39. von Freeden N, Duerr F, Fehr M, Diekmann C, Mandel C, Harms O. Comparison of two cold compression therapy protocols after tibial plateau leveling osteotomy in dogs. Tierarztl Prax Ausg K Kleintiere Heimtiere. 2017;45(4):226–33.

40. Rexing J, Dunning D, Siegel AM, Knap K, Werbe B. Effects of cold compression, bandaging, and microcurrent electrical therapy after cranial cruciate ligament repair in dogs. Vet Surg. 2010;39(1):54–8.

41. Rogatko CP, Baltzer WI, Tennant R. Preoperative low level laser therapy in dogs undergoing tibial plateau levelling osteotomy: a blinded, prospective, randomized clinical trial. Vet Comp Orthop Traumatol. 2017;30(1):46–53.

42. Kennedy KC, Martinez SA, Martinez SE, Tucker RL, Davies NM. Effects of low-level laser therapy on bone healing and signs of pain in dogs following tibial plateau leveling osteotomy. Am J Vet Res. 2018;79(8):893–904.

43. Gammel JE, Biskup JJ, Drum MG, Newkirk K, Lux CN. Effects of low-level laser therapy on the healing of surgically closed incisions and surgically created open wounds in dogs. Vet Surg. 2018;47(4):499–506.

44. Kurach LM, Stanley BJ, Gazzola KM, et al. The effect of low-level laser therapy on the healing of open wounds in dogs. Vet Surg. 2015;44(8):988–96.

45. Posten W, Wrone DA, Dover JS, Arndt KA, Silapunt S, Alam M. Low-level laser therapy for wound healing: mechanism and efficacy. Dermatol Surg. 2005;31(3):334–40.

46. Canapp DA. Select modalities. Clin Tech Small Anim Pract. 2007;22(4):160–5.

47. Garrison DW, Foreman RD. Effects of transcutaneous electrical nerve stimulation (TENS) on spontaneous and noxiously evoked dorsal horn cell activity in cats with transected spinal cords. Neurosci Lett. 1996;216(2):125–8.

48. Barnes K, Faludi A, Takawira C, et al. Extracorporeal shock wave therapy improves short-term limb use after canine tibial plateau leveling osteotomy. Vet Surg. 2019;48(8):1382–90.

49. Leeman JJ, Shaw KK, Mison MB, Perry JA, Carr A, Shultz R. Extracorporeal shockwave therapy and therapeutic exercise for supraspinatus and biceps tendinopathies in 29 dogs. Vet Rec. 2016;179(15):385.

50. Becker W, Kowaleski MP, McCarthy RJ, Blake CA. Extracorporeal shockwave therapy for shoulder lameness in dogs. J Am Anim Hosp Assoc. 2015;51(1):15–19.

51. Dycus DL, Levine D, Marcellin-Little DJ. Physical rehabilitation for the management of canine hip dysplasia. Vet Clin North Am Small Anim Pract. 2017;47(4):823–50.

52. Bhathal A, Spryszak M, Louizos C, Frankel G. Glucosamine and chondroitin use in canines for osteoarthritis: a review. Open Vet J. 2017;7(1):36–49.

53. Gupta RC, Lall R, Srivastava A, Sinha A. Hyaluronic acid: molecular mechanisms and therapeutic trajectory. Front Vet Sci. 2019;6:192.

54. Lee MI, Kim JH, Kwak HH, et al. A placebo-controlled study comparing the efficacy of intra-articular injections of hyaluronic acid and a novel hyaluronic acid-platelet-rich plasma conjugate in a canine model of osteoarthritis. J Orthop Surg Res. 2019;14(1):314.

55. Fahie MA, Ortolano GA, Guercio V, et al. A randomized controlled trial of the efficacy of autologous platelet therapy for the treatment of osteoarthritis in dogs. J Am Vet Med Assoc. 2013;243(9):1291–7.

56. Grubb T, Lobprise H. Local and regional anaesthesia in dogs and cats: overview of concepts and drugs (Part 1). Vet Med Sci. 2020;6(2):209–17.

57. Sepehripour S, Dheansa BS. Is there an advantage in onset of action with mixing lignocaine and bupivacaine? J Plast Reconstr Aesthet Surg. 2017;70(12):1782.

58. DeRossi R, Frazilio FO, Jardim PH, Martins AR, Schmidt R, Negrini-Neto JM. Evaluation of thoracic epidural analgesia induced by lidocaine, ketamine, or both administered via a lumbosacral approach in dogs. Am J Vet Res. 2011;72(12):1580–5.

59. Wilkie DA, Kirby R. Methemoglobinemia associated with dermal application of benzocaine cream in a cat. J Am Vet Med Assoc. 1988;192(1):856.

60. Paneta M, Waring WS. Literature review of the evidence regarding intravenous lipid administration in drug-induced cardiotoxicity. Expert Rev Clin Pharmacol. 2019;12(7):591–602.

61. Oliveira RL, Soares JH, Moreira CM, Silva CP, Carrasco LP, Souza HJ. The effects of lidocaine-prilocaine cream on responses to intravenous catheter placement in cats sedated with dexmedetomidine and either methadone or nalbuphine. Vet Anaesth Analg. 2019;46(4):492–5.

62. van Oostrom H, Knowles TG. The clinical efficacy of EMLA cream for intravenous catheter placement in client-owned dogs. Vet Anaesth Analg. 2018;45(5):604–8.

63. Crisi PE, De Santis F, Giordano MV, et al. Evaluation of eutectic lidocaine/prilocaine cream for jugular blood sampling in cats. J Feline Med Surg. 2021;23:185–9.

64. Joudrey SD, Robinson DA, Kearney MT, Papich MG, da Cunha AF. Plasma concentrations of lidocaine in dogs following lidocaine patch application over an incision compared to intact skin. J Vet Pharmacol Ther. 2015;38(6):575–80.

65. Weil AB, Ko J, Inoue T. The use of lidocaine patches. Compend Contin Educ Vet. 2007;29(4):208–10, 12, 14–16.

66. Ko JC, Maxwell LK, Abbo LA, Weil AB. Pharmacokinetics of lidocaine following the application of 5% lidocaine patches to cats. J Vet Pharmacol Ther. 2008;31(4):359–67.

67. Carpenter RE, Wilson DV, Evans AT. Evaluation of intraperitoneal and incisional lidocaine or bupivacaine for analgesia following ovariohysterectomy in the dog. Vet Anaesth Analg. 2004;31(1):46–52.

68. Buback JL, Boothe HW, Carroll GL, Green RW. Comparison of three methods for relief of pain after ear canal ablation in dogs. Vet Surg. 1996;25(5):380–5.

69. Abelson AL, McCobb EC, Shaw S, et al. Use of wound soaker catheters for the administration of local anesthetic for post-operative analgesia: 56 cases. Vet Anaesth Analg. 2009;36(6):597–602.

70. Reader RC, McCarthy RJ, Schultz KL, et al. Comparison of liposomal bupivacaine and 0.5% bupivacaine hydrochloride for control of postoperative pain in dogs undergoing tibial plateau leveling osteotomy. J Am Vet Med Assoc. 2020;256(9):1011–19.

71. Lascelles BD, Rausch-Derra LC, Wofford JA, Huebner M. Pilot, randomized, placebo-controlled clinical field study to evaluate the effectiveness of bupivacaine liposome injectable suspension for the provision of post-surgical analgesia in dogs undergoing stifle surgery. BMC Vet Res. 2016;12(1):168.

72. NOCITA® Insert. Bupivacaine Liposome Injectable Suspension. https://nocita.aratana.com/
73. Accola PJ, Bentley E, Smith LJ, Forrest LJ, Baumel CA, Murphy CJ. Development of a retrobulbar injection technique for ocular surgery and analgesia in dogs. J Am Vet Med Assoc. 2006;229(2):220–5.
74. Castejon-Gonzalez AC, Reiter AM. Locoregional anesthesia of the head. Vet Clin North Am Small Anim Pract. 2019;49(6):1041–61.
75. Stathopoulou TR, Pinelas R, Haar GT, Cornelis I, Viscasillas J. Description of a new approach for great auricular and auriculotemporal nerve blocks: a cadaveric study in foxes and dogs. Vet Med Sci. 2018;4(2):91–7.
76. Castaneda-Herrera FE, Buritica-Gaviria EF, Echeverry-Bonilla DF. Anatomical evaluation of the thoracolumbar nerves related to the transversus abdominis plane block technique in the dog. Anat Histol Embryol. 2017;46(4):373–7.
77. Schroeder CA, Snyder LB, Tearney CC, Baker-Herman TL, Schroeder KM. Ultrasound-guided transversus abdominis plane block in the dog: an anatomical evaluation. Vet Anaesth Analg. 2011;38(3):267–71.
78. Skouropoulou D, Lacitignola L, Centonze P, Simone A, Crovace AM, Staffieri F. Perioperative analgesic effects of an ultrasound-guided transversus abdominis plane block with a mixture of bupivacaine and lidocaine in cats undergoing ovariectomy. Vet Anaesth Analg. 2018;45(3):374–83.
79. Schroeder CA, Schroeder KM, Johnson RA. Transversus abdominis plane block for exploratory laparotomy in a Canadian lynx (Lynx canadensis). J Zoo Wildl Med. 2010;41(2):338–41.
80. Portela DA, Romano M, Briganti A. Retrospective clinical evaluation of ultrasound guided transverse abdominis plane block in dogs undergoing mastectomy. Vet Anaesth Analg. 2014;41(3):319–24.
81. Sun Q, Liu S, Wu H, et al. Dexmedetomidine as an adjuvant to local anesthetics in transversus abdominis plane block: a systematic review and meta-analysis. Clin J Pain. 2019;35(4):375–84.
82. Adami C, Studer N. A case of severe ventricular arrhythmias occurring as a complication of nerve-stimulator guided brachial plexus location. Vet Anaesth Analg. 2015;42(2):230–1.
83. Song JH, Shim HY, Lee TJ, et al. Comparison of dexmedetomidine and epinephrine as an adjuvant to 1% mepivacaine in brachial plexus block. Korean J Anesthesiol. 2014;66(4):283–9.
84. Campoy L, Bezuidenhout AJ, Gleed RD, et al. Ultrasound-guided approach for axillary brachial plexus, femoral nerve, and sciatic nerve blocks in dogs. Vet Anaesth Analg. 2010;37(2):144–53.
85. Bartel AK, Campoy L, Martin-Flores M, et al. Comparison of bupivacaine and dexmedetomidine femoral and sciatic nerve blocks with bupivacaine and buprenorphine epidural injection for stifle arthroplasty in dogs. Vet Anaesth Analg. 2016;43(4):435–43.
86. Trein TA, Floriano BP, Wagatsuma JT, et al. Effects of dexmedetomidine combined with ropivacaine on sciatic and femoral nerve blockade in dogs. Vet Anaesth Analg. 2017;44(1):144–53.
87. Costa-Farre C, Blanch XS, Cruz JI, Franch J. Ultrasound guidance for the performance of sciatic and saphenous nerve blocks in dogs. Vet J. 2011;187(2):221–4.

Further reading

Campoy L, Read MR. *Small Animal Regional Anesthesia and Analgesia*. Ames, IA: Wiley-Blackwell, 2013.
Otero PE, Portela DA. *Manual of Small Animal Regional Anesthesia*, 2nd edn. Buenos Aires, Argentina: Intermedicine Editorial, 2019.

Chapter 7

Section II: Drug formulary

Dario A. Floriano and Amanda M. Shelby

The perianesthetic drugs covered in this chapter are commonly used in anesthetic protocols during the anesthetic process or are medications that are used in the perianesthetic period. Each drug is listed in detail, alphabetically, and drug tables comparing common, categorical medications such as common induction agents, nonopioid sedatives, opioids, and blood pressure support are provided.

I. Acepromazine maleate *phenothiazine*

A. DOSE AND DURATION

- See Table 1

B. CLINICAL APPLICATIONS

- All phenothiazines have a wide range of central and peripheral effects. In human medicine, they are classified as antipsychotic drugs or neuroleptics and are still used in the treatment of psychiatric disturbances. In veterinary medicine, they are widely used for sedation and premedication
- Because the drug is long-lasting, postoperative recoveries are often smooth
- Provides antiemetic action against opioid-induced emesis
- No analgesic properties
- Antihistamine
- Exerts a significant dose-dependent MAC-sparing effect on inhalant anesthetics (up to 48%) [1]
- Acepromazine possesses antiarrhythmic, antispasmodic, and hypothermic properties
- Causes a reduction in platelet aggregation but hemostasis is not altered
- Splenic engorgement after alpha-1-adrenergic receptor blockade, shortly after acepromazine administration, results in a reduction of the HCT [2].

Small Animal Anesthesia Techniques, Second Edition. Edited by Amanda M. Shelby and Carolyn M. McKune.
© 2023 John Wiley & Sons, Inc. Published 2023 by John Wiley & Sons, Inc.
Companion website: www.wiley.com/go/shelby/anesthesia2

Table 1   Nonopioid sedatives/premedications

Drug name	Classification	Dosage	Onset/duration
Acepromazine maleate	Phenothiazine tranquilizer	Healthy patients in combination with opioid: 0.01–0.05 mg/kg IM 0.01–0.03 mg/kg is routinely given IV preoperatively, and 0.005 mg/kg postoperatively for sedation	Slow onset (after IV injection it make take up to 15 min, up to 30 min when given IM). Peak effects are seen at 30–60 min. Clinical sedation lasts for 4–6 h but episodes of animals, especially dogs of giant breeds, depressed for several days are reported. This drug may last substantially longer in patients with hepatic dysfunction
Dexmedetomidine	Alpha-2 agonist	Premedication: 0.002–0.01 mg/kg IV, 0.003–0.015 mg/kg IM CRI 1 μg/kg/h IV for sedation and analgesia	Relatively short onset when given IM (10–20 min), duration of up to 2–3 h
Diazepam	Benzodiazepine	Premedication: dogs and cats 0.1–0.4 mg/kg IV, IM Seizures: 0.5–1 mg/kg IV or rectally CRI: 0.2–0.5 mg/kg/h	In dogs half-life is less than 1 h In cats half-life can be up to 5 h
Midazolam	Benzodiazepine	Premedication [193]/ sedation: 0.1–0.3 mg/kg IM, IV Seizures: 0.5–1 mg/kg IV	Rapid onset with a duration clinically of 30–45 min, although as dose is increased, behavioral effects may last up to 2 h in the dog [194] As usual, cats are unpredictable with their pharmacokinetics; while hepatic clearance may be so rapid elimination could not be accurately assessed [195], there is also huge variability amongst felines in this regard [196]
Xylazine	Alpha-2 agonist	0.5–2 mg/kg IM, 0.2–1 mg/kg IV	Quick onset when given IM (10–15 min) with duration of 30–120 min depending on dose and route

CRI, constant-rate infusion; IM, intramuscular; IV, intravenous.

C. PHARMACOLOGY

- Acepromazine acts predominantly by blocking dopamine D2 receptors, but other effects derive from the ability to block alpha-1-adrenergic, muscarinic, serotoninergic, and histamine (H1) receptors
- Inhibition of dopaminergic receptors of the brain causes sedation and, in combination with opioids, produces a state characterized by sedation and analgesia, known as neuroleptanalgesia [3,4]
- Increase in doses may cause extrapyramidal signs
- Alpha-1-adrenergic blockade results in decrease in SVR, peripheral vasodilation and decrease in blood pressure [5]. Healthy animals rarely display severe decreases in blood pressure but the impact on hemodynamics must be taken into account and caution is warranted in cardiovascularly unstable patients [6]
- Heart rate is usually unchanged but following the reductions in SV, CO, and afterload that result in hypotension, periods of mild tachycardia may be observed [2]
- Clinical doses of acepromazine may cause a mild decrease in respiratory rate, but this is often associated with an increase in tidal volume with minute ventilation usually unchanged
- Metabolized in the liver; conjugated and nonconjugated metabolites are excreted in the urine

D. CONTRAINDICATIONS/PRECAUTIONS

- Hypovolemic or hypotensive patients
- Patients with severe liver dysfunction
- Splenectomy
- Caution in patients with HCM, valvular stenosis or DCM

E. PRACTICAL NOTES

- Commonly diluted to 1 mg/mL with 0.9% saline or sterile water
- Tablets for oral use are also available
- No reversal agent available
- Commonly used via OTM route in the chill protocol at 0.01–0.05 mg/kg to be given 30–60 min before hospital visit by owner [7]

II. Albuterol *intermediate acting beta-2-adrenergic agonist*

A. DOSE AND DURATION

- Two puffs of 90 µg/puff by metered dose inhaler (inhalation), separated by 1–5 min
- Peak effect is 30–60 min after administration
- 4 h duration

B. CLINICAL APPLICATIONS

- Bronchodilator, helpful in reducing V/Q mismatch

C. PHARMACOLOGY

- Selective beta-2-agonist which will relax smooth muscle tissue (both bronchiole and uterine) without stimulating the heart via beta-1 receptor effects

D. CONTRAINDICATIONS/PRECAUTIONS

- Patients with cardiac disease (such as preexisting tachyarrhythmia) as it may cause increases in HR at higher plasma concentrations
- Caution in patients at end-stage pregnancy
- Can cause a decrease in K+ and hyperglycemia
- Muscle tremors may result from beta receptor stimulation

E. PRACTICAL NOTES

- Use a chamber that facilitates proper particle dispersion for full effect
- When administering to an intubated patient, a significant amount of the drug (50–70%) will reside within the ET tube [8]. Therefore, the doses delivered may be increased when administering albuterol to an intubated patient
- Protect from light

III. Alfaxalone *synthetic neuroactive steroid with anesthetic properties*

A. DOSE AND DURATION

- See Table 2

B. CLINICAL APPLICATIONS

- Because it is relatively short-acting and noncumulative, it is used for intravenous induction of anesthesia and maintenance by bolus injection or constant-rate infusion
- It is commonly used IM in association with other sedatives, benzodiazepines, or dissociative agents for chemical restraint of aggressive or noncompliant animals. However, due to low concentration, large volumes may be necessary and, therefore, the IM route is often limited to small patients
- Premedication with sedatives, opioids, and benzodiazepine results in significant dose reductions [9,10], enhancement of sedation and prolongation of recumbency [11], and allows smoother intubation in both dogs and cats [12]
- Recovery is variable; incidences of agitation and noise sensitivity are reported, especially in cats, and seem to be more common than with propofol anesthesia [13]

Table 2   Induction agents

Induction agent	Classification	Dosage	Duration
Alfaxalone	Synthetic neuroactive steroid	1–4 mg/kg IV to effect (over 60 seconds) as a single bolus CRI: 4.2–6 mg/ kg/h [197,198]	Single bolus duration is dependent on dose. In dogs a single dose of 2 mg/kg IV is reported to last about 6 min, 10 mg/kg about 26 min [199,200]
Etomidate	Imidazole derivative	0.5–2.0 mg/kg IV to effect	Promptly redistributed away from the brain, although metabolism may take 2–5 h
Ketamine	NMDA antagonist and dissociative anesthetic	Induction dosage in sedated patient: 3–5 mg/kg IV IM induction dosage of 5–10 mg/kg Buccal dose 5–20 mg/ kg for sedation/ immobilization Loading dose for CRI: 0.5–1 mg/kg, CRI: 0.12–1.8 mg/kg/h	Duration is dependent on route of administration, but single IV boluses are expected to last less than 15 min with an onset of 60–90 sec
Pentobarbital	Barbiturate	Anesthetic dose: 20–30 mg/kg IV To control seizures: 3–15 mg/ kg IV slowly Manufactured at 390 mg/mL as euthanasia agent; dose for euthanasia is 120 mg/kg IV	Effect terminates rapidly, but may take up to 8 h to clear from the body
Propofol	Injectable sedative-hypnotic anesthetic	2.0–6.0 mg/kg IV 2–4 mg/kg IV to effect in patients with appropriate premedication TIVA: 6–24 mg/kg/h IV	10–20 min as a single bolus; prolonged exposure to propofol (e.g., as a CRI) can result in prolonged duration of sedation, especially in cats [201]
Tiletamine and zolazepam (Telazol®)	Injectable anesthetic combination of dissociative agent and benzodiazepine	For induction of anesthesia: 2–4 mg/ kg IV; 6–10 mg/kg IM For maintenance of anesthesia: 6–13 mg/kg IM	Surgical anesthesia <30 min, but it may take up to 4 h before drug effect subsides completely

CRI, constant-rate infusion; IM, intramuscular; IV, intravenous; NMDA, N-methyl-D-aspartate; TIVA, total intravenous anesthesia.

- Alfaxalone is used without complication in young animals (under 12 weeks of age) [14] and to induce anesthesia in dogs prior to cesarean section [15]
- No pain on injection noted [16]
- Decreases cerebral blood flow, intracranial pressure, and cerebral metabolic oxygen demand [17]
- Dose-dependent cardiovascular depression with decrease in arterial blood pressure, cardiac output and systemic vascular resistance may occur with dose-dependent delivery [18]. However, clinically used doses do not elicit hypotension when given slowly to effect [19] and result in a cardiovascular stable anesthesia
- Alfaxalone causes dose-dependent respiratory depression. Apnea is the most common side-effect, especially when administered quickly [20]
- Alfaxalone administration was evaluated to be appropriate for allowing assessment of laryngeal motion in nonbrachycephalic and brachycephalic dogs [21]
- An overdose of 10 times prolonged recovery with obtunded mentation and cardiorespiratory depression for several hours without being lethal [22]

C. PHARMACOLOGY

- Acts primarily on the GABA receptors. The hyperpolarization of the postsynaptic membrane that follows is responsible for altering the pathways responsible for arousal and awareness
- Alfaxalone is rapidly metabolized in the liver and the metabolites are then eliminated by the hepatic/fecal and renal routes
- Plasma clearance is rapid with no accumulation after repeated administration [23]
- In contrast to the previous version (Saffan®, which was formulated with castor oil as vehicle and withdrawn from the market due to hyperemia and histamine release), the current formulation is diluted in cyclodextrins (HPCD) and does not cause anaphylactoid reactions
- Administration of repetitive doses in cats does not appear to result in plasma accumulation or increase in recovery times

D. CONTRAINDICATIONS/PRECAUTIONS

- Patients with known sensitivity to this drug

E. PRACTICAL NOTES

- Half of premedicated cats can be intubated with a coinduction technique using 0.5 mg/kg IV alfaxalone, followed by 0.08 mg/kg midazolam IV [24]. If one is not able to intubate, additional alfaxalone is administered
- Often in small patients, volumes of alfaxalone are minimal. Alfaxalone is diluted with saline for reasonable dose delivery

IV. Amantadine *oral NMDA antagonist analgesic*

A. DOSE AND DURATION

- 3–5 mg/kg PO every 24 h; however, newer pharmacokinetic studies suggest that administrations every 12 h may be needed [25]

B. CLINICAL APPLICATIONS

- Generally ineffective when used alone, but in combination with an opioid or NSAID, may be useful as an adjunctive therapy for chronic pain, such as osteoarthritis [26]
- NMDA antagonist with oral bioavailability
- It is expected to produce analgesia when pain and central sensitization are already present; therefore, it may be ineffective in the treatment of acute pain

C. PHARMACOLOGY

- Acts as an NMDA antagonist to block modulation of pain
- Amantadine seems to have potentiating effects on dopaminergic and anticholinergic activity
- Local anesthetic properties are reported through blockage of the sodium channels
- Amantadine is primarily eliminated via renal mechanisms

D. CONTRAINDICATIONS/PRECAUTIONS

- Due to amantadine's effects on release and reuptake of dopamine, caution is warranted for use in patients receiving other drugs that may alter neurotransmitter release (e.g., tramadol). These combinations could lead to development of the serotonin syndrome, a fatal syndrome characterized by CNS stimulation, tremors, tachycardia, tachypnea, and hypertension
- Amantadine's half-life may be increased in patients with renal impairment

E. PRACTICAL NOTES

- Several weeks of treatment may be required to obtain results in pain relief

V. Aminocaproic acid

A. DOSE AND DURATION

- 27 mg/kg diluted in 15 mL saline; give this over 30 min postoperatively

B. CLINICAL APPLICATIONS

* Traditionally, this drug is used for greyhounds to decrease postoperative bleeding after sedation or anesthesia [27,28]

C. PHARMACOLOGY

* Synthetic antifibrinolytic
* Effect is likely due to the formation of a reversible complex with plasminogen (which would otherwise activate to plasmin); halting this activation prevents fibrin lysis and results in a more stable clot formation [29]

D. CONTRAINDICATIONS/PRECAUTIONS

* In theory, this drug might result in thrombosis

E. PRACTICAL NOTES

* Conventionally, oral therapy at 100 mg/kg is also sent home with owners for the next 3–5 days

VI. Amiodarone *class 3 antiarrhythmic drug*

A. DOSE AND DURATION

* 5 mg/kg IV [30], IO

B. CLINICAL APPLICATIONS

* Antiarrhythmic drug used for treatment of tachyarrhythmias; specifically ventricular tachycardia and ventricular fibrillation during CPR when unresponsive to other therapies [31]

C. PHARMACOLOGY

* Exact mechanism of action is unknown but it is believed to increase the action potential duration

D. CONTRAINDICATIONS/PRECAUTIONS

* Risk of toxicity is documented in humans at 2.2 g in 24 h [32,33]. Dose of toxicity for veterinary species is unknown
* Allergic reactions as well as hypotension possible in dogs

E. PRACTICAL NOTES

- The price of this drug has fallen considerably, but it is not without side-effects
- Antiarrhythmic agents are considered as adjunctive therapy in refractory cases of ventricular fibrillation or pulseless VT, but electrical defibrillation is the recommended primary treatment of choice

VII. Atenolol *beta-1-adrendergic antagonist*

A. DOSE AND DURATION

- 0.1–0.5 mg/kg IV slowly (over 5 min) q 12 h

B. CLINICAL APPLICATIONS

- Slows sinus rate and acts as an antihypertensive
- Negative inotrope and negative chronotrope
- May cause bradycardia and bradyarrhythmias

C. PHARMACOLOGY

- Little to no hepatic metabolism; eliminated by the kidneys

D. CONTRAINDICATIONS/PRECAUTIONS

- Uncontrolled heart failure patients
- Patients with existing bradyarrhythmias
- Use conservatively in patients with renal failure
- Asthmatic patients

E. PRACTICAL NOTES

- Commonly used in patients with HCM or hyperthyroidism
- This drug is not typically used under anesthesia to decrease the sinus HR

VIII. Atipamezole *alpha-2 antagonist*

A. DOSE AND DURATION

- See Table 3

B. CLINICAL APPLICATIONS

- Causes vasodilation and may result in hypotension, especially when administered IV
- May result in excitement or rapid arousal
- May produce gastrointestinal side-effects, such as vomiting or diarrhea

Table 3   Reversal agents

Reversal agent	Reversal for	Dosage	Onset/duration
Atipamezole	Alpha-2 agonists (e.g., dexmedetomidine)	When the 0.5 mg/mL formulation of dexmedetomidine is reversed, atipamezole IM is used as a reversal at equal volume to the dexmedetomidine administered in dogs. In cats, atipamezole IM, at equal to ½ volume of the dexmedetomidine (0.5 mg/ mL) solution is administered for reversal Without the alpha-2 agonist administered, doses of 0.1–0.25 mg/kg are reported	Peak effect is reached within 25 min when used to reverse alpha-2 agonists, and duration is 2–3 h
Flumazenil	Reversal of benzodiazepines	0.02–0.1 mg/kg IV	Quick onset; 30–60 min duration
Naloxone	Used to reverse opioids	0.01–0.04 mg/kg IV CRI to reverse long-duration opioids: 0.005 mg/kg/h	Quick onset, 45–60 min duration
Neostigmine	Reversal of nondepolarizing NMBA (atracurium, cisatracurium, pancuronium)	0.01–0.03 mg/kg IV given slowly over 20 min	Onset is within 5–10 min Duration is 4–6 h
Yohimbine	Reversal of alpha-2 agonists; specific for xylazine	0.1 mg/kg IM, IV	2 h

IM, intramuscular; IV, intravenous; NMBA, neuromuscular blocking agent; PNS, peripheral nerve stimulator.

C. PHARMACOLOGY

- A highly selective antagonist of alpha-2 agonists by binding to the alpha-2 receptors
- There appears to be no effect at other receptor sites, including benzodiazepine, opioid, beta-adrenergic, dopaminergic, GABA, histaminergic, and muscarinic receptors [34]
- Onset of peak effect is quicker when this drug is used without an alpha-2 agonist

D. CONTRAINDICATIONS/PRECAUTIONS

- IV injection results in severe hypotension due to action at the peripheral alpha-2 agonist receptors

E. PRACTICAL NOTES

- If alpha-2 agonists are the sole means of analgesia and pain is anticipated after recovery, consider administering other analgesics prior to reversal
- Signs of reversal occur in 5–10 min following IM injection, although peak effect is longer

IX. Atracurium *nondepolarizing neuromuscular blocking agent*

A. DOSE AND DURATION

- See Table 4

B. CLINICAL APPLICATIONS

- Administered to paralyze a patient generally for a procedural purpose, such as an ophthalmological procedure where the ocular globe needs to be central

C. PHARMACOLOGY

- Exerts actions at the neuromuscular junction, where this drug competes with acetylcholine to bind the nicotinic receptor without depolarizing it. This prevents muscle contractions of skeletal muscle (paralysis)
- Metabolized by Hoffman elimination and ester hydrolysis in plasma (metabolism is dependent upon patient's pH and body temperature); therefore, multiple doses do not become cumulative

Table 4   Neuromuscular blocking agents (NMBA)

NMB	Classification	Dosage	Onset/duration
Atracurium	Short-acting nondepolarizing NMBA	0.1–0.2 mg/kg slow IV	Onset occurs within 3–5 min; effect lasts 20–30 min
Cisatracurium	Short-acting nondepolarizing NMBA	0.1 mg/kg IV bolus, CRI 0.03–0.24 mg/kg/h IV	Rapid onset; effects last 20–35 min
Pancuronium	Nondepolarizing NMBA	0.022–0.1 mg/kg IV	Onset is within 5 min, and duration is 40–60 min [202]

NMB are indicated where muscle paralysis is required. They are most commonly used for ophthalmology procedures when the eyes must remain central.
CRI, constant-rate infusion; IV, intravenous.

D. CONTRAINDICATIONS/PRECAUTIONS

- Patients with a history of adverse reactions (histamine release)

E. PRACTICAL NOTES

- Before administration, a mechanical ventilator is appropriately set to maintain ventilation for the patient. Diligent monitoring of the patient to ensure adequate ventilation prior to extubation is also required
- Monitor paralysis with a train of four (TOF) on a peripheral nerve stimulator; during recovery, at least two twitches should be present before reversal of the drug (see Table 3 for reversal agents)
- Recovery – monitoring with a capnograph and pulse oximeter is beneficial during recovery. Patients may relapse or have residual paralytic effects and are continuously monitored until completely recovered
- Results in histamine release when given rapidly in high doses (resulting in hypotension and tachycardia)
- Some anesthetists will administer this drug as a CRI
- Protect from light and refrigerate drug

X. Atropine *anticholinergic, parasympatholytic agent*

A. DOSE AND DURATION

- See Table 5

B. CLINICAL APPLICATIONS

- Prevent or treat perianesthetic bradycardia, sinoatrial arrest or incomplete AV block
- IM and IV are the preferred routes because of the faster absorption and shorter onset
- Bronchodilation
- Prevent the cardiovascular effect of cholinergic drugs used when reversing neuromuscular blockade such as neostigmine and edrophonium

Table 5   Anticholinergics

Drug	Classification	Dose	Duration
Atropine	Naturally occurring tertiary amine anticholinergic	0.02–0.04 mg/kg IM, IV, SC CPR: 0.04–mg/kg IV in the closest catheter to the heart	20–30 min for cardiovascular effects, although effects on other systems may last longer
Glycopyrrolate	Semisynthetic quaternary ammonium-derived anticholinergic	0.01 mg/kg IV, IM, SC	30–45 min for cardiovascular effects, although with a slower onset (may take up to 5–10 min)

CPR, cardiopulmonary resuscitation; IM, intramuscular; IV, intravenous; SC, subcutaneous.

- May cause sedation, when administered systemically, as it crosses the blood–brain barrier. Effect is negligible when clinical doses are administered. Ataxia, seizures stimulation or drowsiness can occur
- Topical administration in the eye induces mydriasis and, in cats, can increase intraocular pressure (IOP) caused by drainage angle closure. Blurred vision, photophobia, cycloplegia, and pupillary dilation are possible
- The blockade of M3 receptors causes inhibition of salivation

C. PHARMACOLOGY

- Competitive, reversible antagonist of the muscarinic acetylcholine receptors types M1, M2, M3, M4, and M5 at the postganglionic parasympathetic neuroeffector sites
- Antagonizing the parasympathetic nervous system helps to prevent bradycardia, but also decreases GI motility and salivation, and causes mydriasis. The blockade of M3 receptors causes a decrease in gastrointestinal and urinary tract motility resulting in ileus and urinary retention

D. CONTRAINDICATIONS/PRECAUTIONS

- May increase the incidence of arrhythmias, tachycardia, increased myocardial workload, and oxygen consumption
- Caution using anticholinergics following the administration of alpha-2 agonists during the hyperdynamic phase. Increasing the heart rate during the period of vasoconstriction and reflexive bradycardia will cause an increase in myocardial oxygen consumption, predisposing the patient to potential life-threatening arrhythmias
- Narrow angle glaucoma
- Thyrotoxicosis-induced tachycardia
- Cardiac insufficiency-associated tachycardia
- Gastrointestinal obstruction
- Paralytic ileus
- Myasthenia gravis (unless used to reverse adverse muscarinic effects)
- Gastrointestinal infections
- Autonomic neuropathy
- Atropine and glycopyrrolate may enhance the actions of sympathomimetics and may antagonize the actions of metoclopramide
- Very high doses can inhibit gastric acid secretion
- Overall, this drug can result in a dry mouth, dysphagia, constipation, and vomiting

E. PRACTICAL NOTES

- For bradycardia under anesthesia, start with 0.02 mg/kg IV to avoid excessive tachycardia
- Paradoxical parasympathomimetic activity (bradyarrhythmias such as second-degree AV block Mobitz I) can develop in the first phase after the administration or when low doses are administered. The proposed cause is an initial blockade of presynaptic peripheral M1 receptors that normally inhibit acetylcholine release. This causes a transient increase in acetylcholine prior to the postsynaptic M2 receptor blockade

- Greater increases in heart rate (excess tachycardia) may be observed in patients with high preexisting vagal tone
- Antihistamines, procainamide, quinidine, meperidine, benzodiazepines, and phenothiazines may enhance the activity of atropine (and glycopyrrolate)

XI. Bupivacaine (standard formulation) *local anesthetic*

A. DOSE AND DURATION

- See Table 6

B. CLINICAL APPLICATIONS

- Used for local regional analgesia blocks

Table 6   Common local anesthetics

Local anesthetic	Dosage	Toxic dose	Onset/duration
Bupivacaine	Regional: 2 mg/kg in dogs, 1 mg/kg in cats Epidural dosage: 0.5–1.0 mg/kg Liposomal encapsulated bupivacaine: Dog: recommended dose is 5.3 mg/kg or 0.4 mL/kg Cat: the approved dose for onychectomy is 5.3 mg/kg per forelimb (0.4 mL/kg per forelimb), for a total dose of 10.6 mg/kg per cat	Dogs: 3 mg/kg Cats: 2 mg/kg Liposomal encapsulated bupivacaine: unknown	5–20 min onset (in human patients, epidural analgesia has an onset of about 10 min [203], regionally 5–20 min [204]). Duration 4–6 h Liposomal encapsulated bupivacaine: duration up to 72 h from a single dose administration
Lidocaine	Dogs: 0.5–2 mg/kg IV (which may be repeated) or as regional/infiltrative block CRI: 1–6 mg/kg/h (often 1–3 mg/kg/h for analgesic benefit, 3+ mg/kg/h for antiarrhythmic benefit) Cats: regional/infiltrative block 0.5–1.5 mg/kg	Dogs: 6 mg/kg Cats: 3 mg/kg	Regional effects: 60–90 min, quick onset (2–5 min regionally) IV bolus effects: up to 45 min, which may be increased in anesthetized compared to awake animals [205]
Mepivacaine	Dogs: do not exceed 3 mg/kg Cats: do not exceed 1.5 mg/kg	Dogs: 6 mg/kg Cats: 3 mg/kg	1.5–3 h duration with quick onset (2–5 min regionally)
Proparacaine 0.5%	Two drops administered 1 min apart	Unknown	Dogs: up to 55 min Cats: up to 30 min [206]

Table 6 *(Continued)*

Local anesthetic	Dosage	Toxic dose	Onset/duration
Ropivacaine	Dog maximum dose: 3 mg/kg Cat maximum dose: 1.5 mg/kg Epidural: 1 mg/kg of 0.5% sol. (0.2 mL/kg)	Unknown	Slow onset of action and duration, similar to bupivacaine, when low concentrations are used (0.25–0.5%) Onset is faster, similar to mepivacaine, when higher concentrations are used (0.75%)

Toxic signs for doses are as follows, and gradually progress with increasing toxic dose: first signs of toxicity are usually GI in nature (nausea, vomiting). As the toxicity worsens, neurologic signs evolve (tremors, twitches, seizures). As toxicity progresses, cardiovascular depression and arrest will follow. These later signs occur at much higher doses than what is listed.
CRI, constant-rate infusion; IV, intravenous.

C. PHARMACOLOGY

- All local anesthetics share a common chemical structure that includes a lipophilic, benzene ring and a hydrophilic amine group. This compound is then linked to either an ester or an amide
- pKa8.1. pKa determines the amount of ionized and unionized fraction of drug present in the plasma. At high pKa, the proportion of local anesthetic is greater as the ionized, charged hydrophilic form at physiologic pH (7.4), and the onset of action will be slower. In contrast, at low pKa, a greater proportion of the nonionized lipid-soluble form is present at physiologic pH. Onset of action is more rapid at a low pKa
- % Ionized at physiological pH: 83
- Lipid solubility (the main determinant of potency and onset of action) is 30
- % Protein binding 95; protein binding influences the duration of action. Only the unbound fraction of drug is pharmacologically active. The higher protein binding, the longer the duration of action
- Baricity is the property affecting the distribution and spread of the local anesthetic solution after intrathecal administration. When injected into the subarachnoid space, hypobaric solutions will migrate to nondependent areas, while hyperbaric solutions will migrate to dependent areas. Isobaric solutions will migrate to both sides of the spinal cord, causing bilateral spinal block. Bupivacaine routinely used in veterinary medicine is isobaric but hypo- and hyperbaric solutions are available

D. CONTRAINDICATIONS/PRECAUTIONS

- IV administration, as this medication has high cardiotoxicity potential
- Local anesthetic toxicity generally affects first the gastrointestinal system, causing nausea, vomiting, and inappetence, then the musculoskeletal system, causing muscle weakness and ataxia; continued dosing will lead to CNS toxicity, resulting in seizures and obtundation. As dosing continues, cardiovascular toxicity ensues, including hypotension, bradycardia or even ventricular arrthmias, and possible

cardiovascular collapse. It is important to recognize that many of these toxic effects would go unnoticed (outside the cardiovascular effects) in the anesthetized patient.

E. PRACTICAL NOTES

- Loss of motor function when used in epidural or brachial plexus block
- Highly protein bound (caution with dosage in hypoalbuminemic animals)
- If multiple blocks are used, ensure total dosage for patient does not exceed the toxic dose
- In an epidural, preservative-free formulations are recommended
- Do not dilute concentration to less than 2.5 mg/mL or block may lose effectiveness
- The addition of dexmedetomidine at 0.5 µg/mL of the volume for the local block volume will extend the duration of bupivacaine
- NaCO$_3$ can be added to local anesthetic solutions to increase the pH, resulting in less sting upon injection when administering to conscious patients. Increasing the pH may also increase the lipid-soluble fraction, providing a more rapid onset of action and prolonged duration of sensory blockage
- For many years, mixing lidocaine and bupivacaine was recommended, but this methodology was based on erroneous assumptions for the onset of action of bupivacaine, and is starting to lose favor [35,36]. The authors do not mix lidocaine and bupivacaine

XII. Bupivacaine (liposomal encapsulated) *local anesthetic*

A. DOSE AND DURATION

- See Table 6

B. CLINICAL APPLICATIONS

- Prolonged-release liposomal encapsulated bupivacaine formulation approved by the FDA in 2016 for postoperative analgesia lasting up to 72 h for cranial cruciate ligament surgery in dogs by applying into the tissue layers during closure
- Drug is often diluted 1:1 with 0.9% saline to increase volume
- Useful off-label in practically any surgical wound closure, respecting the labeled dose
- Useful in TAP blocks at the labeled dose (see Chapter 7, p.261)

C. PHARMACOLOGY

- Liposomal encapsulated bupivacaine is a sterile, preservative-free, white to off-white aqueous suspension that comes in a concentration of 13.3 mg/mL
- Full prescribing summary as reference found at: www.elancolabels.com/us/nocita

D. CONTRAINDICATIONS/PRECAUTIONS

- At this time, it is recommended to avoid laser therapy following administration of liposomal encapsulated bupivacaine, due to concerns over destruction of the liposomal encapsulation

E. PRACTICAL NOTES

- Liposomal encapsulated bupivacaine is infiltrated in the tissues surrounding the surgical site using a moving-needle injection technique in order to infiltrate deep and superficial layers of the surgical site
- Before withdrawing the product into a syringe, the vial should be inverted several times (avoid shaking) to resuspend the particles
- According to the manufacturer, unopened vials should be stored in the refrigerator at a temperature of 36–46 °F, or at room temperature of 68–77 °F for up to 4 h after withdrawal from vial. However, off-label reports suggest storage up to 4 days after puncture of the vial at room temperature or refrigerated [37]

XIII. Buprenorphine (standard formulation) *partial mu agonist opioid*

A. DOSE AND DURATION

- See Table 7

B. CLINICAL APPLICATIONS

- Provides mild to moderate analgesia and sedation or euphoria, especially in cats, making them more cooperative; however, has minimal sedation in dogs when used alone
- Does not cause vomiting or histamine release
- Has a ceiling effect

C. PHARMACOLOGY

- Potent semisynthetic and highly lipophilic opioid derivative of thebaine
- The authors agree with the statement made by Steagall et al: "Some authors consider buprenorphine a unique drug with a complex pharmacologic profile. The drug binds avidly to, and dissociates slowly from, opioid receptors, but does not elicit a maximal clinical response, because it is not a classic 'full agonist' like morphine" [38]
- Metabolized by the liver
- Reversible with naloxone

Table 7   Opioids

Opioid	Classification	Dosage	Onset/duration
Buprenorphine	Partial mu agonist	Standard preparation 0.01–0.03 mg/kg IM, IV, or in cats, oral transmucosal (OTM) Epidural 0.003–0.006 mg/kg; preservative-free formulations are recommended when available High concentration formulation buprenorphine (HCFB) (1.8 mg/mL) is labeled for cats at 0.24 mg/kg q 24 h for up to 3 days SC for the control of postoperative pain associated with surgical procedures [207,208] Sustained-release (SR) buprenorphine: 0.12 mg/kg cats, 0.2 mg/kg dogs [209,210]	Onset varies by route of administration, but due to its pharmacologic profile, onset is generally considered delayed [211] Duration of traditional formulation (0.3 mg/mL): while duration is also affected by route of administration, generally buprenorphine is thought to last 6–8 h. When administered epidurally, duration has been reported as up to 24 h Onset of HCFB is delayed; the drug should be administered at least 1 h prior to desired effect Onset time of SR buprenorphine has not been studied. Buprenorphine SR is reported to provide 72 h worth of analgesia
Butorphanol	Kappa agonist, mu antagonist	0.1–0.4 mg/kg IM, SC, IV	Duration of 30–90 min (canine) [212] –300 min (feline) [213]
Fentanyl	Full mu agonist	IV: bolus 2–10 µg/kg CRI: 2–42 µg/kg/h Postoperative CRI: 2–5 µg/kg/h Transdermal delivery: 25 µg/h for patients under 10 kg, 50 µg/h for patients 10–20 kg, 75 µg/h for patients 20–30 kg, and 100 µg/h for patients greater than 30 kg	Duration of IV bolus in dogs and cats: 20–45 min Transdermal onset takes up to 12–24 h; duration of 48 h or more after onset. Plasma concentrations start to decline at 72 h after application in dogs [214]
Hydromorphone	Full mu agonist	0.05–0.1 mg/kg IV 0.1–0.2 mg/kg IM CRI: 0.02–0.04 mg/kg/h	Duration of 4 h

Table 7 (Continued)

Opioid	Classification	Dosage	Onset/duration
Meperedine	Full mu agonist	Canine: 5–10 mg/kg IM Feline: 3–5 mg/kg IM	Duration of 45 min
Methadone	Full mu agonist opioid but also possesses NMDA antagonist properties	0.1–0.5 mg/kg IV, IM, SC	Duration of 4–6 h
Morphine	Prototype mu agonist opioid, to which all other opioids are compared. Morphine also works at delta and kappa receptors	0.1–1.0 mg/kg SC, IM CRI: 0.1–0.3 mg/kg/h IV Epidural: 0.1 mg/kg preservative-free formulation	Onset of action may take up to 30 min Duration of IM systemic, single dose administration is 2–4 h; epidural duration is 12–24 h
Remifentanil	Full mu agonist	IV: bolus 0.002–0.005 mg/kg CRI: 2–42 µg/kg/h, with one dose-finding study suggesting 24 µg/kg/h may be most suitable for cats undergoing routine OHE [215]	Duration is seconds regardless of duration of exposure; must be given as a CRI
Sufentanil	Full mu agonist	Loading dose of 0.1–0.7 µg/kg, followed by an infusion at 0.5–0.72 µg/kg/h IV [216,217]	Sufentanil has a more rapid onset and shorter duration of action than fentanyl in people [218]
Tramadol	Central acting analgesic with weak mu opioid receptor agonist	Canine: 2.5–5 mg/kg PO Feline: 2 mg/kg PO	4–12 h

CRI, constant-rate infusion; IM, intramuscular; IV, intravenous; NMDA, N-methyl-D-aspartate; OHE, ovariohysterectomy; PO, per os (by mouth); SC, subcutaneous.

D. CONTRAINDICATIONS/PRECAUTIONS

- Patients which are hypersensitive to buprenorphine
- Causes miosis in the canine and mydriasis in the feline

E. PRACTICAL NOTES

- Controlled, Schedule III
- OTM is ideal for fractious cats especially when combined with ketamine. This route is questionable in dogs, due to the low bioavailability of the drug
- In cats, buprenorphine has been shown to be as effective as morphine in treating moderate to severe pain [39]

- Difficult to reverse due to extremely high affinity for mu receptor
- Protect from light

XIV. Buprenorphine *high-concentration formulation of buprenorphine [1.8 mg/mL]*

A. DOSE AND DURATION

- See Table 7

B. CLINICAL APPLICATIONS

- Reliable analgesia with subcutaneous route of administration, once daily, for cats

C. PHARMACOLOGY

- High-concentration formulation buprenorphine is still a potent semisynthetic and highly lipophilic opioid derivative, but concentration is higher at 1.8 mg/mL
- Biphasic rapid and slow absorption kinetics, which account for its prolonged duration of effect when given SC [40]
- Available as a multi-use 10 mL vial, stored at room temperature, offering 28 days shelf-life from first broach

D. CONTRAINDICATIONS/PRECAUTIONS

- Patients which are hypersensitive to buprenorphine
- Patients acutely painful and requiring immediate analgesia (this drug takes approximately 60 min for onset)

E. PRACTICAL NOTES

- This drug may last longer than 24 h in some feline patients [41]
- Studies have examined intravenous and OTM routes of administration, but neither route has the prolonged duration found with SC administration of the drug [40]
- FDA-approved buprenorphine injection for long-lasting pain relief in cats
- Off-label applications are occurring. Dose in dogs appears to be 0.12 mg/kg SC or IV with an onset of greater than 60 min and duration of up to 6 (IV)–16 h (SC) [41]

XV. Buprenorphine SR *sustained-release (SR) buprenorphine*

A. DOSE AND DURATION

- See Table 7

B. CLINICAL APPLICATIONS

- It is reported to provide up to 72 h of analgesia [42,43]. In previous studies, antinociception produced by 0.12 mg/kg of buprenorphine SR was similar to that produced by buccal administration of the regular formulation of buprenorphine [44]

C. PHARMACOLOGY

- Formulation consists of buprenorphine hydrochloride in an SR delivery matrix of a water-insoluble polymer that precipitates in body fluids and forms a depot for SR of the active drug after SC administration

D. CONTRAINDICATIONS/PRECAUTIONS

- Patients which are hypersensitive to buprenorphine
- Patients acutely painful and requiring immediate analgesia as onset is likely slow

E. PRACTICAL NOTES

- Non-FDA-approved formulation of buprenorphine

XVI. Butorphanol *mu antagonist, kappa agonist opioid*

A. DOSE AND DURATION

- See Table 7

B. CLINICAL APPLICATIONS

- Mild visceral pain relief [45,46], sedation, and antitussive effects with reduced bronchospasms
- Minimal cardiovascular and respiratory side-effects

C. PHARMACOLOGY

- Semisynthetic agonist (k)/antagonist (m)
- Metabolized by the liver

D. CONTRAINDICATIONS/PRECAUTIONS

- Any animal with a previous sensitivity to this drug

E. PRACTICAL NOTES

- Can be used as partial reversal for full agonists at 0.1 mg/kg IV

- Protect from light
- Controlled, Schedule IV substance

XVII. Calcium gluconate *calcium supplement*

A. DOSE AND DURATION

- Treatment is a recommended dose of 5–15 mg/kg of elemental calcium slowly over 10–30 min
- As a constant-rate infusion, 2.5–3.5 mg/kg/h of elemental calcium is targeted
- See "Pharmacology" of this drug

B. CLINICAL APPLICATIONS

- Treatment for hyperkalemia, hypocalcemia, and Ca^{2+} channel blocker toxicity
- Acts as a positive inotrope, improving contractility of the myocardium, which may improve CO and BP
- Administer after large amounts of blood products (e.g., if more than one unit of blood is administered)

C. PHARMACOLOGY

- There are two different formulations of calcium available:
  - Calcium gluconate 10% (9.3 mg of elemental calcium/ml): 0.54–1.6 mL/kg of calcium gluconate over 10–30 min or 0.27–1.5 mL/kg/h
  - Calcium chloride 10% (27.3 mg of elemental calcium/mL): 0.18–0.55 mL/kg of calcium chloride over 10–30 min or 0.092–0.128 mL/kg/h

D. CONTRAINDICATIONS/PRECAUTIONS

- When supplementing calcium, continuous monitoring of the ECG is important. Oversupplementation will cause bradycardia and possibly cardiac arrest
- Calcium supplementation is contraindicated in patients with hypercalcemia
- Administer separately from blood products and other drugs which may chelate calcium
- Will precipitate with sodium bicarbonate

E. PRACTICAL NOTES

- Hyperkalemia: calcium gluconate 0.54–1.6 mL/kg over 10–30 min may be "cardio-protective"
- Always administer slowly. Place an ECG on patient and monitor HR, especially for bradycardia, during administration
- Protect from light
- If administering calcium supplements, blood gas and electrolyte values must be monitored closely, particularly the ionized calcium value

XVIII. Carprofen *NSAID*

A. DOSE AND DURATION

- See Table 8

Table 8   Nonsteroidal antiinflammatory drugs (NSAIDs)

Name	Classification	Dosage	Onset/duration
Carprofen	Selectively inhibits COX–2	Dog: 2.2 mg/kg BID or 4.4 mg/kg SID PO, SC, IV The authors cannot recommend carprofen in cats due to its unpredictable metabolism in this species	12–24 h
Deracoxib	Selective COX-2 inhibitor	Postoperative pain in dogs: 3–4 mg/kg Osteoarthritis pain in dogs: 1–2 mg/kg	24 h
Grapiprant	Antagonist of the prostaglandin E2 receptor 4	Dogs: 2 mg/kg PO SID Cats: not approved for use in cats; however, pharmacokinetics of 2 mg/kg PO and safety/toxicokinetic profiles at 3, 9, 15 mg/kg have been evaluated [219,220], with dosages of less than 15 mg/kg resulting in no adverse effects	24 h
Ketoprofen	Nonselectively inhibits both COX-1 and COX-2	Cats and dogs: initial dose 2 mg/kg followed by 1.0 mg/kg for up to 5 days	24 h
Meloxicam	COX-2 preferential	Dog: 0.2 mg/kg SC as the first dose, following doses 0.1 mg/kg PO Cats: 0.1 mg/kg SC or PO once. This dosage is recommended in compliance with the FDA's black box warning about repeated dosing of meloxicam in this species	24 h
Robenacoxib	Selective COX-2 inhibitor	Dog: 2 mg/kg SC SID for maximum 3 days; tablet dose 2 mg/kg PO for maximum 3 days Cats: 2 mg/kg SC SID for maximum 3 days; tablet dose 1 mg/kg PO for maximum 3 days	24 h

NSAIDs are used for decreasing inflammation and pain due to inflammatory mediators and osteoarthritis. It is important to allow 3–5 days' "wash out" between NSAIDs or following administration of steroids.

BID, bis in die (twice a day); COX, cyclooxygenase; FDA, Food and Drug Administration; IV, intravenous; PO, per os (by mouth); SC, subcutaneous; SID, semel in die (once a day).

B. CLINICAL APPLICATIONS

- Used to manage pain and inflammation associated with osteoarthritis and acute pain associated with soft tissue and orthopedic surgery in dogs
- Carprofen is recognized for its analgesic efficacy for up to 72 h postoperatively in canine ovariohysterectomies [47]

C. PHARMACOLOGY

- Highly selective for COX-2 inhibition
- COX-2 inhibition by NSAIDs is thought to be responsible for the antipyretic, analgesic, and antiinflammatory actions of NSAIDs. However, concurrent inhibition of COX-1 may result in many of the unwanted effects of NSAIDs, including gastric ulceration and renal toxicity
- Carprofen acts primarily to reduce the biosynthesis of prostaglandins by inhibiting cyclooxygenase (COX-1, and preferentially COX-2). Inhibition of prostaglandins that regulate blood flow to the gastric mucosa and stimulate bicarbonate and mucus production may result in loss of GI protective mechanisms
- NSAIDs are biotransformed in the liver to inactive metabolites that are excreted either by the kidney via glomerular filtration and tubular secretion or by the bile

D. CONTRAINDICATIONS/PRECAUTIONS

- Although carprofen's use as part of a premedication prior to the inflammatory event (as opposed to postoperative administration) provides preemptive and better analgesia, caution is advised if using this drug preoperatively
- Carprofen may reduce the diuretic effects of furosemide and increase serum levels of digoxin. Use with caution in patients with severe cardiac failure
- Laboratory interactions – in dogs, carprofen may lower total T4 and TSH levels in dogs, but apparently does not affect free concentrations of T4
- The risk or severity of hypotension may be increased when carprofen is combined with acepromazine
- GI ulceration is the most common life-threatening effect while vomiting is the most common adverse effect
- May compromise renal blood flow
- Potentially serious idiosyncratic hepatopathies, characterized by acute hepatic necrosis, have been reported in some dogs [48]
- Avoid use of NSAIDs, especially those that are COX-2 selective, in patients with GI surgical incisions or suspected ulcers, as they may inhibit GI healing [49]
- Use with caution in patients already receiving highly protein-bound drugs (e.g., warfarin, heparin)

E. PRACTICAL NOTES

- Injectable and oral formulation are available
- The authors cannot recommend carprofen in cats due to its unpredictable metabolism in this species

XIX. Cisatracurium *nondepolarizing neuromuscular blocking agent*

A. DOSE AND DURATION

- See Table 4

B. CLINICAL APPLICATIONS

- Used for patients requiring paralysis

C. PHARMACOLOGY

- Nondepolarizing neuromuscular blocking agent
- The drug is a refined form of one of the 10 stereoisomers of atracurium
- Has action at the neuromuscular junction where it competes with ACh to bind the cholinergic receptor, preventing muscle contractions of skeletal muscle (paralysis)
- Cleared primarily by Hoffmann elimination (metabolism is dependent upon patient's pH and body temperature)

D. CONTRAINDICATIONS/PRECAUTIONS

- Before administration, a mechanical ventilator is appropriately set to maintain ventilation for the patient. Diligent monitoring of the patient to ensure adequate ventilation prior to extubation is also required
- Monitor paralysis with a train of four (TOF) on a peripheral nerve stimulator; during recovery, at least two twitches should be present before reversal of the drug (see Table 3 for reversal agents)

E. PRACTICAL NOTES

- Often used for ophthalmological procedures so the eye remains central
- Recovery – monitoring with a capnograph and pulse oximeter is beneficial during recovery. Patients may relapse or have residual paralytic effects and are continuously monitored until completely recovered
- Some anesthetists will administer this drug as a CRI
- Protect from light and refrigerate drug
- Minimal cardiovascular side-effects (cisatracurium does not induce histamine release)

XX. Dantrolene *muscle relaxant*

A. DOSE AND DURATION

- 0.5–2 mg/kg IV
- Duration 8 h

B. CLINICAL APPLICATIONS

- Treatment of malignant hyperthermia (MH)
- Used in feline urethral spasm (0.5–2 mg/kg q 12 h)

C. PHARMACOLOGY

- Skeletal muscle relaxant which works by binding to the ryanodine receptor, depressing the intrinsic mechanisms of contraction potentially by decreasing intracellular calcium concentration
- Poor water solubility

D. CONTRAINDICATIONS/PRECAUTIONS

- Can cause drowsiness and dizziness
- Hepatoxicity is possible; use with caution in patients with hepatic disease
- Results in muscle weakness

E. PRACTICAL NOTES

- No discernible effects on respiratory and cardiovascular systems
- Protect from light
- Once reconstituted per manufacturer's instructions, only stable for 6 h
- Frequency of MH is rare, and the drug is moderately expensive. If there is preemptive suspicion that a patient may have an MH episode, this drug is obtained by an internet search

XXI. Deracoxib *NSAID, selective COX-2 inhibitor*

A. DOSE AND DURATION

- See Table 8

B. CLINICAL APPLICATIONS

- Used for controlling pain and inflammation of osteoarthritis
- Used for postoperative pain from surgical procedures, specifically dentals and orthopedic procedures

C. PHARMACOLOGY

- Highly selective for COX-2 inhibition
- COX-2 inhibition by NSAIDs is thought to be responsible for the antipyretic, analgesic, and antiinflammatory actions of NSAIDs. However, concurrent inhibition of COX-1 may result in many of the unwanted effects of NSAIDs, including gastric ulceration and renal toxicity

- Inhibits one or more steps in the metabolism of arachidonic acid (AA) and possesses both analgesic and antiinflammatory properties
- Deracoxib acts primarily to reduce the biosynthesis of prostaglandins by inhibiting cyclooxygenase (COX-1 and COX-2). Inhibition of prostaglandins that regulate blood flow to the gastric mucosa and stimulate bicarbonate and mucus production may result in loss of GI protective mechanisms
- NSAIDs are biotransformed in the liver to inactive metabolites that are excreted either by the kidney via glomerular filtration and tubular secretion or by the bile

D. CONTRAINDICATIONS/PRECAUTIONS

- Use with caution in patients already receiving highly protein-bound drugs (e.g., warfarin, heparin)
- For patients with renal failure, use at the lowest effective dose or avoid
- Preemptive evaluation of liver function and liver enzymes, as well as periodic rechecks of liver values, are warranted in any patient where long-term use is indicated. Rare side-effect of hepatic toxicity can occur in dogs
- Patients predisposed to or experiencing intraoperative hypotension may have compromised renal blood flow. It is the authors' recommendation to avoid this drug for the first 24 h post anesthesia in these patients
- Avoid use of NSAIDs, especially those that are COX-2 selective, in patients with gastrointestinal surgical incisions or suspected ulcers, as they may inhibit GI healing [49]
- NSAIDs may antagonize the antihypertensive effects of ACE inhibitors

E. PRACTICAL NOTES

- Vomiting is the most common adverse effect
- GI ulceration is the most common life-threatening adverse effect

XXII. Desflurane *inhalant anesthetic*

A. DOSE AND DURATION

- See Table 9

B. CLINICAL APPLICATIONS

- Desflurane is characterized by a more rapid induction due to its very low solubility in the blood. This characteristic also means there are rapid changes in anesthetic depth when the vaporizer is adjusted, and recovery is quicker than with isoflurane and sevoflurane
- Suitable for anesthesia induction via facemask or induction chamber
- Inhalant maintenance of anesthesia

Table 9 Common inhalants

Inhalant	MAC in dog and cat	Duration	Blood/gas partition coefficient	Oil/gas partition coefficient	Vapor pressure (mmHg)
Desflurane	Ranging from 7.2% (canine) to 9.8% (feline)	Short (i.e., shorter than isoflurane and sevoflurance)	0.42	18.70	700
Isoflurane	Well conserved between species at 1.2 (canine)–1.4% (feline)	Based on exposure (longer duration than sevoflurane or desflurane)	1.4	91	240
Sevoflurane	Well conserved between species at 2.3 (canine)–2.6% (feline)	Based on exposure (shorter acting than isoflurane)	0.68	47	160

MAC, minimum alveolar concentration.

C. PHARMACOLOGY

- Desflurane is a clear, colorless, and odorless liquid with a boiling point close to room temperature
- The exact mechanism of action by which inhalant anesthetic agents cause general anesthesia is not precisely known, but they seem to influence the electrical activity of the CNS by acting on the lipid bilayer of the cell membrane, altering cerebral metabolism and perfusion
- Most important effects include prevention of movement, which is likely mediated at the level of the spinal cord, dose-dependent cardiovascular and respiratory depression, decreased systemic vascular resistance (thus vasodilation and hypotension), increased cerebral blood flow (and therefore possible increase in intracranial pressure), depression of body temperature regulating centers, and muscular relaxation

D. CONTRAINDICATIONS/PRECAUTIONS

- Patients with preexisting extreme hypotension, cardiovascular derangements or reason for inability to handle vasodilation
- In susceptible individuals, inhalant anesthesia may trigger a clinical syndrome known as malignant hyperthermia (MH). MH is a cellular hypermetabolic state that, if not treated quickly, causes death. Although it is mostly reported in human patients and pigs, other species have also been reported to be affected
- The National Institute for Occupational Safety and Health Administration (NIOSH) recommends that no worker should be exposed to ceiling concentrations greater than 2 ppm of any halogenated anesthetic agent over a sampling period not to exceed 1 h
- Caution in patients with increased intracranial pressure or head trauma

E. PRACTICAL NOTES

- Desflurane requires a precision vaporizer with an external heat source and electricity to function

XXIII. Desmopressin (DDAVP) *arginine vasopressin (AVP) analogue*

A. DOSE AND DURATION

- 1–4 µg/kg SC [50]
- Duration of 2–4 h; additional dosage within 12–24 h will not result in a greater effect

B. CLINICAL APPLICATIONS

- Although this drug is used to treat central diabetes insipidus, it is also useful in patients with von Willebrand disease to increase the release of von Willebrand factor (factor VIII)

C. PHARMACOLOGY

- Synthetic analogue of AVP with minimal pressor effects (V_1), but significant antidiuretic effects (V_2), causing reabsorption of water in the kidney
- The V_2 effects are what triggers endothelial cells to release von Willebrand factor
- Results in less vasoconstriction than vasopressin

D. CONTRAINDICATIONS/PRECAUTIONS

- Hypercoagulable patients
- Monitor blood pressure in hypertensive patients after administration (although pressor activity is minimal, it is still present)

E. PRACTICAL NOTES

- Effects are short-lived but drug is useful for administration prior to a surgical event in a patient with von Willebrand disease

XXIV. Dexamethasone sodium phosphate (SP) *corticosteroid*

A. DOSE AND DURATION

- 0.1–2.0 mg/kg IV or IM
- Duration: 12–24 h (varies based on dosage)

B. CLINICAL APPLICATIONS

- Antiinflammatory, immunosuppressive
- May reduce intracranial pressure (ICP) and edema
- Used as an injectable alternative for a patient who missed their oral dosage of corticosteroids (i.e., prior to anesthesia)

C. PHARMACOLOGY

- Fluorinated derivative of prednisolone
- Water soluble, allowing for a variety of routes of administration
- While this drug technically has no mineralocorticoid activity, it does appear to result in a clinical effect when administered at 1/7th the dose of glucocorticoids, in animals presently on oral glucocorticoid supplementation

D. CONTRAINDICATIONS/PRECAUTIONS

- Do not use in patients currently receiving NSAIDs
- Caution in diabetics and patients with renal insufficiencies
- Do not use in patients with GI ulcers or GI compromise, as it may cause GI ulcers
- Long-term use results in adrenocortical dependency; if a patient has received dexamethasone, especially at high doses, an Addisonian crisis may manifest under anesthesia (see Chapter 5) if this drug is abruptly withdrawn prior to the anesthetic event. Patients tapered slowly off the drug are unlikely to have this effect
- Immunosuppressive features may precipitate delayed wound healing and promote secondary infections

E. PRACTICAL NOTES

- Protect from light
- An increase in urination and water consumption may result from a high dosage of this drug
- Commonly referred to as dexamethasone SP 4 mg/mL

XXV. Dexmedetomidine *alpha-2 agonist*

A. DOSE AND DURATION

- See Table 1
- Intranasal: a study showed that 0.02 mg/kg dexmedetomidine produced effective sedation with less bradycardia and more profound sedation compared to IM administration in healthy dogs and may be considered as an alternative route for administration in dogs [51], similar to previous studies in rabbits [52]
- 125 μg/m^2 of dexmedetomidine oromucosal gel is useful (potentially for administration by owners), prior to veterinary visits, in reducing signs of stress (vocalizations, avoidance behaviors, panting, trembling, urination, defecation) in dogs [53]

B. CLINICAL APPLICATIONS

- Dexmedetomidine is commonly used both as a sole sedative for minor procedure and in combination with opioids as a premedication for general anesthesia or to improve the quality of sedation
- Dexmedetomidine has multiple routes and modalities of administration (including epidurally or as a constant-rate infusion), is not controlled, provides substantial analgesia and moderate to profound sedation (especially when combined with opioids), making it one of the most versatile drugs for anesthesia a veterinarian has available
- This drug is often used with the intent of extending the duration of a local regional block, when added to the local anesthetic solution used for regional anesthesia at 0.001mg/kg. However, efficacy of this varies by study [54–56]

C. PHARMACOLOGY

- Dexmedetomidine is the active enantiomer of the racemic mixture medetomidine, and a potent sedative and analgesic drug
- Dexmedetomidine is the most selective alpha-2-adrenergic receptor agonist and has almost completely replaced xylazine for the same purposes. The selectivity for alpha-2-adrenergic receptors is higher (1620:1) than xylazine, making dexmedetomidine more potent than xylazine
- Presynaptic alpha-2-adrenergic receptors: inhibits release of norepinephrine and attenuates the sympathetic drive from the CNS
- Postsynaptic alpha-2-adrenergic receptors: effect similar to alpha-1-adrenergic receptor actions resulting in vasoconstriction
- After IV, IM, SC routes and across transmucosal membranes, the bioavailability is high and the onset of sedation rapid
- Sedation, analgesia, muscle relaxation, and centrally mediated cardiovascular effects (central bradycardia, hypotension)
- Analgesic and sedative effects have the same duration
- The action on the alpha-2 receptors in the CNS causes dose-dependent degree of sedation up to a plateau, after which higher doses only increase length of sedation and side-effects. Animals deeply sedated can abruptly arise and demonstrate responses to external stimuli. The combination with opioids reduces these responses and produces deep sedation; indeed, these drugs may be synergistic when given together [57]
- Analgesia is exerted by dampening the afferent inputs at various point of the nociceptive pathway. When administered epidurally or intrathecally (preservative-free formulations preferred for this purpose), it provides excellent analgesia for a direct action on the receptors in the dorsal horn of the spinal cord
- Metabolized by the liver

D. CONTRAINDICATIONS/PRECAUTIONS

- Cardiovascular (CV) diseases including valvular regurgitation or arrhythmias are by far the most pressing contraindication to use of dexmedetomidine (see "Alfaxalone," p.280 in this formulary, as an alternative IM injectable for sedation in the patient with valvular disease)

- Cardiovascular effects are marked and biphasic: blood pressure is initially markedly increased, with profound bradycardia caused by a baroceptor reflex following peripheral vasoconstriction. In the second phase, a less profound bradycardia is evident and due to the suppression of the central cardiovascular center, followed by possible hypotension due to a decrease in CO
- Bradyarrhythmias, including second-degree AV block, escape rhythms and accelerated idioventricular rhythms (AIVR) are frequent in both dogs and cats. In practice, the authors use anticholinergic to treat the bradycardia related to alpha-2-adrenergic receptor agonists only when hypotension exists (i.e., the second phase of the cardiovascular effects). If the patient is within the first phase of cardiovascular effects (i.e., blood pressure is normal to high), administration is often reversed when hypotension or bradyarrhythmias are present. Alternatively, recent work suggests that lidocaine, initially as a 2 mg/kg bolus IV and followed with a constant-rate infusion (CRI) of 3–6 mg/kg/h for 30 min, may counteract dexmedetomidine-induced bradycardia [58]
- Respiratory effects are related to the depth of sedation achieved and, unless the sedation is very deep, the reduction in respiratory rate is compensated by the increase in tidal volume, allowing the maintenance of a normal minute ventilation
- Increase in urine output is caused by central inhibition of ADH secretion and hyperglycemia as a result of the decrease in serum level of insulin
- Dexmedetomidine is contraindicated in patients with renal insufficiencies, anuria, or a blocked urinary system
- Dexmedetomidine is contraindicated in patients with liver function disease
- Avoid in geriatric, pregnant, pediatric, sick, or debilitated patients

E. PRACTICAL NOTES

- Patients will often develop a transient hyperglycemia after administration
- Most effective when administered to a patient that is allowed 5–10 min in a quiet, darkened room, with minimal stimulus
- Monitor the patient after premedication and ensure reversal dose has been calculated and is available if needed
- The reversal, atipamezole (see p. 285 in this formulary), is given IM, to avoid rapid vasodilation
- Vasoconstriction may cause pale or blue MMC, and the pulse oximeter may have difficulty obtaining a measurement
- Low doses work nicely as premedication in cats with HCM
- In a study comparing the two, dexmedetomidine was more likely to cause vomiting than xylazine in cats [59]. If vomiting is undesirable, consider premedication with maropitant (see p. 337 in this formulary) [60]

XXVI. Dextrose *supplement*

A. DOSE AND DURATION

- IV bolus for profound hypoglycemia 250 mg/kg or 0.5 mL/kg of 50% dextrose (diluted 1:4 with isotonic fluids)

- Fluid additives: add appropriate amount to fluids, to yield a 2.5 5% solution (see Appendix D, Dilution equations, p.397)
- Often given as a component of a CRI to prolong duration of supplementation

B. CLINICAL APPLICATIONS

- Increases serum blood glucose, providing energy stores for cellular metabolism
- Prevention of hypoglycemia in prone patients such as neonates
- Treatment of diabetic ketoacidosis
- Adjunctive treatment for hyperkalemia (see Chapter 3, p.78)

C. PHARMACOLOGY

- Dextrose is a molecule made from corn identical to blood glucose ($C_6H_{12}O_6$), a monosaccharide, and type of carbohydrate

D. CONTRAINDICATIONS/PRECAUTIONS

- Extremely hypertonic, requiring dilution prior to administration
- Hyperglycemic patients

E. PRACTICAL NOTES

- Common dilutions for anesthesia are 2.5–5% in crystalloid solutions
- Monitor blood glucose from an independent catheter
- High concentrations of dextrose cause tissue irritation (especially when given perivascular) due to its hypertonic nature. 1:3 or 1:4 dilutions are recommended when administered via peripheral veins

XXVII. Diazepam *benzodiazepine*

A. DOSE AND DURATION

- See Table 1

B. CLINICAL APPLICATIONS

- Unreliable sedative in healthy animals but useful as central muscle relaxant and anticonvulsant
- Used as coinduction agent to reduce the dose of primary induction drug needed [61]
- Appetite stimulant, especially in cats
- Administered in combination with ketamine or tiletamine to counteract the muscle rigidity of the dissociative agents
- Antianxiety effects

C. PHARMACOLOGY

- Sedative effects occur by enhancing the $GABA_A$ receptor's affinity for the inhibitory neurotransmitter GABA within the CNS. Benzodiazepines are considered to have an indirect effect by potentiating the activity of endogenous GABA neurotransmitter, leading to a wide safety margin and minimal depression of ventilation, cardiac output, and oxygen delivery
- Muscle relaxant and anticonvulsant properties derive from action on spinal interneurons
- Highly protein bound
- Metabolized by the liver with production of active metabolites that can persist for several hours after administration
- Poorly water soluble; is supplied for injection in a solution that contains organic solvents such as propylene glycol and ethanol

D. CONTRAINDICATIONS/PRECAUTIONS

- Can cause pain on IM injection and thrombophlebitis after intravenous injection [62]
- Muscle tissue necrosis can develop following IM injection [63]
- Crosses the placental barrier and may result in respiratory depression in neonates
- Patients with liver function insufficiencies may have prolonged effect
- Avoid in patients with hepatic encephalopathy
- In contrast to humans and dogs, diazepam has been reported to induce severe hepatic side-effects in cats, particularly after repeated doses [64]

E. PRACTICAL NOTES

- Propylene glycol-based and highly lipid soluble, making it incompatible with many drugs and painful on IM or SC injection as well as inconsistently absorbed
- Is light sensitive and will bind to soft plastics, such as infusion lines
- Reversible with flumazenil (see Table 3)

XXVIII. Diphenhydramine *antihistamine*

A. DOSE AND DURATION

- 0.5–2.0 mg/kg IM, IV or PO (tablet form)
- Duration of 6–8 h

B. CLINICAL APPLICATION

- Part of the premedication for conditions that predispose the patient to histamine release: mast cell tumors, anaphylaxis, and heart worm extractions
- Some clinicians administer preemptively before blood transfusions

C. PHARMACOLOGY

- Blockade of histamine1 (H1) receptors

D. CONTRAINDICATIONS/PRECAUTIONS

- May result in sedation but this is unpredictable

E. PRACTICAL NOTES

- In patients with histamine release, there are decreased symptoms of reaction; however, this will not reverse a reaction. It will simply prevent histamine molecules released from binding to the receptor sites. In life-threatening histamine release that occurs with a severe allergic reaction, diphenhydramine alone will be insufficient

XXIX. Dobutamine *positive inotrope*

A. DOSE AND DURATION

- See Table 10

B. CLINICAL APPLICATIONS

- Patients with weak cardiac contractility

C. PHARMACOLOGY

- Beta-1 stimulation increases myocardial contractility to improve SV and CO [65]
- Mild beta-2 agonist stimulation results in some smooth muscle relaxation (this may cause decrease in BP although CO is likely increased), although its affinity for beta-2 receptors is approximately 10-fold less than that of beta-1 [65]
- Short-acting, so typically administered as a CRI
- Sympathomimetic
- Mild chronotropic, arrhythmogenic and vasodilator effects which increase oxygen consumption [65]

C. CONTRAINDICATIONS/PRECAUTIONS

- High doses may cause hypertension, tachycardia, and arrhythmias
- Contraindicated in patients with HCM, ventricular hypertrophy, ventricular arrhythmias, endogenous catecholamine overproduction
- Beta-blockers (e.g., propranolol) may antagonize the cardiac effects of dobutamine

D. PRACTICAL NOTES

- Common dilution for administration is 1–2 mg/mL
- Refrigeration is recommended after broaching vial

Table 10. Blood pressure support

Drug name	Classification	Dosage	Duration	Contractility	Vasoconstriction
Dobutamine	Positive inotrope	CRI: 2–20 µg/kg/h IV	1–2 min; thus, usually administered as a CRI	+++	Minimal/none
Dopamine	Catecholamine and positive Inotrope	CRI: 2–20–µg/kg/min IV	1–2 min; thus, usually administered as a CRI	++	++ at high doses
Ephedrine	Sympathomimetic	0.06–0.1 mg/kg IV 0.1–0.25 mg/kg IM	Half-life is up to 6 h, clinical effect 30–45 min	+	+
Epinephrine	Catecholamine and sympathomimetic	For CPR (see Appendix B, p.393): Low dose: 0.01 mg/kg IV High dose: 0.1 mg/kg IV IT dose: 10x standard low IV dose is recommended For intraoperative hypotension in CRI: 0.006–0.06 mg/kg/h IV For anaphylaxis treatment: 0.02 mg/kg IM or IN [221]	Very quick onset and short duration due to rapid metabolism (less than 2 min when administered IV). Need frequent redosing or CRI for a prolonged effect	+++	+++
Nitroprusside	Peripheral vasodilator	0.1–2 µg/kg/min (ideal to use less than 0.5 mg/kg/h)	1–3 min	–	–
Norepinephrine	Catecholamine and vasopressor	0.006–0.09 µg/kg/min	1–2 min	+	+++
Phenylephrine	Vasopressor	0.002–0.005 mg/kg IV, CRI 0.5–2 µg/kg/min	A single bolus may last up to 20 min	–	+++
Vasopressin	Vasopressor	Bolus 0.2–0.8 units/kg IV with the higher dose appropriate for CPR; CRI 0.02–0.04 units/kg/h	10–20 min	–	+++

CPR, cardiopulmonary resuscitation; CRI, constant-rate infusion; IM, intramuscular; IN, intranasal; IV, intravenous.

XXX. Dopamine *endogenous catecholamine and positive inotrope*

A. DOSE AND DURATION

- See Table 10

B. CLINICAL APPLICATIONS

- Used to improve blood pressure through increased contractility of the heart and to provide mild vasoconstriction

C. PHARMACOLOGY

- Dopamine, which is also present as an endogenous catecholamine, is an immediate precursor to norepinephrine [65]
- Action at various receptors, including alpha, beta, and dopaminergic, depends on dose (although exact doses are controversial)
- Low doses (<3 µg/kg/min) provide higher affinity for dopaminergic receptors D1 and D2. This may improve hemodynamics by vasodilating capillary beds in renal, mesenteric, coronary, and cerebral regions. Because of this, outside the OR it is sometimes used as adjunctive therapy for treatment of oliguric renal failure or acute heart failure
- At mid-range doses (3–10 µg/kg/min), beta-1 and beta-2 receptors are the most stimulated, often maximizing myocardial contractility and increasing organ perfusion, renal blood flow, and urine production
- At higher doses, vasoconstriction and increase in SVR caused by alpha-1-adrenergic receptor stimulation. Blood pressure increases and renal and peripheral blood flow may decrease
- Dopamine has an indirect sympathomimetic activity in stimulating the release of endogenous norepinephrine from adrenergic receptors

D. CONTRAINDICATIONS/PRECAUTIONS

- Patients with endogenous catecholamine overproduction (e.g., pheochromocytomas)
- Patients with ventricular tachyarrhythmias, HCM, ventricular hypertrophy
- Severe hypertension develops when dopamine is used in conjunction with oxytocin [66]
- The effects of dopamine may be prolonged and enhanced in patients in which monoamine oxidase (MAO) inhibitors (i.e., selegiline) were administered
- Concomitant use of ephedrine with beta-blockers may decrease the effects of both drugs
- Tachycardia, tachyarrhythmias, and hypertension may occur from the coadministration of anticholinergic and dopamine

E. PRACTICAL NOTES

- Note that it is controversial as to whether cats express dopaminergic receptors; while there is some evidence to support putative D1-like or D1 receptor existence in feline kidneys [67], its use in feline renal failure patients is less reliable than in canine renal failure patients

- Common dilutions are 1–2 mg/mL
- Dilutions are used within 24 h and discarded if solution changes color
- Refrigerate bottle after first broaching
- Protect bottle and dilutions from light
- High doses or administration of undiluted product can cause arrhythmias, hypertension, and tachycardia
- Extravasation can cause necrosis of perivascular tissue [68]

XXXI. Doxapram *respiratory stimulant*

A. DOSE AND DURATION

- 2–5 mg/kg IV or 1–2 drops under tongue of newborn
- Usually administered only once, as additional dosages may have decreased effectiveness

B. CLINICAL APPLICATIONS

- Used to stimulate respiration typically in neonates or for laryngeal examination
- May increase CO

C. PHARMACOLOGY

- Stimulates respiration by action on the carotid chemoreceptors, resulting in an increase in tidal volume rather than respiratory rate
- Contains benzyl alcohol (cautious use in cats)

D. CONTRAINDICATIONS/PRECAUTIONS

- Repeated dosages may result in undesirable CNS stimulation
- Protect from light

E. PRACTICAL NOTES

- Authors' preference is to avoid unnecessary use of doxapram as it causes undesirable CNS stimulation

XXXII. Ephedrine *synthetic noncatecholamine inotropic and vasopressor agent*

A. DOSE AND DURATION

- See Table 10

B. CLINICAL APPLICATIONS

- Used to temporarily increase blood pressure and heart rate
- Vasoconstriction and increases in heart rate, coronary blood flow, and blood pressure result in increase in CO
- Presumed splenic contraction may increase hemoglobin concentration and thus oxygen-carrying capacity

C. PHARMACOLOGY

- Directly stimulates alpha and beta receptors to increase vascular tone through mild vasoconstriction and an increase in myocardial contractility, thus increasing CO and stroke volume
- Indirectly stimulates alpha, beta-1- and beta-2-adrenergic receptors by causing the release of endogenous norepinephrine. Tachyphylaxis is observed due to depletion of norepinephrine stores [69]
- Similar to other adrenergic agents, bronchodilation derives from the beta-2 stimulation
- Sympathomimetic

D. CONTRAINDICATIONS/PRECAUTIONS

- When used at higher doses, more profound bradycardia may result reflexively from the significant and prolonged increase in arterial blood pressure
- Crosses the blood–brain barrier and acts as a CNS stimulant; adequate anesthesia of the patient should be ensured prior to administration
- The drug is excreted in milk and may have deleterious effects on nursing animals
- Ephedrine may reduce renal blood flow and glomerular filtration rate due to regional vasoconstriction
- Patients with heart disease where increasing myocardial workload would be detrimental, such as HCM
- Increased effects can derive from the coadministration of multiple sympathomimetics
- The effects of ephedrine can be prolonged and enhanced in patients where MAO inhibitors (i.e., selegiline) are previously administered
- The urinary excretion of ephedrine and its duration of activity can be prolonged when urinary alkalinizers (e.g., sodium bicarbonate, citrates, carbonic anhydrase inhibitors) are administered
- Concomitant use of ephedrine with beta-blockers may decrease the effects of both drugs

E. PRACTICAL NOTES

- This drug has an advantage for locations which cannot provide constant rate infusions, as it is easily administered as a single bolus
- Repeating the dose once is acceptable; repeat bolus (e.g., more than twice) or a CRI is not recommended

- Drug is relatively short-acting with an appreciable clinical effect
- Protect from light
- Effect is dependent on norepinephrine stores; in patients with depleted norepinephrine stores, there is less of an effect

XXXIII. Epinephrine (adrenaline) *endogenous catecholamine*

A. DOSE AND DURATION

- See Table 10

B. CLINICAL APPLICATIONS

- Cardiac resuscitation
- Treatment for anaphylaxis
- Adjunct to local anesthetics (LA) to extend the duration of the local block by causing vasoconstriction and therefore decreasing the systemic absorption of the LA, which decreases the dose of LA required, prolongs its effect and decreases the probability of systemic toxicity. Used in this manner, it may also decrease bleeding in the area blocked

C. PHARMACOLOGY

- Naturally occurring catecholamine
- Prototype sympathomimetic
- Direct stimulation of beta- and alpha-adrenergic receptor results in cardiac chronotropic, inotropic and vasopressor dose-dependent effects
- Has action on alpha and beta receptors, resulting in increased blood pressure and systemic vascular resistance, decreased airway resistance, bronchodilation, tachycardia and possible ventricular arrhythmias

D. CONTRAINDICATIONS/PRECAUTIONS

- Patients with hypertension and tachycardia
- Can cause ventricular fibrillation
- Caution should be exercised in cases of hypovolemia
- Caution when using as a CRI, as healthy human volunteers demonstrated increased heart rate, plasma insulin, and glucose levels, and decreased mean arterial pressure and diastolic pressure [70]
- Do not use as an adjuvant for a local block performed in a distal region, as it may cause necrosis or sloughing of tissue
- Increased effects can derive from the coadministration of multiple sympathomimetics
- The effects of epinephrine can be prolonged and enhanced in patients where MAO inhibitors (i.e., selegiline) are previously administered
- Effect can be potentiated by certain antihistamines (diphenhydramine)

- Beta-blockers (propranolol) can reverse the effects of smooth muscle relaxation in the bronchi and alveoli that epinephrine exerts through stimulation of beta-receptors and exacerbate the vasoconstrictive and hypertensive effects caused by alpha-receptor stimulation

E. PRACTICAL NOTES

- Low doses, given slowly IV, can lead to a smoother rise in systolic pressure and a decrease in diastolic pressure and decrease in SVR, due to beta-2 stimulation
- High doses will result in vasoconstriction, hypertension, tachycardia, and possibly ventricular arrhythmias. Also, increases in pulmonary vascular resistance reflect the agonism at level of pulmonary vascular alpha-1-adrenergic receptors that predominates over beta effects
- Decreased airway resistance, bronchodilation, and reversal of hypotension are the main characteristics that make this catecholamine effective in reducing anaphylactic symptoms
- The 2012 RECOVER guidelines suggest 0.01 mg/kg for cardiac arrest every 2–5 min and 0.1 mg/kg only after prolonged periods of nonresponsive resuscitation efforts [30]
- Protect from light

XXXIV. Eutectic mixture of lidocaine and prilocaine *topical local anesthetic*

A. DOSE AND DURATION

- Dosage: minimal amount to cover area of anticipated insult
- Duration: dependent on contact time, but may exceed 2 h [71]
- Onset of action depends on contact with skin, generally 45–60 min. Heat may decrease onset time

B. CLINICAL APPLICATIONS

- Topical anesthetic used for desensitization of skin often for IV catheter placement or blood draw

C. PHARMACOLOGY

- Contains lidocaine 2.5% and prilocaine 2.5% (both local anesthetics) which penetrate the skin's full thickness
- Minimal to immeasurable systemic absorption

D. CONTRAINDICATIONS/PRECAUTIONS

- May cause vasoconstriction [72]

E. PRACTICAL NOTES

- Recommendations for application include clipping hair first
- Authors find that covering area where cream is applied with plastic such as an examination glove to "trap" body heat may decrease onset up to a total time of 10–20 min
- Works well to assist in the placement of IV catheters or drawing of blood in neonates or critical patients to avoid or minimize sedation

XXXV. Esmolol *beta receptor antagonist*

A. DOSE AND DURATION

- 0.2–0.5 mg/kg IV, CRI 0.5–10 mg/kg/h
- Duration of 10 min or less as a bolus

B. CLINICAL APPLICATIONS

- Prevention of tachycardia and hypertension

C. PHARMACOLOGY

- Beta-1 antagonist which is rapid in onset, resulting in decreased HR, of a short duration, unless given as a CRI
- Metabolized by plasma esterase

D. CONTRAINDICATIONS/PRECAUTIONS

- High doses result in myocardial depression, reduction in CO, and bradycardia
- Bradyarrhythmias such as AV blocks and escape rhythms
- Hypovolemic patients [73]
- Beta antagonists are not used if there is a suspected catecholamine-induced nidus for hypertension or tachycardia (e.g., pheochromocytoma), unless appropriate alpha blockade is already present; unopposed alpha stimulation may prove fatal

E. PRACTICAL NOTES

- IV administration only
- May cause pain on injection
- Useful in cases of thyrotoxicosis
- Used for pheochromocytomas where α blockade is already achieved
- Protect from light

XXXVI. Etomidate *induction agent*

A. DOSE AND DURATION

- See Table 2

B. CLINICAL APPLICATIONS

- Induction agent ideal for patient with structural or arrhythmogenic cardiovascular disease due to its minimal cardiovascular and respiratory depression characterized by absent changes in HR, SV, MAP or CO after administration
- Ideal induction agent for neurologic or neurosurgical patients because of a reduction in cerebral blood flow, ICP and decreased $CMRO_2$ consumption

C. PHARMACOLOGY

- Imidazole derivative used for hypnotic properties in cats and dogs
- $GABA_A$ agonist, resulting in CNS depression and hypnosis
- Contains propylene glycol which can cause pain during intravenous administration
- Water soluble
- Rapidly metabolized both in the liver and by plasma esterases
- Highly protein bound

D. CONTRAINDICATIONS/PRECAUTIONS

- Avoid in critically ill patients due to suspected adrenal exhaustion. Inhibits adrenal steroidogenesis and stress response to surgery at 1/100th of the dose required to induce anesthesia, due to a dose-dependent inhibition of cholesterol conversion to cortisol. This effect may last 4–8 h
- Patients with Addison disease
- Etomidate is hyperosmotic when compared to plasma and causes hemolysis. For this reason, prolonged administration of etomidate is avoided. May also cause irritation upon injection and if accidental perivascular administration occurs
- Does not provide analgesia
- Patients (especially cats) with renal failure, due to propylene glycol and resultant hemolysis

E. PRACTICAL NOTES

- Minimal effects on ventilation
- When given without sedation or in a healthy patient, etomidate can cause myoclonus and vomiting at induction and requires high doses
- Best when given in sedated patients or with a dose of midazolam 0.2 mg/kg IV

XXXVII. Famotidine *H2 receptor antagonist*

A. DOSE AND DURATION

- Dogs and cats: 0.5–1.0 mg/kg IV, SC, IM, oral formulations available
- Duration: 8–12 h

B. CLINICAL APPLICATIONS

- Premedication in patients with mast cell tumors (MCT), patients prone to histamine release or gastric ulcers, patients at risk of regurgitation or irritation of the gastrointestinal tract
- Routine and indiscriminate use of gastroprotectants in clinical practice is discouraged by the ACVIM [74]; however, the goal with use prior to general anesthesia is to neutralize the pH of stomach contents, in case of possible regurgitation and aspiration. Due to the remarkably common occurrence of regurgitation [75–77], use prior to anesthesia may be common especially in certain procedures
- While pantoprazole (see p.349) may result in more effective neutralization of gastric pH [78], it takes up to 36 h to reach effective concentrations, as opposed to 60 min for famotidine [79]. Therefore, famotidine is often utilized in emergency procedures where the patient has not been on a proton pump inhibitor and requires gastrointestinal protection

C. PHARMACOLOGY

- Blocks H2 receptors
- Minimizes occupation of H2 receptors in cases of histamine release
- Multidose vial contains benzyl alcohol as a preservative

D. CONTRAINDICATIONS/PRECAUTIONS

- None clinically relevant

E. PRACTICAL NOTES

- Protect from light

XXXVIII. Fentanyl *full mu agonist opioid*

A. DOSE AND DURATION

- See Table 7

B. CLINICAL APPLICATIONS

- Intraoperative management of noxious stimuli, postoperative analgesic
- Common component of a neuroleptic induction
- MAC-sparing agent when used as a CRI during anesthesia for canine patients

C. PHARMACOLOGY

- Short-acting synthetic mu-agonist opioid; it is more potent than morphine but considered to have equal efficacy to morphine

- Metabolized by the liver
- Controlled, Schedule II

D. CONTRAINDICATIONS/PRECAUTIONS

- May cause bradycardia and hypoventilation (caution in patients with head trauma or increased ICP if not supporting ventilation)
- May cause sedation and nausea
- Causes miosis in the canine and mydriasis in the feline
- Heat can increase the rate of delivery and absorption of transdermal fentanyl patches and may result in skin irritation
- Some formulations of transdermal fentanyl patches cannot be cut. If patch is dispensing more fentanyl than the patient requires, cover half the patch (allow half the patch to have contact with the skin)

E. PRACTICAL NOTES

- Ideal for older or cardiovascular compromised canine patients to reduce MAC
- While the canine patient experiences considerable MAC-sparing effects from fentanyl, the feline does not consistently have MAC reduction. Studies done in cats with a chemical derivative of fentanyl (remifentanil; see p. 357) clearly demonstrate an analgesic benefit for cats in spite of lack of MAC reduction in the same population [80]
- "Wooden chest" phenomena are described in human patients subsequent to the use of fentanyl and other opioids. This refers to muscle rigidity of the thorax and abdomen, preventing adequate ventilation. While not commonly seen in veterinary species, should this occur, reversal of the opioid, neuromuscular blockade, and mechanical ventilation may be necessary
- Reversible with naloxone (opioid antagonist; see p.344)
- For fentanyl patches, hair must be shaved over the area where the patch will be attached and the skin cleaned

XXXIX. Flumazenil *benzodiazepine antagonist*

A. DOSE AND DURATION

- See Table 3

B. CLINICAL APPLICATIONS

- Reversal of benzodiazepines

C. PHARMACOLOGY

- Benzodiazepine competitive antagonist at the GABA receptor

D. CONTRAINDICATIONS/PRECAUTIONS

- Can result in rapid arousal when reversing benzodiazepines

E. PRACTICAL NOTES

- Some feline patients experience prolonged sedation from benzodiazepines, and require reversal with flumazenil. At time of publication, flumazenil is relatively inexpensive and suggested to keep on hand for any practice handling felines
- To reverse benzodiazepines, calculate full dose of reversal and dilute 10-fold. Give slowly IV until desired reversal effect is achieved
- Protect from light

XL. Furosemide *diuretic*

A. DOSE AND DURATION

- 0.5–2.0 mg/kg IM or IV
- Variable depending on formulation, but generally considered to have a duration of 1 (canine) [81]–2.5 (feline) [82] h (note: in some patients with altered physiology, this drug may last longer)

B. CLINICAL APPLICATIONS

- Pulmonary edema, congestive heart failure (CHF), volume overload

C. PHARMACOLOGY

- Loop diuretic
- Inhibits the Na-K-2Cl cotransporter (NKCC)-2 in the ascending limb of the loop of Henle, reducing extracellular fluid volume expansion [83]
- Precipitates in acidic solutions

D. CONTRAINDICATIONS/PRECAUTIONS

- Dehydrated patients; monitor patient hydration when using this drug
- Patients with electrolyte imbalances (such as hyponatremia)
- Do not use in patients which are anuric
- High dosages in the feline may result in ototoxicity [84]
- Electrolyte imbalances, constipation, dehydration, and eventually lack of urine production are possible complications of repeated administration of furosemide

E. PRACTICAL NOTES

- Slight vasodilation occurs, which will increase renal perfusion and decrease preload, although the mechanism behind this is not fully understood [83]

- Monitor electrolytes when using this drug
- Protect from light

XLI. Gabapentin *anticonvulsant, nonopioid analgesic*

A. DOSE AND DURATION

- Dogs: 10–30 mg/kg PO, q 8 or q 12 h
- Cats: while doses of 10–30 mg/kg PO q 8–12 h doses are reported [85], it is common to give a 100 mg/capsule (often mixed with a small amount of wet food) orally [86]

B. CLINICAL APPLICATIONS

- Adjunctive therapy for refractory seizures
- Used for the treatment of chronic and neuropathic pain
- Used as an adjunctive analgesic for postoperative pain management
- Sedation, specifically beneficial for reducing fear responses associated with handling and examination in cats and dogs

C. PHARMACOLOGY

- The exact mechanism of analgesia is not fully understood, but is believed to involve inhibition of presynaptic GABA release, action at the locus coeruleus, and effects on spinal noradrenaline [87]
- Gabapentin's main effect is attributed to the inhibition of the N-type voltage-dependent neuronal calcium channels. Calcium influx into the neurons is reduced and therefore also the action potential propagation and the release of excitatory neuro-transmitters, such as glutamate and substance P. Through this mechanism gabapentin is thought to prevent allodynia and hyperalgesia
- Gabapentin is structurally similar to GABA but does not appear to interfere with GABA receptors
- While often dosed every 12–24 h, pharmacokinetic studies in the canine suggest that the dosage frequency may more suitably be every 4–6 h [88]
- Gabapentin has a high bioavailability after oral administration and the peak of action is achieved after 2 h [88]
- It is not significantly metabolized, with minimal hepatic metabolism, and is eliminated by the kidney largely unchanged

D. CONTRAINDICATIONS/PRECAUTIONS

- Sedation can be a side-effect
- Seizures may result with abrupt discontinuation of the drug after chronic treatments. Therefore, it is recommended when withdrawing to taper the dose
- Caution in animals with renal disfunction and reduction of dose may be indicated
- Avoid human formulations that contain xylitol

E. PRACTICAL NOTES

- Protect from light
- Transdermal gabapentin is under investigation and may show promise for easier administration as an analgesic in cats but varies greatly based on preparation [89,90]
- May act as an appetite stimulant in cats comparable to mirtazapine [91]

XLII. Grapiprant *noncyclooxygenase-inhibiting NSAID*

A. DOSE AND DURATION

- See Table 8

B. CLINICAL APPLICATIONS

- Analgesic and antiinflammatory
- Treatment of mild to moderate inflammation associated with osteoarthritis in dogs

C. PHARMACOLOGY

- Initial drug of the novel piprant class [92]
- Effects are produced via potent and specific antagonism of the prostaglandin E2 receptor 4
- It does not inhibit the production of other prostanoids, nor does it interfere with the maintenance of normal homeostatic function [92]

D. CONTRAINDICATIONS/PRECAUTIONS

- Common clinical side-effects include mild diarrhea, appetite loss, and vomiting

E. PRACTICAL NOTES

- Suitable for chronic but not acute pain [92]; do not administer for postoperative surgical pain and select another NSAID if surgery remains a possibility (i.e., for control of pain for a ruptured cruciate with a surgical repair option)
- In cats, pharmacokinetic studies show that this drug has potential to reach comparable plasma levels to that of the dog, effective for analgesia, at 2 mg/kg BID PO [93]. More studies are required before analgesic efficacy in this species is determined
- Work in MDR-1-positive collies suggests grapiprant is well tolerated, although the pharmacokinetics suggested increased drug exposure compared to dogs without this mutation [94]
- Feeding reduces oral absorption of grapiprant [93]

XLIII. Glycopyrrolate *anticholinergic*

A. DOSE AND DURATION

* See Table 5

B. CLINICAL APPLICATIONS

* Used to treat or prevent bradycardia in the perioperative period
* Used to counteract the cholinergic effects of neuromuscular blockade antagonists such as neostigmine [95]
* Used to reduce salivation

C. PHARMACOLOGY

* Synthetic quaternary ammonium compound
* Glycopyrrolate is an antimuscarinic with similar actions to atropine, but has four times the potency of atropine
* Glycopyrrolate is completely ionized and has poor lipid solubility. For this reason, it does not cross, or crosses only marginally, the blood–brain or blood–placenta barriers or penetrate into the eye [96]
* Rapidly eliminated from the serum after IV administration and virtually no drug remains in the serum 30 min to 3 h after dosing
* Only a small amount is metabolized, with most being excreted unchanged in the urine
* Promotes bronchodilation and smooth muscle relaxation via M2 and M3 receptor antagonism

D. CONTRAINDICATIONS/PRECAUTIONS

* Caution using anticholinergics following the administration of alpha-2 agonists during the hyperdynamic phase [97]. Increasing the heart rate during the period of vasoconstriction and reflexive bradycardia will cause an increase in myocardial oxygen consumption, predisposing the patient to potential life-threatening arrhythmias.
* In dogs, the LD_{50} for glycopyrrolate is reported to be 25 mg/kg IV. In the cat, the LD_{50} after IM injection is reported to be 283 mg/kg. Because of its quaternary structure, minimal CNS effects should occur after an overdose of glycopyrrolate, when compared to atropine
* Low doses may cause an idiosyncratic bradyarrhythmia and second-degree AV block Mobitz I followed by sinus tachycardia
* Systemic administration of glycopyrrolate has not been associated with changes in pupil diameter or IOP. In contrast, it resulted in a clinically relevant transient decrease in aqueous tear production [96]
* Gastrointestinal motility has been shown to be decreased after glycopyrrolate administration in dogs

E. PRACTICAL NOTES

- The authors prefer using glycopyrrolate as premedication IM in patients with high vagal tone over atropine when available
- The onset of action of glycopyrrolate is slightly slower than that of atropine, usually occurring within a few minutes. However, glycopyrrolate has a longer duration of effects than atropine

XLIV. Hydromorphone *full mu agonist opioid*

A. DOSE AND DURATION

- See Table 7

B. CLINICAL APPLICATIONS

- Sedation
- Premedication for painful procedures
- Intraoperative noxious stimuli management
- Postoperative analgesic

C. PHARMACOLOGY

- Semi-synthetic derivative of morphine
- Perfect efficacy of 1
- Five times the potency of morphine
- Metabolized by the liver

D. CONTRAINDICATIONS/PRECAUTIONS

- When given IM, will likely cause vomiting and panting. Avoid in patients where vomiting would be undesirable
- High doses may cause bradycardia and slight respiratory depression
- May increase ICP secondary to hypoventilation. Avoid in patients with head trauma or increased ICP if ventilation is not supported
- Causes miosis in the canine and mydriasis in the feline
- Histamine release may occur but is unlikely. Avoid, if possible, in patients predisposed to histamine release (MCT, heart worm extractions)
- Patients with severe liver dysfunction may have prolonged duration
- There may be increased incidence of regurgitation and aspiration in patients receiving hydromorphone, especially if they have neurologic disease [98]

E. PRACTICAL NOTES

- Up to 69% of cats may experience hyperthermia secondary to hydromorphone [99,100], especially if intraoperative hypothermia occurs [101]
- Reversible with naloxone (see Table 3)

XLV. Hydroxyethyl starch, "Hetastarch 6%" *colloid fluid*

A. DOSE AND DURATION

- Dogs: IV bolus 2–5 mL/kg, total volume delivered not to exceed 10–20 mL/kg/day
- Cats: IV bolus 2–3 mL/kg, total volume delivered not to exceed 5–10 mL/kg/day
- Hypoproteinemic patient fluid rate: 1–3 mL/kg/h
- Duration: 12–24 h

B. CLINICAL APPLICATIONS

- Used when plasma is not available in patient that are hypoproteinemic
- Used as a volume expander to treat hypotension under anesthesia, although routine and indiscriminate use is falling out of favor

C. PHARMACOLOGY

- Polysaccharide with an average molecular weight of 450,000 daltons
- Most commonly available as a 6% aqueous solution for veterinary use
- Large molecular structure allows retainment in vasculature with a long elimination half-life to expand intravascular volume
- Removed by renal excretion as well as redistribution

D. CONTRAINDICATIONS/PRECAUTIONS

- Use results in hemodilution, which is associated with hypercoagulable effects at low dilutions and hypocoagulable effects at higher dilutions [102]. Additionally, there is a decrease in factor VII, von Willebrand factor and fibrongen, as well as decreased platelet function [103,104]. All these factors contribute to potential coagulopathy
- The role of hetastarch in acute kidney injury (AKI) is actively being investigated. Recent work suggests that in a clinical setting for dogs requiring a fluid bolus, there were no changes over time of urine AKI biomarkers in dogs [105], in contrast to work with gelatin colloid solutions, which produced greater increases in urine biomarkers of AKI and more frequent histopathologic changes in the kidneys when used in hemorrhagic shock model patients [106,107]. In humans with renal insufficiency or sepsis, hydroxyethyl starch is avoided [108]. Until more conclusive large-scale work is available, it is best to avoid in oliguric or anuric renal failure patients, as well as to avoid indiscriminate use of this fluid
- Avoid in patients with pulmonary edema or congestive heart failure
- Avoid in normo- or hypervolemic patients, as it may contribute to volume overload
- Total protein value in patients that received hydroxyethyl starch may decrease but oncotic pressure is generally maintained

E. PRACTICAL NOTES

- Anaphylactoid reactions are low, compared to natural colloid products
- Monitoring colloid oncotic pressure (COP) is advised when hydroxyethyl starch is used

- The authors prefer fresh frozen plasma in patients with renal disease and sepsis
- Generally, this fluid is not suitable as a substitute for maintenance fluids

XLVI. Isoflurane *inhalant anesthetic*

A. DOSE AND DURATION

- See Table 9

B. CLINICAL APPLICATIONS

- Inhalant maintenance of anesthesia
- Anesthesia induction via facemask or induction chamber (authors do not recommend mask or chamber inductions)

C. PHARMACOLOGY

- Isoflurane is a clear, colorless, and volatile liquid at room temperature and sea level
- The exact mechanism of action by which inhalant anesthetic agents cause general anesthesia is not precisely known, but it is likely their influence on the electrical activity of the CNS, mediated at the level of the spinal cord, through actions at the lipid bilayer of the cell membrane
- Most important effects cause CNS depression, prevention of movement likely mediated at the level of the spinal cord, dose-dependent cardiovascular and respiratory depression, decreased systemic vascular resistance (vasodilation) and hypotension, increased cerebral blood flow and intracranial pressure, depression of body temperature regulating centers, and muscular relaxation

D. CONTRAINDICATIONS/PRECAUTIONS

- Patients with preexisting extreme hypotension, cardiovascular derangements or reason for inability to handle vasodilation (i.e., the unstable septic patient)
- Caution in patients with increased intracranial pressure or head trauma
- In susceptible individuals, inhalant anesthesia may trigger a clinical syndrome known as malignant hyperthermia, a cellular hypermetabolic state that if not treated quickly causes death. Although mostly reported in human patients and pigs, other species have also been reported to be affected

E. PRACTICAL NOTES

- Requires a precision vaporizer
- The National Institute for Occupational Safety and Health Administration (NIOSH) recommends that no worker should be exposed to ceiling concentrations greater than 2 ppm of any halogenated anesthetic agent over a sampling period not to exceed 1 h

XLVII. Isolyte®

A. DOSE AND DURATION

- See Table 11

Table 11   Common crystalloid fluids for anesthetic management

Crystalloid	Buffer	pH	Osmolarity (mOsmol/L)	Electrolytes (mEq/L)	Dosage/duration
Isolyte®	Acetate	7.0–7.8	295	Acetate: 27 Chloride: 98 Gluconate: 23 Magnesium: 3 Potassium: 5 Sodium: 141	Dosing in dogs: Routine anesthetic maintenance fluid rates for dogs start at 5 mL/kg/h, with incremental dose reduction following the first hour until maintenance fluid rates are achieved (2–3 mL/kg/h) [222] Shock bolus: 80–90 mL/kg IV; often administered in ¼ dose increments under continuous monitoring and reassessment Treatment of anesthetic hypotension: 5–10 mL/kg IV bolus, which may be repeated Dosing in cats: routine anesthetic maintenance fluid rates for cats start at 3 mL/kg/h, with incremental dose reduction following first hour until maintenance fluid rates are achieved (1–3 mL/kg/h) [222] Shock 60–70 mL/kg IV, often given in ¼ dose increments under continual monitoring and reassessment Treatment of anesthetic hypotension: 3–5 mL/kg IV bolus; repeated up to two times As this fluid approximates extracellular solution, only 20–25% will remain in the intravascular space after an hour or so

(Continued)

Table 11   (*Continued*)

Crystalloid	Buffer	pH	Osmolarity (mOsmol/L)	Electrolytes (mEq/L)	Dosage/duration
Lactated Ringer's solution (LRS)	Lactate	6.0–7.5	273	Calcium: 2.7 Chloride: 109 Lactate: 28 Potassium: 4 Sodium: 130	Same as above
Normosol®	Acetate	6.5–7.6	294	Acetate: 27 Chloride: 98 Gluconate: 23 Magnesium: 3 Potassium: 5 Sodium: 140	Same as above
Plasma-Lyte® 148	Acetate	4.0–8.0	294	Acetate: 27 Chloride: 98 Gluconate: 23 Magnesium: 3 Potassium: 5 Sodium: 140	Same as above
Sodium chloride 0.9%		4.5–7.0	308	Chloride: 154 Sodium: 154	Same as above
Sodium chloride 7.5% (hypertonic saline)			2464	Chloride: 1232 Sodium: 1232	Canine: 3–5 mL/kg Feline: 1–3 mL/kg To reduce intracranial pressure, hypertonic saline can be given at 4 mL/kg over 5 min 7.5% hypertonic saline has a duration of 30–60 min

B. CLINICAL APPLICATIONS

- Preoperative fluid resuscitation
- Intraoperative fluid administration
- Treatment of hypotension due to ineffective circulating volume during anesthesia

C. PHARMACOLOGY

- Crystalloid fluid
- Balanced electrolyte solution
- Replacement solution
- Acetate buffer

D. CONTRAINDICATIONS/PRECAUTIONS

- Caution using high volumes or boluses in patients with congestive heart failure, as excessive volumes may result in pulmonary edema; consider reduced rates and avoid bolus

E. PRACTICAL NOTES

- Safe to administer with blood products

XLVIII. Isoproterenol *beta agonist*

A. DOSE AND DURATION

- 0.01–0.08 µg/kg/min IV
- Duration is short-lived if not given as a CRI

B. CLINICAL APPLICATIONS

- Chronotropic; "pharmacologic pacemaker" for patients with sick sinus syndrome or third-degree AV block

C. PHARMACOLOGY

- Sympathomimetic at beta-1 and beta-2 receptors which increases myocardial contractility and HR, causes bronchodilation and reduces bronchial spasms
- Of all sympathomimetics, isoproterenol is the most potent. It is 2–3 times more potent than epinephrine and 100 times more active than norepinephrine [109]
- No alpha agonist effects
- Metabolized in the liver

D. CONTRAINDICATIONS/PRECAUTIONS

- Causes vasodilation via beta-2 receptors in skeletal muscles
- May result in tachycardia and tachyarrhythmias
- Do not use in conjunction with other catecholamines (e.g., epinephrine); effects may be additive
- Coronary blood flow may be reduced due to a decrease in diastolic blood pressure at the same time as myocardial oxygen consumption increases; caution in patients with known coronary artery disease

E. PRACTICAL NOTES

- Protect vial and dilutions from light
- When diluted with 5% dextrose, stable for 24 h

XLIX. Ketamine *NMDA antagonist and dissociative anesthetic*

A. DOSE AND DURATION

- See Table 2

B. CLINICAL APPLICATIONS

- Used in cats and dogs as a general anesthetic for induction
- Used as part of multidrug combinations for chemical restraint or anesthesia
- Used as a coinduction agent to reduce primary induction drug (often propofol or alfaxalone) requirement
- Used as an adjunctive analgesic
- Has been used in local regional techniques such as epidurals or in regional blocks
- Used as a CRI for MAC reduction (up to 40%) of inhalants in dogs [110] and cats [111]

C. PHARMACOLOGY

- Phencyclidine derivative
- Primary action occurs by antagonism of the NMDA receptors leading to a dissociation of the limbic and thalamocortical systems. Induces a cataleptic state in which the patient does not respond to external stimuli
- Causes indirect stimulation of cardiovascular system through catecholamine reuptake inhibition (increases BP and HR and thus CO, increases myocardial O_2 requirements)
- Canines completely metabolize ketamine; however, the feline metabolizes ketamine to norketamine, an active metabolite which may contribute to altered feline recovery

D. CONTRAINDICATIONS/PRECAUTIONS

- Patients induced with ketamine alone exhibit a catatonic state (mydriasis, nystagmus, swallowing, muscle movement/rigidity). For this reason, administration with a muscle relaxant is recommended
- In privileged sites such as the CNS (secondary to protection of the blood–brain barrier), vasodilation and thus an increase in ICP occurs secondary to ketamine. In patients where increases in ICP are a concern (those with seizures or suspected space-occupying diseases of the cranium), ketamine is avoided
- Increased extraocular muscle tone results in an increase in intraocular pressure (IOP) [112]. Often ketamine is avoided in patients where increased IOP is a concern unless no other induction agent is available, in which case ketamine is administered with a benzodiazepine. Avoid in patients with ocular injuries and glaucoma
- May result in hyperthermia due to increased muscle tone. This is often not an issue in patients where inhalant anesthetics are used for maintenance anesthesia, due to the concurrent hypothermia that inhalant anesthesia induces
- Cats with hypertrophic cardiomyopathy
- Cats with significant renal insufficiency

E. PRACTICAL NOTES

- May result in apneustic breathing pattern
- Painful on IM injection due to low pH
- Administer with a muscle relaxant such as benzodiazepine or alpha-2 agonist

- Induction dose can act as the loading dose for a CRI provided there is not a significant delay in beginning the CRI
- When using ketamine as a coinduction technique, the authors' preference is to administer ketamine about 30 sec before titrating the primary induction agent to effect, due to the slightly longer onset time of ketamine
- "Ketofol" is the combination of ketamine and propofol at 1:1 mixture, traditionally 2 mg of each agent. This combination improves the cardiovascular stability of propofol [113] and the induction quality of ketamine alone. Indeed, there were improved tracheal intubation and induction qualities using ketofol compared to propofol [114]
- Lubricate eyes, although animal may still blink
- Cats and dogs may exhibit emergence delirium
- Controlled, Schedule III

L. Ketoprofen *NSAID*

A. *DOSE AND DURATION*

- See Table 8

B. *CLINICAL APPLICATIONS*

- Recommended for acute pain (up to 5 days) in both dogs and cats

C. *PHARMACOLOGY*

- Nonselective, potent inhibitor of COX-1 and COX-2
- Inhibits one or more steps in the metabolism of arachidonic acid (AA) and possesses both analgesic and antiinflammatory properties
- Acts primarily to reduce the biosynthesis of prostaglandins by inhibiting cyclooxygenase (COX-1 and COX-2). Inhibition of prostaglandins that regulate blood flow to the gastric mucosa and stimulate bicarbonate and mucus production may result in loss of GI protective mechanisms
- COX-2 inhibition by NSAIDs is thought to be responsible for the antipyretic, analgesic, and antiinflammatory actions of NSAIDs. However, concurrent inhibition of COX-1 may result in many of the unwanted effects of NSAIDs, including gastric ulceration and renal toxicity
- NSAIDs are biotransformed in the liver to inactive metabolites that are excreted either by the kidney via glomerular filtration and tubular secretion or by the bile

D. *CONTRAINDICATIONS/PRECAUTIONS*

- Although use as part of the premedication prior to the inflammatory event, as opposed to postoperative administration, provides preemptive and better analgesia, caution is advised if using this drug preoperatively
- Caution in patients that are hypoproteinemic

- Because of potential antiplatelet effects, care should be exercised when using keto-profen perioperatively

LI. Lactated Ringer's Solution (LRS) *balanced electrolyte, isotonic crystalloid solution*

A. DOSE AND DURATION

- See Table 11

B. CLINICAL APPLICATIONS

- Preoperative fluid resuscitation
- Intraoperative fluid administration
- Treatment of hypotension due to ineffective circulating volume during anesthesia

C. PHARMACOLOGY

- Crystalloid fluid
- Balanced electrolyte solution
- Replacement solution
- Lactate buffer; lactate is broken down by the liver to bicarbonate, resulting in an alkalinizing effect

D. CONTRAINDICATIONS/PRECAUTIONS

- Caution using high volumes or boluses in patients with congestive heart failure, as excessive volumes may result in pulmonary edema; consider reduced rates and avoid bolus
- Contains Ca++: best practice is to avoid administering in the same catheter as blood products, as Ca++ will chelate with anticoagulant in blood products

E. PRACTICAL NOTES

- In hypocalcemic patients, this may be a fluid of choice; however, it is unlikely to increase serum Ca++ of patient
- In hyperkalemic patients, some do not recommend administering LRS as it contains K+; however, content of K+ is unlikely to clinically affect patient [115]

LII. Lidocaine *Na+ channel blocker, local anesthetic*

A. DOSE AND DURATION

- See Table 6

B. CLINICAL APPLICATIONS

- Used systemically to control ventricular arrhythmias and as a MAC reducer in dogs [116]
- Antinociceptive effects when used as an intraoperative CRI in dogs [117]
- Used as IV bolus at 1–1.5 mg/kg prior to intubation to reduce laryngeal response to orotracheal intubation [118]
- Used during CPR for ventricular arrhythmias such as sustained ventricular tachycardia
- Used for topical laryngeal splash block to ease orotracheal intubation in species prone to laryngeal spasms [119] (cats, pigs, and various exotic species)

C. PHARMACOLOGY

- All local anesthetics share a common chemical structure that includes a lipophilic, benzene ring and a hydrophilic amine group. This compound is then linked to either an ester or an amide; in the case of lidocaine, it is an amide
- pKa 7.8. pKa determines the amount of ionized and unionized fraction of drug present in the plasma. At high pKa, greater will be the proportion of local anesthetic in the ionized, charged hydrophilic form at physiologic pH (7.4), and the onset of action will be slower. In contrast, at low pKa, a greater proportion of the nonionized lipid-soluble form will be present at physiologic pH and the onset of action will be more rapid
- % Ionized at physiological pH: 76
- Lipid solubility 3.6. Lipid solubility is the main determinant of potency and onset of action.
- % Protein binding: 64. Protein binding influences the duration of action. Only the unbound fraction of drug is pharmacologically active. The higher the protein binding, the longer the duration of action

D. CONTRAINDICATIONS/PRECAUTIONS

- Cats have increased sensitivity to local anesthetics [120], although the use of lidocaine to desensitize arytenoids prior to intubation and local administration of lidocaine appears safe [121]
- Avoid IV use in patients with bradyarrhythmias such as AV block, sick sinus syndrome, or escape rhythms which are not secondary to dexmedetomidine (see "Practical notes")
- Patients with liver dysfunction or hypoproteinemia may have prolonged effect when given lidocaine IV

E. PRACTICAL NOTES

- Used for regional and epidural (use preservative-free) anesthesia; see Chapter 7
- New evidence suggests that systemic lidocaine may reverse dexmedetomidine-induced bradycardia [58]
- Often preparations for regional blocks contain epinephrine, which will prolong the duration of a lidocaine block [122]. Epinephrine is added to lidocaine to cause vasoconstriction and therefore decrease systemic absorption of the local anesthetic

when used as a local block. This technique can decrease the total dose of local anesthetic required, prolong the effect and decrease the potential for systemic toxicity. This combination is commercially available or frequently is mixed in-house. This combination should never be administered IV. Use with caution in peripheral limbs
- Sodium bicarbonate can be added to local anesthetic solutions to increase the pH, resulting in less sting upon injection when administering to conscious patients
- Mixture of long-acting (bupivacaine or ropivacaine) and short-acting (lidocaine) local anesthetics is no longer recommended; while there is faster onset of blocks, there is also decreased duration [123]

LIII. Mannitol *osmotic diuretic*

A. DOSE AND DURATION

- Reduction of ICP or IOP: 0.25–2.0 g/kg administered slow over 20 min IV (commonly 0.5 g/kg)
- For renal support [124,125]: 0.25–1 g/kg/h as a CRI during anesthesia
- Duration: often given once as a single bolus; elimination half-life is around 70–90 min [126]

B. CLINICAL APPLICATIONS

- Used to reduce ICP following cerebral injury. Commonly given in neurologic patients which demonstrate indications of increased ICP (Cushing reflex, cerebral edema)
- Reduces IOP in cases of glaucoma
- Used as a CRI to increase urinary output
- Used to increase plasma osmolarity

C. PHARMACOLOGY

- Hyperosmotic diuretic which promotes water loss via the kidneys and blocks reabsorption of water by the kidney tubules
- Only means of clearance is by glomerular filtration [109]

D. CONTRAINDICATIONS/PRECAUTIONS

- Patients with intracranial hemorrhage
- Dehydrated patients
- Patient with congestive heart failure
- Anuric renal failure patients
- Use with caution in hypertensive patients

E. PRACTICAL NOTES

- In single-dose vials, at room temperature, crystals form quickly; keep solution in a warmer or run under warm water prior to administration. For this reason, a filter is used when administering this drug

- When administering this drug, ensure appropriate fluid therapy and monitor urine output
- May be used topically for pharyngeal swelling following brachiocephalic surgeries or a traumatic intubation. Place on cotton tip applicators and swab inflamed tissue prior to extubation

LIV. Maropitant *neurokinin-1 receptor antagonist*

A. DOSE AND DURATION

- 1 mg/kg SC or IV slow, 2 mg/kg PO
- Duration of 24 h with peak plasma concentration reached after minutes of IV injection, 1 h after SC injections, and 2 h following PO administration

B. CLINICAL APPLICATIONS

- Approved by the FDA as antiemetic for dogs and cats [127], although this does not translate to an increase in postoperative appetite [128]
- In addition, maropitant may provide adjunctive analgesia for visceral pain [129]
- MAC-sparing effect (15–25% reduction) is reported in dogs and cats in which general anesthesia was maintained with sevoflurane [130–132]

C. PHARMACOLOGY

- The antinociceptive action is thought to be dependent on the antagonism of NK1 receptors located in the central and peripheral nervous system (specifically in the brain, spinal cord, and viscera) [133]
- Blocks the binding of the endogenous neurotransmitter substance P that is known to cause emesis [133]
- The drug is highly protein bound and caution should be exercised in animals receiving drugs that are also protein bound (e.g., NSAIDs). It is metabolized primarily by the liver and less than 1% is eliminated unchanged in urine or feces
- Novel work suggests there may be a role for NK-1 and associated substance P antagonism in pain modulation, as substance P is found in multiple areas of the pain pathways, including sensory afferents, dorsal root ganglia, dorsal horn, and ascending projections of the spinal cord and higher brain centers involved in pain perception [133,134]

D. CONTRAINDICATIONS/PRECAUTIONS

- Patients with possible gastrointestinal outflow obstruction when not going immediately to surgery or endoscopy
- Caution in patients with liver failure; it is appropriate to reduce the dose if used in these patients
- May cause hypotension, which was more significant for patients who were anesthetized than those who were not [135]

E. PRACTICAL NOTES

- While some clinicians use maropitant to reduce nausea, only 25% of canine patients experience this result, as opposed to 90% of patients receiving ondansetron [136]
- Pain on injection appears to be related to drug formulation [137]. Pain is primarily with SC injection; refrigerating the solution ensures more active ingredient remains bound in the cyclodextrin carrier, effectively reducing pain during injection
- While undocumented in the literature, the authors note that patients with mechanical obstruction to outflow of the GI tract may profusely regurgitate during induction, when maropitant has been used to prevent vomiting (i.e., patients retain fluid in the GI tract which would have otherwise been expelled). As the airway is typically unprotected while induction is occurring, this can lead to aspiration pneumonia. Emptying the stomach with a nasogastric tube and neutralizing gastric pH are appropriate in patients who have been administered maropitant but ultimately will have surgery for obstruction of the GI tract

LV. Meloxicam *NSAID*

A. DOSE AND DURATION

- Dog: 0.2 mg/kg SC as the first dose, following doses 0.1 mg/kg PO
- Cats: 0.1 mg/kg SC or PO once. This dosage is recommended in compliance with the FDA's black box warning about repeated dosing of meloxicam in this species
- Single dose duration of 24 h

B. CLINICAL APPLICATIONS

- Common NSAID for small-breed dogs and cats
- Used perioperatively and has been recognized for its analgesic efficacy for up to 20 h post surgery, including following canine ovariohysterectomies

C. PHARMACOLOGY

- Blocks the action of cyclooxygenase to provide antiinflammatory, analgesic, and antipyretic effects
- COX-2 preferential
- Metabolized by oxidation in cats; this is the preferred route of metabolism for drugs used in this species, as cats do not glucuronidate effectively

D. CONTRAINDICATIONS/PRECAUTIONS

- Patients with gastrointestinal disease, bleeding disorders, and renal insufficiencies
- Patients who have undergone a surgery where the GI tract was breached

E. PRACTICAL NOTES

- If given prior to anesthesia (either with the premedication or orally in the morning), ensure the patient is normotensive throughout the anesthetic period. If one cannot be

certain, do not administer meloxicam until the animal is stabilized in the postoperative period
* Injectable and oral formulations and a transmucosal spray are available

LVI. Meperidine *full agonist opioid*

A. DOSE AND DURATION

* Dog: 3–5 mg/kg IM
* Cat: 3–5 mg/kg IM
* Duration of 45–60 min

B. CLINICAL APPLICATIONS

* Mild analgesia and sedation
* Useful as premedication specifically in young patients

C. PHARMACOLOGY

* Full mu agonist
* Synthetic
* Metabolized by the liver
* Has anticholinergic-like effects (e.g., increase in HR)
* May block sodium channels, similar to local anesthetics
* May also possess alpha-2 agonist receptor activity

D. CONTRAINDICATIONS/PRECAUTIONS

* Histamine release possible (especially when given IV), which may result in hypotension and facial edema (for this reason, it is limited to IM administration)
* Vomiting may occur
* Avoid in patients prone to histamine release (MCT, heart worm extractions)
* Patients receiving monoamine oxidase inhibitors (MAOI) (e.g., selegiline)
* Patients with head trauma or increased ICP if ventilation is not supported

E. PRACTICAL NOTES

* Causes miosis in the canine and mydriasis in the feline
* Reversible with naloxone
* Synergistic action with sedatives may cause profound sedation
* Excitement possible when used alone
* Ideal for young patients with patent ductus arteriosus (PDA) or portosystemic shunt (PSS) as premedication as it provides analgesia while helping to maintain heart rate
* This drug is extremely short-acting and thus has limited usefulness in most veterinary practices; a longer acting opioid should be included postoperatively

- In human patients, the combination of a meperidine and an MAOI has reportedly caused serotonin syndrome – a potentially fatal reaction. While this is not documented in veterinary medicine, the possibility exists
- Controlled drug, Schedule II

LVII. Mepivacaine *local anesthetic*

A. DOSE AND DURATION

- See Table 6

B. CLINICAL APPLICATIONS

- Used for regional and epidural (use preservative-free) anesthesia

C. PHARMACOLOGY

- All local anesthetics share a common chemical structure that includes a lipophilic, benzene ring and a hydrophilic amine group. This compound is then linked to either an ester or an amide; in the case of mepivacaine, it is an amide
- pKa 7.72. pKa determines the amount of ionized and unionized fraction of drug present in the plasma. At high pKa, greater will be the proportion of local anesthetic in the ionized, charged hydrophilic form at physiologic pH (7.4), and the onset of action will be slower. In contrast, at low pKa, a greater proportion of the nonionized lipid-soluble form will be present at physiologic pH and the onset of action will be more rapid
- % Ionized at physiological pH: 61
- Lipid solubility 2; lipid solubility is the main determinant of potency and onset of action
- % Protein binding: 77; protein binding influences the duration of action. Only the unbound fraction of drug is pharmacologically active. The higher the protein binding, the longer the duration of action

D. CONTRAINDICATIONS/PRECAUTIONS

- Avoid IV use due to potential for cardiotoxicity
- Cats have increased sensitivity to local anesthetics

E. PRACTICAL NOTES

- Slightly longer lasting than lidocaine, shorter duration than bupivacaine
- Useful for dental blocks due to quick onset and length of duration
- Sodium bicarbonate can be added to local anesthetic solutions to increase the pH, resulting in less sting upon injection when administering to conscious patients
- Mixture of long-acting (bupivacaine or ropivacaine) and short-acting (lidocaine or mepivacaine) local anesthetics is no longer recommended because they produce unpredictable clinical results [123]

LVIII. Methadone *full agonist opioid*

A. DOSE AND DURATION

* See Table 7

B. CLINICAL APPLICATIONS

* Used for preemptive analgesia within the premedication, especially when vomiting should be avoided
* Used for perianesthetic analgesia

C. PHARMACOLOGY

* Synthetic derivative of morphine
* Perfect efficacy of 1
* Equal potency with morphine
* Full mu agonist opioid but also possesses NMDA antagonist properties
* Metabolized by the liver

D. CONTRAINDICATIONS/PRECAUTIONS

* May increase ICP secondary to hypoventilation. Avoid in patients with head trauma or increased ICP if ventilation is not supported
* Causes miosis in the canine and mydriasis in the feline
* Patients with severe liver dysfunction may have prolonged duration
* High doses may result in bradycardia and respiratory depression

E. PRACTICAL NOTES

* At the time of writing, methadone is remarkably expensive
* Reversible by naloxone
* Ideal for painful patients where vomiting needs to be avoided (patients with increased ICP, IOP, GI foreign bodies, etc.)
* Ideal postoperative analgesic where nausea or sedation is undesirable
* May reduce central sensitization due to its NMDA antagonist properties
* Controlled substance, Schedule II

LIX. Midazolam *benzodiazepine*

A. DOSE AND DURATION

* See Table 1

B. CLINICAL APPLICATIONS

- Used as a premedication; most predictable in sick, calm, geriatric or neonatal patients
- Commonly mixed with other sedatives or anesthetics for the chemical restraint of uncooperative animals [138]
- Used as an anticonvulsant in the treatment of seizures (IV, rectal; however, multi-center work has documented superiority of intranasal administration during canine status epilepticus, as opposed to rectal diazepam administration [139])
- Coinduction agent used to reduce doses of other injectable anesthetics [140–142] and provide muscle relaxation
- Antianxiety action
- Appetite stimulant in some laboratory species [143] and cats [144]. Although this has not been documented in the dog, it stands to reason that, like diazepam, it may result in appetite stimulation [145]

C. PHARMACOLOGY

- Aqueous solution with a pH of 3.5. Not painful on IV injection. Does not cause thrombophlebitis. Once administered, at physiologic pH, the drug becomes lipid soluble and able to cross the blood–brain barrier to cause its central effects. This unique solubility characteristic provides a very rapid onset of action after administration
- High bioavailability after enteral and parenteral administration due to high lipophilicity results in a very rapid onset of action
- Highly protein bound. Because only the unbound portion of the drug crosses the blood–brain barrier, changes in plasma protein concentrations may affect response to a given dose
- Sedative effects occur by enhancing the GABA$_A$ receptor's affinity for the inhibitory neurotransmitter GABA within the CNS. Benzodiazepines are considered to have an indirect effect by potentiating the activity of endogenous GABA neurotransmitter, leading to a wide safety margin and minimal depression of ventilation, CO, and oxygen delivery
- Muscle relaxant and anticonvulsant properties derive from action on spinal interneurons
- Metabolized by the liver
- The impact on the cardiovascular system is minimal [146]
- Rapidly absorbed after IM administration

D. CONTRAINDICATIONS/PRECAUTIONS

- Unpredictable sedative properties if used alone in healthy patients where agitation or excitement may become evident
- Avoid in patients with hepatic encephalopathy or PSS
- Avoid use for cesarean sections; crosses the placental barrier and may result in respiratory depression in neonates
- Use with other CNS depressant may increase the risk of respiratory depression

E. PRACTICAL NOTES

- Reduces the dose of propofol needed for total intravenous anesthesia (TIVA) [142]
- Reversal agent is flumazenil (see Table 3)
- Can be administered a variety of routes: intranasal [138,147], oral, and rectal, in addition to the traditional IM and IV routes
- Effective sedation for most small mammals and avian species
- Undergoes photodegradation and should be kept protected from the light
- Works well intranasal in a variety of small exotic animal species [52,147]
- Some cats experience profound sedation from midazolam. It is suspected that cats may eliminate 1-hydroxymidazolam more slowly than expected [148]. While traditionally flumazenil is used to reverse this drug, one case report documents the necessity for intravenous lipid emulsion to resolve the overt sedation of one cat [148]
- Controlled drug, Schedule IV

LX. Morphine *full mu agonist opioid*

A. DOSE AND DURATION

- See Table 7

B. CLINCAL APPLICATIONS

- Premedication, sedation, intraoperative management, and postoperative analgesia
- Used by some veterinarians intraarticular to target the peripheral mu opioid receptors
- Decreases MAC up to 45% [149]

C. PHARMACOLOGY

- Phenanthrene alkaloid of opium
- Engages presynaptic and postsynaptic receptor sites in the CNS, as well as on primary afferent neurons
- Prototype mu agonist opioid, to which all other opioids are compared. Morphine also works at delta and kappa receptors
- Metabolized in the liver to several metabolites; the active metabolite (which results in analgesia) is morphine-6-glucuronide

D. CONTRAINDICATIONS/PRECAUTIONS

- Vomiting and panting, as well as other signs of nausea (excessive salivation), likely when given IM. Often avoided in patients where vomiting and retching will increase ICP and IOP. However, maropitant administered prior to morphine was successful in reducing incidence of vomiting [150,151]
- May result in histamine release, especially with high doses given rapidly IV
- Respiratory depression and bradycardia are possible at high doses
- Initially increases peristaltic motility followed by prolonged period of GI stasis, which may result in constipation

- Morphine, among other opioids, causes contracture of the sphincter of Oddi (common biliary duct), increasing gall bladder pressure [152]
- Causes miosis in the canine and mydriasis in the feline. For this reason, in some ophthalmological procedures (lens luxation), morphine is avoided
- Patients predisposed to histamine release (MCT, heart worm extraction)

E. PRACTICAL NOTES

- The highly overstated phenomenon of excitement in cats has been reported. The study responsible for this rumor used doses of up to 20 mg/kg to cause dysphoria [153]. Most cats actually experience euphoria secondary to morphine administration at clinical doses
- Systemic and epidural morphine results in release of antidiuretic hormone. The authors advise gentle bladder expression or catheterization of any animal which receives morphine epidurally prior to recovery, as well as good nursing care documenting normal urination
- When given alone, possible dysphoria, excitement, and increased responsiveness to noise may result
- Reversible with naloxone (see Table 3)
- Controlled substance, Schedule II

LXI. Naloxone *opioid antagonist*

A. DOSE AND DURATION

- See Table 3

B. CLINICAL APPLICATIONS

- Used to reverse opioid full and partial agonists
- Commonly used to reverse opioid effects when they contribute to a prolonged or dysphoric recovery

C. PHARMACOLOGY

- Nonselective opioid antagonist
- Antagonizes both exogenous and endogenous opioids
- Metabolized by the liver

D. CONTRAINDICATIONS/PRECAUTIONS

- Use could result in inadequate analgesia
- May result in hypertension and excitement
- Short duration may necessitate repeated dosing, depending on duration of the opioid reversed

E. PRACTICAL NOTES

- Reversal of opioid agonists may leave the patient painful! Always have alternative analgesia on board prior to beginning reversal
- Calculate dose and dilute 1:10 with saline; give in increments until desired reversal is achieved for nonemergent situations
- Emergency situation or anesthetic arrest: full dose of naloxone is given IV when an opioid was administered and repeated every hour for the duration of opioid agonist

LXII. Neostigmine *nondepolarizing neuromuscular blocking antagonist*

A. DOSE AND DURATION

- See Table 3

B. CLINICAL APPLICATIONS

- Reversal of nondepolarizing NMB agents (atracurium, cisatracurium, and pancuronium)

C. PHARMACOLOGY

- Inhibits acetylcholinesterase, to increase the amount of the neurotransmitter acetylcholine at the neuromuscular junction (favoring binding of acetylcholine)
- If a nondepolarizing neuromuscular blocking agent is not on board prior to administration of neostigmine, there will be presynaptic effects (resulting in muscle fasciculations)
- Inhibition is reversible, as the drug acts as a competitive substrate substitute for acetylcholine and acetylcholinesterase interactions [109]
- Poorly lipid soluble

D. CONTRAINDICATIONS/PRECAUTIONS

- May result in bradycardia
- Increases smooth muscle tone of the bladder; for this reason, it is often avoided, when possible, in patients with urinary or GI obstruction
- Results in peristalsis (diarrhea) and increased secretions

E. PRACTICAL NOTES

- Does not cross the blood–brain barrier or placenta
- Give anticholinergic (atropine or glycopyrrolate) prior to giving neostigmine to prevent the muscarinic effects which may otherwise result in bradycardia

LXIII. Nitroprusside *alpha antagonist*

A. DOSE AND DURATION

- CRI 0.03–0.3 mg/kg/h (ideal to use less than 0.03 mg/kg/h) IV
- Duration of a single dose is 1–3 min, short half-life

B. CLINICAL APPLICATIONS

- Vascular smooth muscle relaxant used as a peripheral vasodilator for acute/severe hypertension
- Used in patients with acute heart failure secondary to mitral regurgitation and in patients with refractory congestive heart failure (CHF)
- Used to treat hypertension secondary to unmanaged pheochromocytoma

C. PHARMACOLOGY

- Causes peripheral vasodilation (arterial and venous) through liberation of nitric oxide (NO) at the level of the vascular endothelium and underlying smooth muscle, resulting in a significant reduction of total peripheral resistance and a decrease in blood pressure. The HR increases in response to the hypotension. Finally, CO mildly decreases
- Metabolized to cyanogen, which results in cyanide or thiocyanate toxicity after prolonged therapy

D. CONTRAINDICATIONS/PRECAUTIONS

- Renal insufficiencies and failure (which prolong drug duration)
- Risk of cyanide and thiocyanate toxicity
- Signs of toxicity are tachycardia, hyperventilation, metabolic acidosis, and seizures
- Toxicity is treated with thiosulfate [154] (6 mg/kg/h IV in dogs)
- Avoid in patients with raised ICP
- Avoid in patients whose hypertension is compensatory (such as with a Cushing reflex)
- The hypotensive effects of nitroprusside may be enhanced by concomitant administration of general anesthetics or other hypotensive agents (e.g., beta-blockers, ACE inhibitors, etc.)
- Synergistic effects (increased CO and reduced wedge pressure) may result if dobutamine is used with nitroprusside

E. PRACTICAL NOTES

- To administer this drug, dilute with D5W. See Appendix D for dilution equations
- Being remarkably light sensitive, dilutions are only stable for 24 h if protected from all light. Wrap entire dilution and delivery line with light-blocking material such as aluminum foil, vet wrap or brown plastic bags

LXIV. Norepinephrine *endogenous catecholamine, vasopressor*

A. DOSE AND DURATION

- See Table 10

B. CLINICAL APPLICATIONS

- Pressor treatment of choice for patients with sepsis
- Helpful for nonresponsive hypotension as a result of vasodilation

C. PHARMACOLOGY

- Endogenous neurotransmitter released from postganglionic sympathetic nerves
- Agonist at alpha-1-, alpha-2-, and beta-1-adrenergic receptors with predominating alpha-1 receptor-mediated effects when used at clinical doses
- Potent and results in profound arterial and venous vasoconstriction

D. CONTRAINDICATIONS/PRECAUTIONS

- Conflicting opinions exist about administration of this drug during pregnancy, as vasoconstriction of uterine vessels may decrease perfusion to the fetus
- Patients with hypertension

E. PRACTICAL NOTES

- Very low doses (0.025 µg/kg/min), beta-1-adrenergic receptor-mediated effects predominate, resulting in increases in HR and CO and decreases in systemic vascular resistance
- At higher dose rates (greater than 0.5–1.5 µg/kg/min), norepinephrine causes dose-dependent increases in systolic, diastolic, and mean arterial blood pressures, CO, and systemic and pulmonary vascular resistance. This may ultimately reduce CO and increase myocardial oxygen consumption due to the increase in afterload
- Vasoconstriction may result in decreased perfusion. Increasing lactate levels may indicate that the drug is worsening perfusion in spite of improved BP
- Tachycardia is less likely when compared with administration of epinephrine; indeed, bradycardia may result from profound vasoconstriction
- Extravasation of the drug can cause necrosis due to regional vasoconstriction and ischemia. Monitor the patency of the intravenous catheter before administration. Ideally, the drug should be given through a central line

LXV. Normosol® *balanced electrolyte, isotonic crystalloid solution*

A. DOSE AND DURATION

- See Table 11

B. CLINICAL APPLICATIONS

- Preoperative fluid resuscitation
- Intraoperative fluid administration
- Treatment of hypotension due to ineffective circulating volume during anesthesia

C. PHARMACOLOGY

- Crystalloid fluid
- Balanced electrolyte solution
- Replacement solution
- Acetate buffer

D. CONTRAINDICATIONS/PRECAUTIONS

- Caution if using high volumes or boluses in patients with congestive heart failure, as excessive volumes may result in pulmonary edema; consider reduced rates and avoid bolus
- There is a report of a single dog becoming hypotensive secondary to bolus of Normosol-R

E. PRACTICAL NOTES

- Safe to administer with blood products

LXVI. Pancuronium *nondepolarizing neuromuscular blocking agent*

A. DOSE AND DURATION

- See Table 4

B. CLINICAL APPLICATIONS

- Provides paralysis so often used to implement mechanical ventilation or ophthalmic procedures to keep the pupil central

C. PHARMACOLOGY

- Original NMBA with a steroid molecule base
- Exerts action at the neuromuscular junction where it competes with ACh to bind the cholinergic receptor, preventing contractions of skeletal muscle (paralysis)
- Repeated doses will accumulate, so redosing is discouraged
- Dependent on renal excretion, as most is eliminated unchanged in the urine (>80%)

D. CONTRAINDICATIONS/PRECAUTIONS

- Patients with renal insufficiency or failure
- Inhibition of cardiac muscarinic receptors (especially those of the sinoatrial node) may result in an increase in HR, blood pressure, and CO; although this is rarely of clinical concern, alternative NMBAs may be selected for a patient with underlying cardiac disease

E. PRACTICAL NOTES

- Longer duration of action than atracurium
- Does not result in histamine release
- Must be refrigerated

LXVII. Pantoprazole *proton pump inhibitor*

A. DOSE AND DURATION

- 0.7–1 mg/kg IV slow every 12–24 h

B. CLINICAL APPLICATIONS

- Used to increase pH of gastric acid to decrease incidence of esophagitis, should regurgitation occur during anesthesia or sedation
- Used to increase pH of gastric acid for treatment of gastroesophageal reflux disease

C. PHARMACOLOGY

- Irreversible inhibitor of the hydrogen-potassium adenosine triphosphatase proton pump [155]
- Weak base that becomes unprotonated in the presence of physiologic pH of blood and suppresses gastric acid production
- Requires reconstitution, after which stability is pH dependent (degradation increases as pH decreases)
- 98% serum protein bound, primary binding to albumin
- Metabolized via the liver through the cytochrome P450 system
- Eliminated via excretion in the urine and feces through the biliary system

D. CONTRAINDICATIONS/PRECAUTIONS

- Caution if coadministering oral medications that require targeted gastric pH ranges for effectiveness (i.e., slow release, protective coated drugs) as PPIs increase gastric pH. These drugs may need to be avoided or doses adjusted
- Use of PPIs with NSAIDs may increase risk of NSAID-induced intestinal injury and ulceration [156]

E. PRACTICAL NOTES

- Effective clinical benefit of PPIs likely requires daily administration for several days [74]
- Per manufacturer, requires reconstitution with 0.9% NaCl to a 4 mg/mL solution and can be stored at room temperature for 24 h
- PPIs are consistently superior to histamine type-2 receptor antagonists (i.e., famotidine) at increasing gastric pH and preventing exercise-induced gastritis in dogs and cats [78,79]; however, limited pharmacokinetic data on IV usage in the dog and cat is available. The data available suggests it takes up to 36 h to see the effectiveness of PPIs [74]; in a patient who is not currently on a PPI, famotidine remains the more effective choice at increasing gastric pH immediately prior to anesthesia
- Thrombophlebitis is associated with IV administration in people, according to FDA data
- Requires protection from light

LXVIII. Pentobarbital sodium *barbiturate*

A. DOSE AND DURATION

- See Table 2

B. CLINICAL APPLICATIONS

- Short-acting barbiturate that, due to its longer residence time and low therapeutic index, has been replaced as a general anesthetic by other agents
- Used in the treatment and control of seizures
- Euthanasia solution

C. PHARMACOLOGY

- CNS depression caused by activation of GABA receptors
- Highly protein bound
- Redistributes quickly (effect terminates shortly after administration), but hepatic metabolism and renal clearance are necessary for elimination

D. CONTRAINDICATIONS/PRECAUTIONS

- As with most induction agents, crosses the placental barrier. Not recommended for C-sections with viable fetuses
- Cardiovascular and respiratory depression are common
- If used as an anesthetic, excitement may occur during recovery
- Patients with hypoalbuminemia or liver insufficiencies will have profound and prolonged effects
- Use with caution in patients with renal insufficiencies
- Do not use to treat seizures secondary to lidocaine toxicity

E. PRACTICAL NOTE

- Controlled drug, Schedule II
- The very alkalotic pH of pentobarbital will cause sloughing if extravasation of the drug occurs
- Sometimes used to control seizures following myelograms

LXIX. Phenoxybenzamine *alpha receptor blocker*

A. DOSE AND DURATION

- 0.5–0.6 mg/kg PO q 12 h for ideally 14–20 days before surgery

B. CLINICAL APPLICATIONS

- Administer prior to surgical removal of pheochromocytomas, to establish effective circulating volume, secondary to α reduction in chronic vasoconstriction because of catecholamine release from the pheochromocytoma

C. PHARMACOLOGY

- Nonselective, irreversible alpha receptor blockade
- Inhibition of neuronal and extraneuronal uptake of catecholamines
- Long-acting
- Metabolized in the liver
- Excreted in the urine and bile

D. CONTRAINDICATIONS/PRECAUTIONS

- Arrhythmias are still possible during excision of the pheochromocytoma; it is advisable to consider beta blockade if α receptor blockade is successful, and arrhythmias are still evident
- Sedation may result from a reduction in sympathetic outflow at the level of the CNS

E. PRACTICAL NOTES

- Reduction in mortality associated with pheochromocytomas, with preoperative administration [157]
- Some owners report overt sedation in their pets while on this drug, so counseling owners as to this side-effect is advisable to ensure the drug is consistently administered

LXX. Phenylephrine *vasopressor*

A. DOSE AND DURATION

- See Table 10

B. CLINICAL APPLICATIONS

- Used to treat hypotension
- Used intranasally (1% nasal solution is available) to reduce bleeding after a rhinoscopy, via local vasoconstriction
- Topical 10% eye drops are occasionally used as part of a phacoemulsification procedure

C. PHARMACOLOGY

- Potent, direct-acting alpha-1 agonist with no beta activity that results in smooth muscle contraction, causing vasoconstriction
- Increases blood pressure by an increase in systemic vascular resistance

D. CONTRAINDICATIONS/PRECAUTIONS

- Constriction of veins is greater than that of arteries
- Likely to result in hypertension with a reflex bradycardia
- Avoid in patients with preexisting hypertension and valvular cardiovascular disease (e.g., MR)
- Extravasation may result in sloughing or necrosis of surrounding skin

E. PRACTICAL NOTES

- Expect hypertension under anesthesia in patients topically administered this drug prior to phacoemulsification
- Useful to manage hypotension in patients where increasing HR or workload is undesirable (i.e., patients with HCM or valvular stenosis)
- Because profound vasoconstriction results in decreased perfusion, some prefer to monitor lactate levels. Increasing lactate levels may indicate that this drug is worsening perfusion in spite of improved BP
- Protect from light

LXXI. Plasma-Lyte® 148 *balanced electrolyte, isotonic crystalloid solution*

A. DOSE AND DURATION

- See Table 11

B. CLINICAL APPLICATIONS

- Preoperative fluid resuscitation
- Intraoperative fluid administration
- Treatment of hypotension due to ineffective circulating volume during anesthesia

C. PHARMACOLOGY

- Crystalloid fluid
- Balanced electrolyte solution
- Replacement solution
- Acetate buffer

D. CONTRAINDICATIONS/PRECAUTIONS

- Caution if using high volumes or boluses in patients with congestive heart failure, as excessive volumes may result in pulmonary edema; consider reduced rates and avoid bolus

E. PRACTICAL NOTES

- Safe to administer with blood products

LXXII. Potassium chloride (KCl) *electrolyte supplement*

A. DOSE AND DURATION

- Rate of administration not to exceed 0.5 mEq/kg/h
- Relatively short-lived if not administered as a part of a CRI

B. CLINICAL APPLICATIONS

- Treatment of patients with hypokalemia

C. PHARMACOLOGY

- As the primary intracellular cation, K+ is vital to many physiologic processes (nerve transmission, muscular contraction, renal function, and normal intracellular tonicity, to name a few)
- The gradient between intracellular and extracellular K+ is maintained by an active ion transport system
- In normal homeostasis, the K+ absorbed from the gastrointestinal tract exceeds what is lost through the kidneys. When this balance is not maintained, patients will become hypokalemic and require K+ supplementation

D. CONTRAINDICATIONS/PRECAUTIONS

- Potassium is necessary to prevent muscle weakness, but extreme caution is used when providing supplementation by any route other than oral
- Hyperkalemia is fatal in a high enough dosage
- Caution in patients with renal insufficiencies
- Never use bolus fluids supplemented with potassium

E. PRACTICAL NOTES

- Place ECG on patient and monitor for changes if using potassium supplementation
- ECG changes associated with hyperkalemia include bradyarrhythmia, spiked T waves, prolonged P–R interval, absent P waves, widened QRS complexes, and asystole; ventricular tachycardia can also be seen
- Monitor serum potassium levels every 30 min during supplementation during anesthesia

LXXIII. Proparacaine 0.5% *local anesthetic*

A. DOSE AND DURATION

- See Table 6

B. CLINICAL APPLICATIONS

- Used mostly for ophthalmologic procedures

C. PHARMACOLOGY

- Na+ channel blocker for ophthalmic use

D. CONTRAINDICATIONS/PRECAUTIONS

- When using this drug to measure IOP, false decreases in IOP may occur [158]

E. PRACTICAL NOTES

- Keep refrigerated
- Protect from light

LXXIV. Procainamide *class IA antiarrhythmic*

A. DOSE AND DURATION

- Dogs: 5–10 mg/kg IV followed by an IV CRI 1.5–3.0 mg/kg/h [159]
- Cats: 1–2 mg/kg IV followed by an IV CRI 0.6–1.2 mg/kg/h
- Duration: effects of the injectable product are short-lived without a CRI

B. CLINICAL APPLICATIONS

- Treatment of ventricular tachyarrhythmias

C. PHARMACOLOGY

- Na+ channel blocker for ventricular ectopic beats and ventricular tachyarrhythmias
- Metabolized in the liver and excreted by the kidney

D. CONTRAINDICATIONS/PRECAUTIONS

- Rarely used during anesthesia as this drug may cause cardiovascular depression and hypotension
- Reduce dose in patients with hepatic or renal disease
- Do not administer in cases of ventricular escape rhythms, sick sinus syndrome or third-degree AV block

E. PRACTICAL NOTES

- Some cardiologists believe this drug is more appropriate to treat feline ventricular tachyarrhythmias, although this suggestion is anecdotal
- Useful alternative to lidocaine prior to a balloon valvuloplasty to prevent ventricular arrhythmias
- Useful for ventricular arrhythmias that are refractory to lidocaine

LXXV. Propofol *induction agent*

A. DOSE AND DURATION

- See Table 2

B. CLINICAL APPLICATIONS

- Injectable sedative-hypnotic anesthetic used as an induction agent in dogs and cats because of its smooth inductions and recoveries
- Noncumulative; useful for TIVA as repeat bolus or CRI. Including midazolam may reduce the propofol TIVA dose necessary, without prolonging recovery [142]
- Often used as the maintenance agent of choice for patients with intracranial disease undergoing imaging such as an MRI, with demonstrably improved arterial pressures, decreased requirements for dopamine, and improved recovery scores in addition to the cerebral perfusion advantages when compared to isoflurane [160]
- Used as an anticonvulsant in patients where other efforts have failed [161]

C. PHARMACOLOGY

- Lipid-based emulsion formulation
- Acts via $GABA_A$ receptors
- Rapidly redistributes; metabolized both hepatically and extrahepatically (e.g., in the muscle, lung, and kidney)

- Like many multidose drugs, veterinary approved preserved formulation contains benzyl alcohol. Use with caution as a CRI in species such as cats

D. CONTRAINDICATIONS/PRECAUTIONS

- Decreases ICP, cerebral metabolic rate of oxygen ($CMRO_2$) consumption, and cerebral blood flow (CBF). There is no change in cerebral autoregulation. Systemic reviews in the human medical field find that propofol has lower mean ICP values and higher cerebral perfusion pressure compared to inhaled agents, making this the agent of choice in cases of intracranial disease [162]
- May suppress the sympathetic nervous system to a greater extent than the parasympathetic nervous system. Bradycardia or even asystole may result if given rapidly to patients with high vagal tone
- Systemic vasodilation after administration may result
- Apnea occurs when administered rapidly
- Muscle twitching and paddling (myoclonus) have been observed
- May result in Heinz body formation and toxic changes in RBCs in cats with repeated administration [163,164]
- No analgesia
- Avoid in patients with allergies to eggs
- Avoid in patients with increased triglycerides or cholesterol
- Ventilation status must be carefully maintained and monitored in patients with neurologic disease
- Use only unpreserved formulations of propofol for cat CRIs; CRIs in cats may result in prolonged recoveries

E. PRACTICAL NOTES

- Ideal for patients with diminished liver function, as it is metabolized extrahepatically
- Best administration technique is slowly, to effect
- Preoxygenation for at least 3 min up to the point of intubation may prolong the period from apnea to desaturation at induction [165]
- Ideal alternative to inhalant anesthetic for neurologic patients as TIVA. It is imperative to maintain an airway and administer oxygen
- Animals have demonstrated pain on injection, particularly with the lipid emulsification formulation of propofol [16]

LXXVI. Propranolol *nonselective beta-blocker*

A. DOSE AND DURATION

- Dogs and cats: 0.02–0.1 mg/kg IV slowly to effect
- Duration of 2–6 h

B. CLINICAL APPLICATIONS

- Treatment of tachycardia and supraventricular arrhythmias

C. PHARMACOLOGY

- Beta-1 and beta-2 blocker
- Class II antiarrhythmic
- Extensively protein bound
- Dependent on liver metabolism; undergoes extensive first-pass metabolism

D. CONTRAINDICATIONS/PRECAUTIONS

- Patients with bradycardia or escape beats
- Resulting bradycardia may cause a reduction in CO
- Asthmatic patients
- Use with caution in patients with liver insufficiencies or hypoproteinemia; drug may have profound effect and delayed clearance

E. PRACTICAL NOTES

- Bronchoconstriction may result from beta-2 blockade
- In humans, a decrease in local anesthetic and opioid clearance has been reported with administration of propranolol. It is unknown whether this occurs in animals

LXXVII. Remifentanil *full agonist opioid*

A. DOSE AND DURATION

- See Table 7

B. CLINICAL APPLICATIONS

- Used for intraoperative analgesia and to significantly reduce inhalant requirement when used as a CRI [166]
- Commonly used for patients with liver failure [167], hepatic shunts, or extremely critical patients

C. PHARMACOLOGY

- Full mu agonist
- Highly lipid soluble
- Metabolized by plasma esterase

D. CONTRAINDICATIONS/PRECAUTIONS

- May cause bradycardia and hypoventilation at high doses or following boluses
- Caution in patients with head trauma or increased ICP if ventilation is not supported

E. PRACTICAL NOTES

- Postoperatively, an alternative opioid is likely more suitable for analgesia due to remifentanil's short duration
- Acute opioid tolerance and hyperalgesia are reported for people exposed to remifentanil. These findings could not be confirmed in canine patients exposed to remifentanil [168]
- Formulation available must be reconstituted
- Controlled drug, Schedule II

LXXVIII. Robenacoxib *NSAID*

A. DOSE AND DURATION

- See Table 8

B. CLINICAL APPLICATIONS

- Used to manage postoperative pain associated with OHE/castration or orthopedic surgeries in cats
- Used to manage postoperative pain and inflammation in dogs associated with soft tissue surgeries

C. PHARMACOLOGY

- Inhibits one or more steps in the metabolism of arachidonic acid (AA) and possesses both analgesic and antiinflammatory properties
- Acts primarily to reduce the biosynthesis of prostaglandins by inhibiting cyclooxygenase (COX-1 and COX-2). In particular, robenacoxib is selective for the COX-2 prostaglandin
- NSAIDs are biotransformed in the liver to inactive metabolites that are excreted either by the kidney via glomerular filtration and tubular secretion or by the bile

D. CONTRAINDICATIONS/PRECAUTIONS

- Although use as part of the premedication prior to the inflammatory event, as opposed to postoperative administration, provides preemptive and better analgesia, caution is advised if using this drug preoperatively, especially in dehydrated patients or those with preexisting renal, cardiovascular or hepatic dysfunction
- COX-2 inhibition by NSAIDs is thought to be responsible for the antipyretic, analgesic, and antiinflammatory actions of NSAIDs. However, concurrent inhibition of

COX-1 may result in many of the unwanted effects of NSAIDs, including gastric ulceration and renal toxicity. Robenacoxib is selective for COX-2 inhibition
- Inhibition of prostaglandins that regulate blood flow to the gastric mucosa and stimulate bicarbonate and mucus production may result in loss of GI protective mechanisms; there is evidence to suggest that COX-2 may actually play an important role in GI healing [169]. Therefore, robenacoxib is contraindicated in cases of GI surgery
- GI ulceration is the most common life-threatening effect while vomiting is the most common adverse effect
- May compromise renal blood flow

E. PRACTICAL NOTES

- Injectable and oral formulations are available. Note in cats, the tablet dose is different from the injectable dose. Cats should only receive the manufactured 6 mg tablets for accurate dosing
- Tablets are not scored and should not be halved. When administering prior to anesthesia, diligent monitoring of blood pressure, treatment of hypotension and administration of fluid therapy are recommended
- Subsequent doses can be interchanged with tablet or injectable, paying close attention to dosing
- It is recommended to assess serum biochemical baselines before administration of NSAIDs

LXXIX. Ropivacaine *local anesthetic*

A. DOSE AND DURATION

- See Table 6

B. CLINICAL APPLICATIONS

- Used for local regional analgesia blocks

C. PHARMACOLOGY

- All local anesthetics share a common chemical structure that includes a lipophilic, benzene ring and a hydrophilic amine group. This compound is then linked to either an ester or an amide. In the case of ropivacaine, there is an amide linkage
- pKa 16. pKa determines the amount of ionized and unionized fraction of drug present in the plasma. At high pKa, greater will be the proportion of local anesthetic in the ionized, charged hydrophilic form at physiologic pH (7.4), and the onset of action will be slower. In contrast, at low pKa, a greater proportion of the nonionized lipid-soluble form will be present at physiologic pH and the onset of action will be more rapid
- % Ionized at physiological pH: 83
- Lipid solubility (the main determinant of potency and onset of action) is 14

- % Protein binding: 94; protein binding influences the duration of action. Only the unbound fraction of drug is pharmacologically active. The higher the protein binding, the longer the duration of action

D. CONTRAINDICATIONS/PRECAUTIONS

- Do not administer IV; medication has high cardiotoxicity potential

E. PRACTICAL NOTES

- Possible loss of motor function when used in epidural or nerve blocks, although ropivacaine is associated with less ataxia than other local anesthetics
- If multiple blocks are performed, ensure total dosage for patient does not exceed the toxic dose
- In an epidural, preservative-free formulations are recommended
- Do not dilute concentration to less than 2.5 mg/mL or block may not be effective
- The addition of dexmedetomidine at 0.5 mg/mL of the volume for the local block volume may extend the duration of the block
- $NaHCO_3$ can be added to local anesthetic solutions to increase the pH, resulting in less sting upon injection when administering to conscious patients. Increasing the pH may also increase the lipid-soluble fraction, providing a more rapid onset of action and prolonged duration of sensory blockage
- At concentrations above 0.5%, ropivacaine produces sensory blockade similar to that obtained with bupivacaine, but there is less chance of inducing motor blockade. For this reason, it is considered very suitable for neuraxial analgesia

LXXX. Sevoflurane *inhalant anesthetic*

A. DOSE AND DURATION

- See Table 9

B. CLINICAL APPLICATIONS

- Maintenance of anesthesia
- Anesthesia induction via facemask or induction chamber. Because the odor is not pungent, sevoflurane is the inhalant of choice for this method. However, the authors discourage the use of induction by any inhalant

C. PHARMACOLOGY

- It is clear, colorless and the odor is reported to be pleasant and not irritating to the airways
- Nonflammable and nonexplosive liquid
- The exact mechanism of action by which inhalant anesthetic agents cause general anesthesia is not precisely known, but it is likely their influence on the electrical

activity of the CNS, mediated at the level of the spinal cord, through actions at the lipid bilayer of the cell membrane

- Most important effects include CNS depression, prevention of movement likely mediated at the level of the spinal cord, dose-dependent cardiovascular and respiratory depression, decreased systemic vascular resistance (vasodilation) and hypotension, increased cerebral blood flow and intracranial pressure, depression of body temperature regulating centers, and muscular relaxation
- Less soluble than isoflurane, sevoflurane acts rapidly, with faster induction and emergence than isoflurane, but not as fast as desflurane. Difference between isoflurane and sevoflurane is unlikely to have clinical significance

D. CONTRAINDICATIONS/PRECAUTION

- Patients with preexisting extreme hypotension, cardiovascular derangements or reason for inability to handle vasodilation
- Causes a dose-dependent decrease in cardiovascular and respiratory depression
- CNS depressant
- In susceptible individuals, inhalant anesthesia may trigger a clinical syndrome known as malignant hyperthermia (MH). MH is a cellular hypermetabolic state that, if not treated quickly, causes death. Although it is mostly reported in human patients and pigs, other species have also been reported to be affected
- The National Institute for Occupational Safety and Health Administration (NIOSH) recommends that no worker should be exposed to ceiling concentrations greater than 2 ppm of any halogenated anesthetic agent over a sampling period not to exceed 1 h
- Results in by-products when used with soda lime, including fluoride ions and compound "A" that may be toxic to the kidney. However, nephrotoxicity has not been demonstrated in clinical patients

E. PRACTICAL NOTES

- Requires a precision vaporizer

LXXXI. Sodium bicarbonate (NaHCO₃) *alkalinizing agent*

A. DOSE AND DURATION

- To correct metabolic acidosis: perform base deficit calculation (see Equation 1). Give half of the dose slowly over 20 min IV. Reevaluate blood gas; if the patient still exhibits metabolic acidosis, give the other half of the dose slowly in the same fashion. Target pH correction is no more than 7.20
- For hyperkalemia: 0.5–1.0 mEq/kg slow over 20 min IV
- Duration variable by patient

Equation 1 Calculation of sodium bicarbonate (NaHCO₃) supplementation

Body weight (BW)×base excess (from blood gas)×0.3 = mEq of sodium bicarbonate

B. CLINICAL APPLICATIONS

- Used to treat metabolic acidosis where the underlying cause is low HCO_3
- Used in the treatment of hyperkalemia

C. PHARMACOLOGY

- Acts as a base to increase pH

D. CONTRAINDICATIONS/PRECAUTIONS

- Administration will increase CO_2 production (e.g., $EtCO_2$); anesthetist must ensure adequate ventilation
- Results in alkaline urine
- Reduction in serum potassium levels may cause hypokalemia
- Administration may lead to hypernatremia
- Hyperosmolar
- May result in alkalosis if overdosed
- Patients with respiratory or metabolic alkalosis
- Patients with hypocalcemia
- Patients intolerant of high sodium levels, such as volume overloaded patients or animals with congestive heart failure

E. PRACTICAL NOTES

- Carefully evaluate patient's acid–base status during bicarbonate administration
- HCO_3 is incompatible with many other drugs, including some opioids and inotropes. It is recommended, when possible, to administer in a dedicated line

LXXXII. Sodium chloride 0.9% *crystalloid solution*

A. DOSE AND DURATION

- See Table 11

B. CLINICAL APPLICATIONS

- Preoperative fluid resuscitation
- Intraoperative fluid administration
- Treatment of hypotension due to ineffective circulating volume during anesthesia

C. PHARMACOLOGY

- Crystalloid fluid
- Replacement solution
- Unbuffered

D. CONTRAINDICATIONS/PRECAUTIONS

- Caution when using high volumes or boluses in patients with congestive heart failure, as excessive volumes may result in pulmonary edema; consider reduced rates and avoid bolus
- Patients with severe acidosis

E. PRACTICAL NOTES

- This product is safe to administer with blood products
- Slightly acidifying solution is useful in patients with alkalosis (i.e., pyloric obstruction)

LXXXIII. Sodium chloride 3–23% *hypertonic fluid*

A. DOSE AND DURATION

- See Table 11

B. CLINICAL APPLICATIONS

- Preoperative fluid resuscitation
- Treatment of hypotension due to hypovolemia or excessive vasodilation during anesthesia
- Hypernatremic patients for sodium matching under anesthesia
- Reduction of intracranial pressure

C. PHARMACOLOGY

- Classically used as 7.5% solution
- Resuscitation solution
- Unbuffered

D. CONTRAINDICATIONS/PRECAUTIONS

- Patients with uncontrolled hemorrhage
- Patients with dehydration
- Preexisting electrolyte imbalances such as hyponatremia
- May cause pulmonary edema if patient has preexisting heart disease
- Patients with severe acidosis

E. PRACTICAL NOTES

- Hypertonic fluids are typically reserved for treatment of shock (hypovolemic/hemorrhagic) and are used concurrently with isotonic crystalloids

- There was no survival benefit when 7.5% sodium chloride was administered empirically in the prehospital setting as a low-volume resuscitation fluid, although it was well tolerated [170]
- A review of evidence suggested that both mannitol and hypertonic sodium chloride effectively lower intracranial pressure, with neither fluid standing out as superior. However, a limited number of studies suggest hypertonic sodium chloride may result in fewer treatment failures in patients with refractory intracranial hypertension compared to mannitol [170]
- Benefits of hypertonic sodium chloride include avoiding diuresis and increases in cardiac preload

LXXXIV. Sufentanil *Full mu opioid*

A. DOSE AND DURATION

- See Table 7

B. CLINICAL APPLICATIONS

- Intraoperative management of noxious stimuli as well as analgesic
- MAC-sparing agent when used as a CRI during anesthesia for canine patients [171,172]; MAC sparing in cats is modest at best (6.3% reduction in inhalant) and unlikely to be of clinical significance [173]
- This agent, like fentanyl, may be used as part of a total intravenous technique [174]

C. PHARMACOLOGY

- Short-acting synthetic mu agonist opioid
- Thienyl analogue of the mu agonist fentanyl and approximately 10 times as potent as fentanyl [172]
- The liver and small intestine are the major sites of biotransformation and sufentanil is rapidly metabolized to a number of inactive metabolites [175]
- Sufentanil is highly lipophilic and is readily absorbed through mucosal tissues but with a small volume of distribution due to its extensive protein binding
- Controlled drug, Schedule II

D. CONTRAINDICATIONS/PRECAUTIONS

- Centrally mediated sympathetic stimulation that could result in an increase in blood pressure and heart rate [176]
- Like morphine, sufentanil results in mydriasis in cats [177]
- As with most potent opioids, respiratory depression is a consequence of sufentanil administration [178]

E. PRACTICAL NOTES

- When used as a CRI in combination with lidocaine and ketamine, recovery scores were improved compared with fentanyl, ketamine and lidocaine CRIs [171]
- Sufentanil should be diluted prior to administration to help minimize accidental overdose

LXXXV. Terbutaline *intermediate acting beta-2-adrenergic agonist*

A. DOSE AND DURATION

- 0.01 mg/kg SC or IM, or nebulized 1–2 metered dose from inhaler
- Duration of 4 h

B. CLINICAL APPLICATIONS

- Used as bronchodilator to help reduce V/Q mismatch
- Used to treat asthma

C. PHARMACOLOGY

- Beta-2-adrenergic receptor agonist

D. CONTRAINDICATIONS/PRECAUTIONS

- May cause a decrease in K+
- May cause transient hyperglycemia
- May cause hypotension
- Tremors can result from beta-receptor stimulation in the muscles
- Use with caution in patients with cardiac disease (patients with preexisting tachyarrhythmia); can cause tachycardia
- Caution in end-stage pregnancy, as beta stimulation can relax the uterine tissue
- Cautious use in canine patients who may have acute lung injury as the inotropic effects may recruit damaged pulmonary capillaries, leading to increased lung endothelial permeability [179,180]

E. PRACTICAL NOTES

- When nebulized, use a chamber that facilitates proper particle dispersion for full effect
- When administering this drug to an intubated patient, a significant amount of the drug (50–70%) will remain within the ET tube [8]. Therefore, the doses delivered may need to be increased when administering terbutaline to an intubated patient
- Increase in HR indicates effect
- Protect from light

LXXXVI. Tiletamine and zolazepam *commercialized combination of dissociative anesthetic agent and a benzodiazepine*

A. DOSE AND DURATION

- See Table 2

B. CLINICAL APPLICATIONS

- Used as a general anesthetic; used IV as traditional induction agent
- Used for chemical restraint of large untamed or aggressive patients
- Used as part of multidrug combinations for chemical restraint or anesthesia
- Works well in exotic patients as a means of induction or chemical restraint

C. PHARMACOLOGY

- Combination of a dissociative phencyclidine agent (tiletamine) and a benzodiazepine (zolazepam) as a 1:1 ratio
- Cats have prolonged recoveries due to the slower metabolism of zolazepam. In short procedures, dogs may have rough recoveries because of metabolism of zolazepam before tiletamine
- Controlled drug, Schedule III

D. CONTRAINDICATIONS/PRECAUTIONS [181]

- Adverse effects are heavily dose dependent
- Patients with seizures, head trauma, and increased intracranial pressure
- Patients with ocular injuries and glaucoma
- Patients with hypertrophic cardiomyopathy or tachyarrhythmias
- Cats with hyperthyroidism
- Patients with significant renal insufficiency

E. PRACTICAL NOTES

- Typical reconstitution is 100 mg/mL
- Lube the eyes as minimal blinking may occur
- Patients appear in a catatonic state with central, fixed, and dilated pupils
- Common reconstitutions involve various other anesthetics and analgesics such as 2.5 mL dexmedetomidine (0.5 mg/mL) + 2.5 mL butorphanol (10 mg/mL) administered at 0.005 mL/kg for mild sedation to 0.04 mL/kg for heavy/deep surgical anesthesia

LXXXVII. Tramadol *oral analgesic with weak opioid properties*

A. DOSE AND DURATION

- See Table 7

B. CLINICAL APPLICATIONS

- Oral analgesic, often used for postoperative adjunctive pain
- May result in sedation

C. PHARMACOLOGY

- Acts as a weak mu opioid agonist coupled with inhibition of synaptic reuptake of serotonin and norepinephrine by central neurons
- Has a lower affinity at mu opioid receptors than M1. The metabolite M1 exerts most of its pharmacologic effects as a high-affinity mu receptor agonist. The analgesic effects of tramadol are primarily attributed to its active metabolite M1 in humans, which are inconsistent in dogs [182]
- Cats may produce more opioid M1 metabolite [182], resulting in potentially more antinociception and analgesia for mild-moderate pain although the bitter taste makes routine oral administration difficult
- Controlled drug, Schedule II

D. CONTRAINDICATIONS/PRECAUTIONS

- Avoid use in patients currently on monoamine oxidase inhibitors (e.g., selegiline)
- Caution in patients with renal disease or seizures

E. PRACTICAL NOTES

- The analgesic effects have been controversial in dogs and there is evidence that tramadol does not provide adequate analgesia for postoperative analgesia [183]
- Only available as an oral formulation in the USA; injectable formulations available elsewhere
- Protect from light

LXXXVIII. Trazodone *serotonin receptor antagonist and reuptake inhibitor (SARI)*

A. DOSE AND DURATION

- Dogs: 8 mg/kg PO BID-TID for sedation, although higher doses have been administered
- Cats: 50 mg per cat PO [184]
- Onset 1–2 h following oral delivery

B. CLINICAL APPLICATIONS

- Sedation
- Antianxiety [185]
- Improves tolerance of cage rest postoperatively [186]

C. PHARMACOLOGY

- Triazolopyridine derivative
- 5-HT_{2A} and 5-HT_{2C} receptor antagonist and selective serotonin reuptake inhibitor
- May also reduce circulating levels of serotonin, noradrenaline, dopamine, acetylcholine, and histamine, providing a sedative effect at some doses
- Promotes antianxiety by increasing serotonin concentrations and attenuating the inhibition of GABA neurotransmitters
- Metabolized by the liver, with less than 1% being excreted unchanged in the urine

D. CONTRAINDICATIONS/PRECAUTIONS

- Serotonin syndrome is a potential risk when administered with other selective serotonin reuptake inhibitors (SSRIs), tricyclic antidepressant agents, opioids, and/or certain antimicrobials

E. PRACTICAL NOTES

- Often prescribed as a sedative for owners to administer to dogs prior to arrival to the veterinary hospital to reduce patient anxiety
- In people, it takes 7–21 days to achieve its therapeutic effect [187]. This information may provide owners with a realistic time frame when using this drug to assist with cage rest for an extended period of time
- Due to the risk of serotonin syndrome when coadministered with other medications, the lowest effective dose should be used and pet owners made aware to report undesirable effects
- There are reports in the literature that the 8 mg/kg rectal dose of trazadone [188] is a suitable alternative for patients where oral administration is not practical (i.e., in the immediate postoperative period)

LXXXIX. Vasopressin *vasopressor*

A. DOSE AND DURATION

- See Table 10

B. CLINICAL APPLICATIONS

- CPR as an alternative to epinephrine
- Vasopressor for treatment of hypotension caused by vasodilation

C. PHARMACOLOGY

- Synthetic antidiuretic hormone
- Acts at G-protein coupled vasopressin receptors (V_{1a}) in the vascular endothelium, resulting in vasoconstriction
- Increases renal permeability to water for conservation through the V_{1b} receptor in the collecting duct

D. CONTRAINDICATIONS/PRECAUTIONS

- Patients with hypertension
- Pregnancy due to uterine smooth muscle contraction
- Reflex bradycardia occurs secondary to increased vascular tone

E. PRACTICAL NOTES

- Recommended in refractory CPR or asystole (cardiac arrest) as a one-time dose instead of epinephrine (see Appendix B, "CPR"), as the V_1 receptors remain active in acidic environments, unlike the alpha-1-adrenergic receptors (which are the binding sites for epinephrine [189])
- If IV access is not available during CPR, the intratracheal route of administration is an alternative [190]
- Results in vasoconstriction, especially to the mesenteric vessels, which allows for redistribution of blood flow to other organs
- Doses of vasopressin used to manage hypotension are considered supraphysiologic; this results in profound vasoconstriction of blood vessels in splanchnic circulation and ultimately possible sloughing of the GI mucosa. The authors like to use the lowest effective dose, starting at 0.04 units/kg IV
- Safest when used only in cases refractory to traditional BP management
- Administer only once during CPR due to the drug's prolonged half-life
- Protect from light

XC. Xylazine *alpha-2 agonist*

A. DOSE AND DURATION

- See Table 1

B. CLINICAL APPLICATIONS

- Potent alpha-2-adrenergic receptor agonist used for its sedative and analgesic properties both for minor noninvasive procedures and in the perioperative period during general anesthesia for muscle relaxation
- Used as the muscle relaxant in combination with dissociative anesthetics for induction of anesthesia
- Used as premedication in combination with opioids
- Used as part of a "pre-euthanasia mix" for canine patients by some end-of-life veterinary service providers
- Because of its strong emetic effect in cats, it is occasionally used to induce vomiting after toxins ingestion

C. PHARMACOLOGY

- Has a selectivity for alpha-2/alpha-1 receptors of 160:1
- Presynaptic alpha-2-adrenergic receptors: inhibits release of norepinephrine and attenuates the sympathetic drive from the CNS
- Postsynaptic alpha-2-adrenergic receptors: effect similar to alpha-1-adrenergic receptor actions resulting in vasoconstriction
- The action on the alpha-2 receptors in the CNS causes dose-dependent degree of sedation up to a plateau, after which higher doses only increase length of sedation and side-effects
- Analgesia is exerted by dampening the afferent inputs at various point of the nociceptive pathway. When administered epidurally or intrathecally, this drug provides excellent analgesia because of direct action on the receptors in the dorsal horn of the spinal cord
- Metabolized by the liver

D. CONTRAINDICATIONS/PRECAUTIONS

- Mild to moderate, albeit short-lived, analgesia (other analgesic drugs should be included for noxious procedures)
- Initial hypertension with a reflex bradycardia, after which secondary hypotension is due to a reduction in cardiac output and centrally mediated bradycardia
- Arrhythmias, including second-degree AV block and ventricular escape beats, are common; do not use in canine patients with underlying cardiac disease
- Causes vomiting in 60% of dogs and 60–90% of cats [191]
- Vasoconstriction may cause blue or pale mucous membranes
- Patients often develop a transient hyperglycemia due to insulin resistance
- Diuresis is common. For this reason, avoid in patients with urinary obstruction before unblocking
- Avoid in patients with cardiovascular disease, including valvular regurgitation or arrhythmias

- Avoid in patients with renal insufficiencies or anuria
- Avoid in patients with liver disease
- Avoid in geriatric, diabetic, pregnant, pediatric, sick, or debilitated patients

E. PRACTICAL NOTES

- Animals which are deeply sedated can abruptly arise and demonstrate responses to external stimuli. The combination with opioids reduces these responses and produces deep sedation and anesthesia
- A pulse oximeter may have difficulty obtaining a measurement due to vasoconstriction
- Reversible with yohimbine (see Table 3); reversal should only be given IM
- Not recommended for use when a newer generation alpha-2 agonist is available

XCI. Yohimbine *alpha-2-adrenergic antagonist*

A. DOSE AND DURATION

- See Table 3

B. CLINICAL APPLICATIONS

- Reversal of alpha-2 agonists, specific for xylazine

C. PHARMACOLOGY

- Indole alkaloid derived from the bark of specific species of trees found in South America and Africa
- Selective antagonist at presynaptic alpha-2 receptors

D. CONTRAINDICATIONS/PRECAUTIONS

- May result in hypotension
- This drug will cross the blood–brain barrier. At high doses, it may result in seizures or seizure-like activity (i.e., tremors, skeletal muscle activity) [192]

E. PRACTICAL NOTES

- Reversal of alpha-2 agonists' sedative and analgesic effects; prior to reversal, an alternative analgesic should be systemically administered to the animal

www.wiley.com/go/shelby/anesthesia2

Please go to the companion website for access to videos relating to the book

References

1. Monteiro ER, Coelho K, Bressan TF, Simoes CR, Monteiro BS. Effects of acepromazine-morphine and acepromazine-methadone premedication on the minimum alveolar concentration of isoflurane in dogs. Vet Anaesth Analg. 2016;43(1):27–34.
2. Grasso SC, Ko JC, Weil AB, Paranjape V, Constable PD. Hemodynamic influence of acepromazine or dexmedetomidine premedication in isoflurane-anesthetized dogs. J Am Vet Med Assoc. 2015;246(7):754–64.
3. Bitti FS, Campagnol D, Rangel JP, Nunes Junior JS, Loureiro B, Monteiro ER. Effects of three methadone doses combined with acepromazine on sedation and some cardiopulmonary variables in dogs. Vet Anaesth Analg. 2017;44(2):237–45.
4. Monteiro ER, Rabello TA, Rangel JPP, Nunes JS Jr, Freire CD, Campagnol D. Effects of 3 morphine doses, in combination with acepromazine, on sedation and some physiological parameters in dogs. Can J Vet Res. 2019;83(3):235–40.
5. Rangel JPP, Monteiro ER, Bitti FS, Junior JSN, Campagnol D. Hemodynamic, respiratory and sedative effects of progressively increasing doses of acepromazine in conscious dogs. Vet Anaesth Analg. 2020;47(4):447–53.
6. Martin-Flores M, Mostowy MM, Pittman E, et al. Investigation of associations between preoperative acepromazine or dexmedetomidine administration and development of arterial hypotension or bradycardia in dogs undergoing ovariohysterectomy. J Am Vet Med Assoc. 2019;255(2):193–9.
7. Costa RS Karas A, Borns-Weil S. Chill protocol to manage aggressive and fearful dogs. Clinician's Brief. 2019:63–5.
8. Crogan SJ, Bishop MJ. Delivery efficiency of metered dose aerosols given via endotracheal tubes. Anesthesiology. 1989;70(6):1008–10.
9. Dehuisser V, Bosmans T, Kitshoff A, Duchateau L, de Rooster H, Polis I. Cardiovascular effects, induction and recovery characteristics and alfaxalone dose assessment in alfaxalone versus alfaxalone-fentanyl total intravenous anaesthesia in dogs. Vet Anaesth Analg. 2017;44(6):1276–86.
10. Miller C, Hughes E, Gurney M. Co-induction of anaesthesia with alfaxalone and midazolam in dogs: a randomized, blinded clinical trial. Vet Anaesth Analg. 2019;46(5):613–19.
11. Arenillas M, Aguado D, Canfran S, Sanchez-Lopez A, Gomez de Segura IA. Sedative effects of two doses of alfaxalone in combination with methadone and a low dose of dexmedetomidine in healthy Beagles. Vet Anaesth Analg. 2020;47(4):463–71.

12. Italiano M, Robinson R. Effect of benzodiazepines on the dose of alfaxalone needed for endotracheal intubation in healthy dogs. Vet Anaesth Analg. 2018;45(6):72–8.

13. Maney JK, Shepard MK, Braun C, Cremer J, Hofmeister EH. A comparison of cardiopulmonary and anesthetic effects of an induction dose of alfaxalone or propofol in dogs. Vet Anaesth Analg. 2013;40(3):237–44.

14. O'Hagan B, Pasloske K, McKinnon C, Perkins N, Whittem T. Clinical evaluation of alfaxalone as an anaesthetic induction agent in dogs less than 12 weeks of age. Aust Vet J. 2012;90(9):346–50.

15. Sofyan LM, Martinez-Taboada F. Comparison of alfaxalone verses propofol as anesthetic induction agents in increasing the rate of survival and vigor of neonoates. Vet Evidence. 2021;6(2).

16. Michou JN, Leece EA, Brearley JC. Comparison of pain on injection during induction of anaesthesia with alfaxalone and two formulations of propofol in dogs. Vet Anaesth Analg. 2012;39(3):275–81.

17. Li CX, Kempf D, Howell L, Zhang X. Effects of alfaxalone on cerebral blood flow and intrinsic neural activity of rhesus monkeys: a comparison study with ketamine. Magn Reson Imaging. 2021;75:134–40.

18. Pypendop BH, Barter LS, Pascoe PJ, Ranasinghe MG, Pasloske K. Hemodynamic effects of subclinical, clinical and supraclinical plasma alfaxalone concentrations in cats. Vet Anaesth Analg. 2019;46(5):597–604.

19. Muir W, Lerche P, Wiese A, Nelson L, Pasloske K, Whittem T. Cardiorespiratory and anesthetic effects of clinical and supraclinical doses of alfaxalone in dogs. Vet Anaesth Analg. 2008;35(6):451–62.

20. Amengual M, Flaherty D, Auckburally A, Bell AM, Scott EM, Pawson P. An evaluation of anaesthetic induction in healthy dogs using rapid intravenous injection of propofol or alfaxalone. Vet Anaesth Analg. 2013;40(2):115–23.

21. Norgate D, Ter Haar G, Kulendra N, Veres-Nyeki KO. A comparison of the effect of propofol and alfaxalone on laryngeal motion in nonbrachycephalic and brachycephalic dogs. Vet Anaesth Analg. 2018;45(6):729–36.

22. Bayldon W, Carter JE, Beths T, et al. Accidental alfaxalone overdose in a mature cat undergoing anaesthesia for magnetic resonance imaging. JFMS Open Rep. 2016;2(1):2055116916647740.

23. Ferré PJ, Pasloske K, Whittem T, Ranasinghe MG, Li Q, Lefebvre HP. Plasma pharmacokinetics of alfaxalone in dogs after an intravenous bolus of Alfaxan-CD RTU. Vet Anaesth Analg. 2006;33(4):229–36.

24. Lagos-Carvajal A, Queiroz-Williams P, da Cunha A, Liu CC. Determination of midazolam dose for co-induction with alfaxalone in sedated cats. Vet Anaesth Analg. 2019;46(3):299–307.

25. Norkus C, Rankin D, Warner M, KuKanich B. Pharmacokinetics of oral amantadine in greyhound dogs. J Vet Pharmacol Ther. 2015;38(3):305–8.

26. Lascelles B, Gaynor J, Smith E, et al. Amantadine in a multimodal analgesic regimen for alleviation of refractory osteoarthritis pain in dogs. J Vet Intern Med. 2008;22(1):53–9.

27. Marin LM, Iazbik MC, Zaldivar-Lopez S, et al. Retrospective evaluation of the effectiveness of epsilon aminocaproic acid for the prevention of postamputation bleeding in retired racing Greyhounds with appendicular bone tumors: 46 cases (2003–2008). J Vet Emerg Crit Care. 2012;22(3):332–40.

28. Marin LM, Iazbik MC, Zaldivar-Lopez S, Guillaumin J, McLoughlin MA, Couto CG. Epsilon aminocaproic acid for the prevention of delayed postoperative bleeding in retired racing greyhounds undergoing gonadectomy. Vet Surg. 2012;41(5):594–603.

29. Brown JC, Brainard BM, Fletcher DJ, Nie B, Arnold RD, Schmiedt CW. Effect of aminocaproic acid on clot strength and clot lysis of canine blood determined by use of an in vitro model of hyperfibrinolysis. Am J Vet Res. 2016;77(11):1258–65.

30. Fletcher DJ, Boller M. Updates in small animal cardiopulmonary resuscitation. Vet Clin North Am Small Anim Pract. 2013;43(4):971–87.

31. Berlin N, Ohad DG, Maiorkis I, Kelmer E. Successful management of ventricular fibrillation and ventricular tachycardia using defibrillation and intravenous amiodarone therapy in a cat. J Vet Emerg Crit Care. 2020;30(4):474–80.

32. Baumann H, Fichtenkamm P, Schneider T, Biscoping J, Henrich M. Rapid onset of amiodarone induced pulmonary toxicity after lung lobe resection – a case report and review of recent literature. Ann Med Surg. 2017;21:53–7.

33. Colby R, Geyer H. Amiodarone-induced pulmonary toxicity. JAAPA. 2017;30(11):23–6.

34. Virtanen R, Savola JM, Saano V. Highly selective and specific antagonism of central and peripheral alpha 2-adrenoceptors by atipamezole. Arch Int Pharmacodyn Ther. 1989;297:190–204.

35. Sepehripour S, Dheansa BS. Is there an advantage in onset of action with mixing lignocaine and bupivacaine? J Plast Reconstr Aesthet Surg. 2017;70(12):1782.

36. Collins JB, Song J, Mahabir RC. Onset and duration of intradermal mixtures of bupivacaine and lidocaine with epinephrine. Can J Plast Surg. 2013;21(1):51–3.

37. Carlson AR, Nixon E, Jacob ME, Messenger KM. Sterility and concentration of liposomal bupivacaine single-use vial when used in a multiple-dose manner. Vet Surg. 2020;49(4):772–7.

38. Steagall PV, Monteiro-Steagall BP, Taylor PM. A review of the studies using buprenorphine in cats. J Vet Intern Med. 2014;28(3):762–70.

39. Robertson S, Taylor P, Lascelles B, Dixon M. Changes in thermal threshold response in eight cats after administration of buprenorphine, butorphanol and morphine. Vet Rec. 2003;153(15):462–5.

40. Doodnaught GM, Monteiro BP, Benito J, et al. Pharmacokinetic and pharmacodynamic modelling after subcutaneous, intravenous and buccal administration of a high-concentration formulation of buprenorphine in conscious cats. PLoS One. 2017;12(4):e0176443.

41. Hansford J, Henao-Guerrero N, Machado ML, Pypendop BH. Pharmacokinetics of a high-concentration formulation of buprenorphine (Simbadol) in male dogs. Vet Anaesth Analg. 2021;48(4):509–16.

42. Nunamaker EA, Stolarik DF, Ma J, Wilsey AS, Jenkins GJ, Medina CL. Clinical efficacy of sustained-release buprenorphine with meloxicam for postoperative analgesia in beagle dogs undergoing ovariohysterectomy. J Am Assoc Lab Anim Sci. 2014;53(5):494–501.

43. Barletta M, Ostenkamp SM, Taylor AC, Quandt J, Lascelles BDX, Messenger KM. The pharmacokinetics and analgesic effects of extended-release buprenorphine administered subcutaneously in healthy dogs. J Vet Pharmacol Ther. 2018;41(4):502–12.

44. Catbagan DL, Quimby JM, Mama KR, Rychel JK, Mich PM. Comparison of the efficacy and adverse effects of sustained-release buprenorphine hydrochloride following subcutaneous administration and buprenorphine hydrochloride following oral transmucosal administration in cats undergoing ovariohysterectomy. Am J Vet Res. 2011;72(4):461–6.

45. Camargo JB, Steagall PV, Minto BW, Lorena SE, Mori ES, Luna SP. Post-operative analgesic effects of butorphanol or firocoxib administered to dogs undergoing elective ovariohysterectomy. Vet Anaesth Analg. 2011;38(3):252–9.

46. Warne LN, Beths T, Holm M, Carter JE, Bauquier SH. Evaluation of the perioperative analgesic efficacy of buprenorphine, compared with butorphanol, in cats. J Am Vet Med Assoc. 2014;245(2):195–202.

47. Leece EA, Brearley JC, Harding EF. Comparison of carprofen and meloxicam for 72 hours following ovariohysterectomy in dogs. Vet Anaesth Analg. 2005;32(4):184–92.

48. MacPhail CM, Lappin MR, Meyer DJ, Smith SG, Webster CR, Armstrong PJ. Hepatocellular toxicosis associated with administration of carprofen in 21 dogs. J Am Vet Med Assoc. 1998;212(12):1895–901.

49. Halter F, Tarnawski AS, Schmassmann A, Peskar BM. Cyclooxygenase 2-implications on maintenance of gastric mucosal integrity and ulcer healing: controversial issues and perspectives. Gut. 2001;49(3):443–53.

50. Lethagen S, Harris AS, Nilsson IM. Intranasal desmopressin (DDAVP) by spray in mild hemophilia A and von Willebrand's disease type I. Blut. 1990;60(3):187–91.

51. Micieli F, Santangelo B, Reynaud F, et al. Sedative and cardiovascular effects of intranasal or intramuscular dexmedetomidine in healthy dogs. Vet Anaesth Analg. 2017;44(4):703–9.

52. Santangelo B, Micieli F, Mozzillo T, et al. Transnasal administration of a combination of dexmedetomidine, midazolam and butorphanol produces deep sedation in New Zealand White rabbits. Vet Anaesth Analg. 2016;43(2):209–14.

53. Korpivaara M, Huhtinen M, Aspegren J, Overall K. Dexmedetomidine oromucosal gel reduces fear and anxiety in dogs during veterinary visits: a randomised, double-blind, placebo-controlled clinical pilot study. Vet Rec. 2021:e832.

54. Marolf V, Ida KK, Siluk D, Struck-Lewicka W, Markuszewski MJ, Sandersen C. Effects of perineural administration of ropivacaine combined with perineural or intravenous administration of dexmedetomidine for sciatic and saphenous nerve blocks in dogs. Am J Vet Res. 2021;82(6):449–58.

55. Acquafredda C, Stabile M, Lacitignola L, et al. Clinical efficacy of dexmedetomidine combined with lidocaine for femoral and sciatic nerve blocks in dogs undergoing stifle surgery. Vet Anaesth Analg. 2021;48(6):962–71.

56. Trein TA, Floriano BP, Wagatsuma JT, et al. Effects of dexmedetomidine combined with ropivacaine on sciatic and femoral nerve blockade in dogs. Vet Anaesth Analg. 2017;44(1):144–53.

57. Slingsby LS, Murrell JC, Taylor PM. Combination of dexmedetomidine with buprenorphine enhances the antinociceptive effect to a thermal stimulus in the cat compared with either agent alone. Vet Anaesth Analg. 2010;37(2):16–70.

58. Tisotti T, Valverde A, Hopkins A, O'Sullivan ML, Hanna B, Arroyo L. Use of intravenous lidocaine to treat dexmedetomidine-induced bradycardia in sedated and anesthetized dogs. Vet Anaesth Analg. 2021;48(2):174–86.

59. Thawley VJ, Drobatz KJ. Assessment of dexmedetomidine and other agents for emesis induction in cats: 43 cases (2009–2014). J Am Vet Med Assoc. 2015;247(12):1415–18.

60. Martin-Flores M, Sakai DM, Learn MM, et al. Effects of maropitant in cats receiving dexmedetomidine and morphine. J Am Vet Med Assoc. 2016;248(11):1257–61.

61. Robinson R, Borer-Weir K. The effects of diazepam or midazolam on the dose of propofol required to induce anaesthesia in cats. Vet Anaesth Analg. 2015;42(5):493–501.

62. Graham CW, Pagano RR, Katz RL. Thrombophlebitis after intravenous diazepam – can it be prevented? Anesth Analg. 1977;56(3):409–13.

63. Manor D, Sadeh M. Muscle fibre necrosis induced by intramuscular injection of drugs. Br J Exp Pathol. 1989;70(4):457–62.

64. van Beusekom CD, van den Heuvel JJ, Koenderink JB, Russel FG, Schrickx JA. Feline hepatic biotransformation of diazepam: differences between cats and dogs. Res Vet Sci. 2015;103:119–25.

65. Maack C, Eschenhagen T, Hamdani N, et al. Treatments targeting inotropy. Eur Heart J. 2019;40(44):3626–44.

66. Kittner SJ, Stern BJ, Feeser BR, et al. Pregnancy and the risk of stroke. N Engl J Med. 1996;335(11):768–74.

67. Flournoy W, Wohl J, Albrecht-Schmitt T, Schwartz D. Pharmacologic identification of putative D1 dopamine receptors in feline kidneys. J Vet Pharmacol Ther. 2003;26(4):283–90.

68. Bhosale GP, Shah VR. Extravasation injury due to dopamine infusion leading to dermal necrosis and gangrene. J Anaesthesiol Clin Pharmacol. 2012;28(4):534–5.

69. de Moraes S, de Carvalho FV. On the mechanism of action of tachyphylaxis by ephedrine. Pharmacology. 1968;1(1):53–9.

70. Tulen JH, Moleman P, Blankestijn PJ, Man in't Veld AJ, van Steenis HG, Boomsma F. Psychological, cardiovascular, and endocrine changes during 6 hours of continuous infusion of epinephrine or nor-epinephrine in healthy volunteers. Psychosom Med. 1993;55(1):61–9.

71. Baxter AL, Ewing PH, Young GB, Ware A, Evans N, Manworren RC. EMLA application exceeding two hours improves pediatric emergency department venipuncture success. Adv Emerg Nurs J. 2013;35(1):67–75.

72. Huff L, Hamlin A, Wolski D, et al. Atraumatic care: EMLA cream and application of heat to facilitate peripheral venous cannulation in children. Issues Compr Pediatr Nurs. 2009;32(2):65–76.

73. Ramsey J. Esmolol. Can J Anaesth. 1991;38:155–8.

74. Marks SL, Kook PH, Papich MG, Tolbert MK, Willard MD. ACVIM consensus statement: Support for rational administration of gastrointestinal protectants to dogs and cats. J Vet Intern Med. 2018;32(6):1823–40.

75. Bruniges N, Rioja E. Intraoperative anaesthetic complications in dogs undergoing general anaesthesia for thoracolumbar hemilaminectomy: a retrospective analysis. Vet Anaesth Analg. 2019;46(6):720–8.

76. Costa RS, Abelson AL, Lindsey JC, Wetmore LA. Postoperative regurgitation and respiratory complications in brachycephalic dogs undergoing airway surgery before and after implementation of a standardized perianesthetic protocol. J Am Vet Med Assoc. 2020;256(8):899–905.

77. Galatos AD, Raptopoulos D. Gastro-oesophageal reflux during anaesthesia in the dog: the effect of age, positioning and type of surgical procedure. Vet Rec. 1995;137(20):513–16.

78. Parkinson S, Tolbert K, Messenger K, et al. Evaluation of the effect of orally administered acid suppressants on intragastric pH in cats. J Vet Intern Med. 2015;29(1):104–12.

79. Bersenas AM, Mathews KA, Allen DG, Conlon PD. Effects of ranitidine, famotidine, pantoprazole, and omeprazole on intragastric pH in dogs. Am J Vet Res. 2005;66(3):425–31.

80. Brosnan RJ, Pypendop BH, Siao KT, Stanley SD. Effects of remifentanil on measures of anesthetic immobility and analgesia in cats. Am J Vet Res. 2009;70(9):1065–71.

81. Hirai J, Miyazaki H, Taneike T. The pharmacokinetics and pharmacodynamics of furosemide in the anaesthetized dog. J Vet Pharmacol Ther. 1992;15(3):231–9.

82. Sleeper MM, O'Donnell P, Fitzgerald C, Papich MG. Pharmacokinetics of furosemide after intravenous, oral and transdermal administration to cats. J Feline Med Surg. 2019;21(10):882–6.

83. Huang X, Dorhout Mees E, Vos P, Hamza S, Braam B. Everything we always wanted to know about furosemide but were afraid to ask. Am J Physiol Renal Physiol. 2016;310(10):F958–71.

84. Evans EF, Klinke R. The effects of intracochlear and systemic furosemide on the properties of single cochlear nerve fibres in the cat. J Physiol. 1982;331:409–27.

85. Guedes AGP, Meadows JM, Pypendop BH, Johnson EG, Zaffarano B. Assessment of the effects of gabapentin on activity levels and owner-perceived mobility impairment and quality of life in osteoarthritic geriatric cats. J Am Vet Med Assoc. 2018;253(5):579–85.

86. van Haaften KA, Forsythe LRE, Stelow EA, Bain MJ. Effects of a single preappointment dose of gabapentin on signs of stress in cats during transportation and veterinary examination. J Am Vet Med Assoc. 2017;251(10):1175–81.

87. Hayashida KI, Eisenach JC. Descending noradrenergic inhibition: an important mechanism of gabapentin analgesia in neuropathic pain. Adv Exp Med Biol. 2018;1099:93–100.

88. Kukanich B, Cohen RL. Pharmacokinetics of oral gabapentin in greyhound dogs. Vet J. 2011;187(1):133–5.

89. Slovak JE, Costa AP. A pilot study of transdermal gabapentin in cats. J Vet Intern Med. 2021;35(4):1981–7.

90. Adrian D, Papich MG, Baynes R, Stafford E, Lascelles BDX. The pharmacokinetics of gabapentin in cats. J Vet Intern Med. 2018;32(6):1996–2002.

91. Fantinati M, Trnka J, Signor A, et al. Appetite-stimulating effect of gabapentin vs mirtazapine in healthy cats post-ovariectomy. J Feline Med Surg. 2020;22(12):1176–83.

92. Sartini I, Giorgi M. Grapiprant: a snapshot of the current knowledge. J Vet Pharmacol Ther. 2021;44(5):679–88.

93. Lebkowska-Wieruszewska B, De Vito V, Owen H, Poapholatep A, Giorgi M. Pharmacokinetics of grapiprant, a selective EP4 prostaglandin PGE2 receptor antagonist, after 2 mg/kg oral and i.v. administrations in cats. J Vet Pharmacol Ther. 2017;40(6):e11–e15.

94. Heit MC, Mealey KL, King SB. Tolerance and pharmacokinetics of galliprant administered orally to collies homozygous for MDR1-1delta. J Vet Pharmacol Ther. 2021;44(5):705–13.

95. Howard J, Wigley J, Rosen G, D'Mello J. Glycopyrrolate: it's time to review. J Clin Anesth. 2017;36:51–3.

96. Doering CJ, Lukasik VM, Merideth RE. Effects of intramuscular injection of glycopyrrolate on Schirmer tear test I results in dogs. J Am Vet Med Assoc. 2016;248(11):1262–6.

97. Mason KP, Zgleszewski S, Forman RE, Stark C, DiNardo JA. An exaggerated hypertensive response to glycopyrrolate therapy for bradycardia associated with high-dose dexmedetomidine. Anesth Analg. 2009;108(3):906–8.

98. Ovbey DH, Wilson DV, Bednarski RM, et al. Prevalence and risk factors for canine post-anesthetic aspiration pneumonia (1999–2009): a multicenter study. Vet Anaesth Analg. 2014;41(2):127–36.

99. Machado CE, Dyson DH, Grant Maxie M. Effects of oxymorphone and hydromorphone on the minimum alveolar concentration of isoflurane in dogs. Vet Anaesth Analg. 2006;33(1):70–7.

100. Niedfeldt R, Robertson S. Postanesthetic hyperthermia in cats: a retrospective comparison between hydromorphone and buprenorphine. Vet Anaesth Analg. 2006;33(6):381–9.

101. Posner L, Pavuk A, Rokshar J, Carter J, Levine J. Effects of opioids and anesthetic drugs on body temperature in cats. Vet Anaesth Analg. 2010;37(1):35–43.

102. Boyd CJ, Brainard BM, Smart L. Intravenous fluid administration and the coagulation system. Front Vet Sci. 2021;8:662504.

103. Egli GA, Zollinger A, Seifert B, Popovic D, Pasch T, Spahn DR. Effect of progressive haemodilution with hydroxyethyl starch, gelatin and albumin on blood coagulation. Br J Anaesth. 1997;78(6):684–9.

104. Warren BB, Durieux ME. Hydroxyethyl starch: safe or not? Anesth Analg. 1997;84(1):206–12.

105. Boyd CJ, Sharp CR, Claus MA, Raisis AL, Hosgood G, Smart L. Prospective randomized controlled blinded clinical trial evaluating biomarkers of acute kidney injury following 6% hydroxyethyl starch 130/0.4 or Hartmann's solution in dogs. J Vet Emerg Crit Care. 2021;31(3):306–14.

106. Boyd CJ, Claus MA, Raisis AL, et al. Evaluation of biomarkers of kidney injury following 4% succinylated gelatin and 6% hydroxyethyl starch 130/0.4 administration in a canine hemorrhagic shock model. J Vet Emerg Crit Care. 2019;29(2):132–42.

107. Boyd CJ, Claus MA, Raisis AL, Hosgood G, Sharp CR, Smart L. Hypocoagulability and platelet dysfunction are exacerbated by synthetic colloids in a canine hemorrhagic shock model. Front Vet Sci. 2018;5:279.

108. Rhodes A, Evans LE, Alhazzani W, et al. Surviving Sepsis Campaign: international guidelines for management of sepsis and septic shock: 2016. Intensive Care Med. 2017;43(3):304–77.

109. Stoelting RK, Hillier S, Stoelting RK. Handbook of Pharmacology & Physiology in Anesthetic Practice, 2nd edn. Philadelphia: Lippincott Williams & Wilkins, 2006.

110. Wilson J, Doherty TJ, Egger CM, Fidler A, Cox S, Rohrbach B. Effects of intravenous lidocaine, ketamine, and the combination on the minimum alveolar concentration of sevoflurane in dogs. Vet Anaesth Analg. 2008;35(4):289–96.

111. Pascoe PJ, Ilkiw JE, Craig C, Kollias-Baker C. The effects of ketamine on the minimum alveolar concentration of isoflurane in cats. Vet Anaesth Analg. 2007;34(1):31–9.

112. Kovalcuka L, Birgele E, Bandere D, Williams DL. The effects of ketamine hydrochloride and diazepam on the intraocular pressure and pupil diameter of the dog's eye. Vet Ophthalmol. 2013;16(1):29–34.

113. Kennedy MJ, Smith LJ. A comparison of cardiopulmonary function, recovery quality, and total dosages required for induction and total intravenous anesthesia with propofol versus a propofol-ketamine combination in healthy Beagle dogs. Vet Anaesth Analg. 2015;42(4):350–9.

114. Martinez-Taboada F, Leece EA. Comparison of propofol with ketofol, a propofol-ketamine admixture, for induction of anaesthesia in healthy dogs. Vet Anaesth Analg. 2014;41(6):575–82.

115. Cunha MG, Freitas GC, Carregaro AB, et al. Renal and cardiorespiratory effects of treatment with lactated Ringer's solution or physiologic saline (0.9% NaCl) solution in cats with experimentally induced urethral obstruction. Am J Vet Res. 2010;71(7):840–6.

116. Valverde A, Doherty TJ, Hernandez J, Davies W. Effect of lidocaine on the minimum alveolar concentration of isoflurane in dogs. Vet Anaesth Analg. 2004;31(4):264–71.

117. Vullo C, Tambella AM, Falcone A, Marino G, Catone G. Constant rate infusion of lidocaine, tumescent anesthesia and their combination in dogs undergoing unilateral mastectomy. Animals. 2021;11(5):1280.

118. Panti A, Cafrita IC, Clark L. Effect of intravenous lidocaine on cough response to endotracheal intubation in propofol-anaesthetized dogs. Vet Anaesth Analg. 2016;43(4):405–11.

119. Dyson DH. Efficacy of lidocaine hydrochloride for laryngeal desensitization: a clinical comparison of techniques in the cat. J Am Vet Med Assoc. 1988;192(9):1286–8.

120. Pypendop B, Ilkiw J. Assessment of the hemodynamic effects of lidocaine administered IV in isoflurane-anesthetized cats. Am J Vet Res. 2005;66(4):661–8.

121. Soltaninejad H, Vesal N. Plasma concentrations of lidocaine following laryngeal administration or laryngeal and intratesticular administration in cats. Am J Vet Res. 2018;79(6):614–20.

122. Choquette A, Troncy E, Guillot M, Varin F, Del Castillo JR. Pharmacokinetics of lidocaine hydrochloride administered with or without adrenaline for the paravertebral brachial plexus block in dogs. PLoS One. 2017;12(1):e0169745.

123. Cuvillon P, Nouvellon E, Ripart J, et al. A comparison of the pharmacodynamics and pharmacokinetics of bupivacaine, ropivacaine (with epinephrine) and their equal volume mixtures with lidocaine used for femoral and sciatic nerve blocks: a double-blind randomized study. Anesth Analg. 2009;108(2):641–9.

124. McClellan JM, Goldstein RE, Erb HN, Dykes NL, Cowgill LD. Effects of administration of fluids and diuretics on glomerular filtration rate, renal blood flow, and urine output in healthy awake cats. Am J Vet Res. 2006;67(4):715–22.

125. Bragadottir G, Redfors B, Ricksten SE. Mannitol increases renal blood flow and maintains filtration fraction and oxygenation in postoperative acute kidney injury: a prospective interventional study. Crit Care. 2012;16(4):R159.

126. Cloyd JC, Snyder BD, Cleeremans B, Bundlie SR, Blomquist CH, Lakatua DJ. Mannitol pharmacokinetics and serum osmolality in dogs and humans. J Pharmacol Exp Ther. 1986;236(2):301–6.

127. Hickman M, Cox S, Mahabir S, et al. Safety, pharmacokinetics and use of the novel NK-1 receptor antagonist maropitant (Cerenia) for the prevention of emesis and motion sickness in cats. J Vet Pharmacol Ther. 2008;31(3):220–9.

128. Park LS, Hoelzler MG. Retrospective evaluation of maropitant and perioperative factors affecting postoperative appetite in cats. Can Vet J. 2021;62(9):969–74.

129. Correa JMX, Niella RV, Oliveira JNS, et al. Antinociceptive and analgesic effect of continuous intravenous infusion of maropitant, lidocaine and ketamine alone or in combination in cats undergoing ovariohysterectomy. Acta Vet Scand. 2021;63(1):49.

130. Fukui S, Ooyama N, Tamura J, et al. Interaction between maropitant and carprofen on sparing of the minimum alveolar concentration for blunting adrenergic response (MAC-BAR) of sevoflurane in dogs. J Vet Med Sci. 2017;79(3):502–8.

131. Niyom S, Boscan P, Twedt DC, Monnet E, Eickhoff JC. Effect of maropitant, a neurokinin-1 receptor antagonist, on the minimum alveolar concentration of sevoflurane during stimulation of the ovarian ligament in cats. Vet Anaesth Analg. 2013;40(4):425–31.

132. Boscan P, Monnet E, Mama K, Twedt DC, Congdon J, Steffey EP. Effect of maropitant, a neurokinin 1 receptor antagonist, on anesthetic requirements during noxious visceral stimulation of the ovary in dogs. Am J Vet Res. 2011;72(12):1576–9.

133. Hay Kraus BL. Spotlight on the perioperative use of maropitant citrate. Vet Med. 2017;8:41–51.

134. Marquez M, Boscan P, Weir H, Vogel P, Twedt DC. Comparison of NK-1 receptor antagonist (maropitant) to morphine as a pre-anaesthetic agent for canine ovariohysterectomy. PLoS One. 2015;10(10):e0140734.

135. Chi TT, Hay Kraus BL. The effect of intravenous maropitant on blood pressure in healthy awake and anesthetized dogs. PLoS One. 2020;15(2):e0229736.

136. Kenward H, Elliott J, Lee T, Pelligand L. Anti-nausea effects and pharmacokinetics of ondansetron, maropitant and metoclopramide in a low-dose cisplatin model of nausea and vomiting in the dog: a blinded crossover study. BMC Vet Res. 2017;13(1):244.

137. Deckers N, Ruigrok CA, Verhoeve HP, Lourens N. Comparison of pain response after subcutaneous injection of two maropitant formulations to beagle dogs. Vet Rec Open. 2018;5(1):e000262.

138. Marjani M, Akbarinejad V, Bagheri M. Comparison of intranasal and intramuscular ketamine-midazolam combination in cats. Vet Anaesth Analg. 2015;42(2):178–81.

139. Charalambous M, Bhatti SFM, Van Ham L, et al. Intranasal midazolam versus rectal diazepam for the management of canine status epilepticus: a multicenter randomized parallel-group clinical trial. J Vet Intern Med. 2017;31(4):1149–58.

140. Zapata A, Laredo FG, Escobar M, Agut A, Soler M, Belda E. Effects of midazolam before or after alfaxalone for co-induction of anaesthesia in healthy dogs. Vet Anaesth Analg. 2018;45(5):609–17.

141. Munoz KA, Robertson SA, Wilson DV. Alfaxalone alone or combined with midazolam or ketamine in dogs: intubation dose and select physiologic effects. Vet Anaesth Analg. 2017;44(4):766–74.

142. Liao P, Sinclair M, Valverde A, et al. Induction dose and recovery quality of propofol and alfaxalone with or without midazolam coinduction followed by total intravenous anesthesia in dogs. Vet Anaesth Analg. 2017;44(5):1016–26.

143. Herrod JA, Avelino JA, Schonvisky KM, Lynch JK, Hutchinson EK, Izzi JM. The use of midazolam as an appetite stimulant and anxiolytic in the common marmoset (Callithrix jacchus). J Med Primatol. 2021;50(5):249–58.

144. Ilkiw JE, Suter CM, Farver TB, McNeal D, Steffey EP. The behaviour of healthy awake cats following intravenous and intramuscular administration of midazolam. J Vet Pharmacol Ther. 1996;19(3):205–16.

145. Herron ME, Shofer FS, Reisner IR. Retrospective evaluation of the effects of diazepam in dogs with anxiety-related behavior problems. J Am Vet Med Assoc. 2008;233(9):1420–4.

146. Kropf J, Hughes JML. Effects of midazolam on cardiovascular responses and isoflurane requirement during elective ovariohysterectomy in dogs. Ir Vet J. 2018;71:26.

147. Vesal N, Zare P. Clinical evaluation of intranasal benzodiazepines, alpha-agonists and their antagonists in canaries. Vet Anaesth Analg. 2006;33(3):143–8.

148. Dholakia U, Seddighi R, Odunayo A, Cox SK, Jones EH, Pypendop BH. Prolonged anesthetic recovery after continuous infusion of midazolam in 2 domestic cats (Felis catus). Comp Med. 2019;69(4):321–6.

149. Steffey EP, Eisele JH, Baggot JD, Woliner MJ, Jarvis KA, Elliott AR. Influence of inhaled anesthetics on the pharmacokinetics and pharmacodynamics of morphine. Anesth Analg. 1993;77(2):346–51.

150. Martin-Flores M, Mastrocco A, Lorenzutti AM, et al. Maropitant administered orally 2–2.5 h prior to morphine and dexmedetomidine reduces the incidence of emesis in cats. J Feline Med Surg. 2017;19:876–9.

151. Lorenzutti AM, Martin-Flores M, Litterio NJ, Himelfarb MA, Invaldi SH, Zarazaga MP. A comparison between maropitant and metoclopramide for the prevention of morphine-induced nausea and vomiting in dogs. Can Vet J. 2017;58(1):35–8.

152. Coelho JC, Senninger N, Runkel N, Herfarth C, Messmer K. Effect of analgesic drugs on the electromyographic activity of the gastrointestinal tract and sphincter of Oddi and on biliary pressure. Ann Surg. 1986;204(1):53–8.

153. Sturtevant F, Drill V. Tranquilizing drugs and morphine-mania in cats. Nature. 1957;179(4572):1253.

154. Ivankovich AD, Braverman B, Shulman M, Klowden AJ. Prevention of nitroprusside toxicity with thiosulfate in dogs. Anesth Analg. 1982;61(2):120–6.

155. Mansell P, Robinson K, Minck D, Hurtt ME, Cappon GD. Toxicology and toxicokinetics of oral pantoprazole in neonatal and juvenile dogs. Birth Defects Res B Dev Reprod Toxicol. 2011;92(4):345–52.

156. Marlicz W, Loniewski I, Grimes DS, Quigley EM. Nonsteroidal anti-inflammatory drugs, proton pump inhibitors, and gastrointestinal injury: contrasting interactions in the stomach and small intestine. Mayo Clin Proc. 2014;89(12):1699–709.

157. Herrera M, Mehl M, Kass P, Pascoe P, Feldman E, Nelson R. Predictive factors and the effect of phenoxybenzamine on outcome in dogs undergoing adrenalectomy for pheochromocytoma. J Vet Intern Med. 2008;22(6):1333–9.

158. Sarchahi AA, Eskandari M. Effect of four local anesthetics (tetracaine, proparacaine, lidocaine, and bupivacaine) on intraocular pressure in dogs. Int Ophthalmol. 2019;39(7):1467–74.

159. Chandler JC, Monnet E, Staatz AJ. Comparison of acute hemodynamic effects of lidocaine and procainamide for postoperative ventricular arrhythmias in dogs. J Am Anim Hosp Assoc. 2006;42(4):262–8.

160. Caines D, Sinclair M, Valverde A, Dyson D, Gaitero L, Wood D. Comparison of isoflurane and propofol for maintenance of anesthesia in dogs with intracranial disease undergoing magnetic resonance imaging. Vet Anaesth Analg. 2014;41(5):468–79.

161. Steffen F, Grasmueck S. Propofol for treatment of refractory seizures in dogs and a cat with intracranial disorders. J Small Anim Pract. 2000;41(11):496–9.

162. Chui J, Mariappan R, Mehta J, Manninen P, Venkatraghavan L. Comparison of propofol and volatile agents for maintenance of anesthesia during elective craniotomy procedures: systematic review and meta-analysis. Can J Anaesth. 2014;61(4):347–56.

163. Baetge CL, Smith LC, Azevedo CP. Clinical Heinz body anemia in a cat after repeat propofol administration: case report. Front Vet Sci. 2020;7:591556.

164. Andress JL, Day TK, Day D. The effects of consecutive day propofol anesthesia on feline red blood cells. Vet Surg. 1995;24(3):277–82.

165. McNally E, Robertson S, Pablo L. Comparison of time to desaturation between preoxygenated and nonpreoxygenated dogs following sedation with acepromazine maleate and morphine and induction of anesthesia with propofol. Am J Vet Res. 2009;70(11):1333–8.

166. Akashi N, Murahata Y, Kishida H, Hikasa Y, Azuma K, Imagawa T. Effects of constant rate infusions of dexmedetomidine, remifentanil and their combination on minimum alveolar concentration of sevoflurane in dogs. Vet Anaesth Analg. 2020;47(4):490–8.

167. Anagnostou TL, Kazakos GM, Savvas I, Papazoglou LG, Rallis TS, Raptopoulos D. Remifentanil/ isoflurane anesthesia in five dogs with liver disease undergoing liver biopsy. J Am Anim Hosp Assoc. 2011;47(6):e103–9.

168. Ruiz-Lopez P, Navarrete-Calvo R, Morgaz J, et al. Determination of acute tolerance and hyperalgesia to remifentanil constant rate infusion in dogs undergoing sevoflurane anaesthesia. Vet Anaesth Analg. 2020;47(2):183–90.

169. Foral PA, Nystrom KK, Wilson AF, Christensen CM. Gastrointestinal-related adverse effects of COX-2 inhibitors. Drugs Today. 2003;39(12):939–48.

170. Pigott A, Rudloff E. Traumatic brain injury – a review of intravenous fluid therapy. Front Vet Sci. 2021;8:643800.

171. Van Wijnsberghe AS, Marolf V, Claeys S, Sandersen C, Ida KK. Effects of fentanyl-lidocaine-ketamine versus sufentanil-lidocaine-ketamine on the isoflurane requirements in dogs undergoing total ear canal ablation and lateral bulla osteotomy. Vet Anaesth Analg. 2020;47(5):595–603.

172. Polis I, Moens Y, Gasthuys F, Hoeben D, Tshamala M. Anti-nociceptive and sedative effects of sufentanil long acting during and after sevoflurane anaesthesia in dogs. J Vet Med A Physiol Pathol Clin Med. 2004;51(5):242–8.

173. Brosnan RJ, Pypendop BH, Stanley SD. Phenylpiperidine opioid effects on isoflurane minimum alveolar concentration in cats. J Vet Pharmacol Ther. 2020;43(6):533–7.

174. Mendes GM, Selmi AL. Use of a combination of propofol and fentanyl, alfentanil, or sufentanil for total intravenous anesthesia in cats. J Am Vet Med Assoc. 2003;223(11):1608–13.

175. Pypendop BH, Brosnan RJ, Majewski-Tiedeken CR, Stanley SD, Ilkiw JE. Pharmacokinetics of fentanyl, alfentanil, and sufentanil in isoflurane-anesthetized cats. J Vet Pharmacol Ther. 2014;37(1):13–17.

176. Gaumann DM, Yaksh TL, Tyce GM, Stoddard S. Sympathetic stimulating effects of sufentanil in the cat are mediated centrally. Neurosci Lett. 1988;91(1):30–5.

177. Sharpe LG. Separate neural mechanisms mediate sufentanil-induced pupillary responses in the cat. J Pharmacol Exp Ther. 1991;256(3):845–9.

178. Dierssen M, Ruiz F, Florez J, Hurle MA. Ca2+ channel modulation by dihydropyridines modifies sufentanil-induced respiratory depression in cats. Eur J Pharmacol. 1991;198(2–3):149–55.

179. Briot R, Bayat S, Anglade D, Martiel JL, Grimbert F. Increased cardiac index due to terbutaline treatment aggravates capillary-alveolar macromolecular leakage in oleic acid lung injury in dogs. Crit Care. 2009;13(5):R166.

180. Lee JW. beta2 adrenergic agonists in acute lung injury? The heart of the matter. Crit Care. 2009;13(6):1011.

181. Kucharski P, Kielbowicz Z. Dissociative anaesthesia in dogs and cats with use of tiletamine and zolazepam combination. What we already know about it. Pol J Vet Sci. 2021;24(3):451–9.

182. Dominguez-Oliva A, Casas-Alvarado A, Miranda-Cortes AE, Hernandez-Avalos I. Clinical pharmacology of tramadol and tapentadol, and their therapeutic efficacy in different models of acute and chronic pain in dogs and cats. J Adv Vet Anim Res. 2021;8(3):404–22.

183. Budsberg SC, Torres BT, Kleine SA, Sandberg GS, Berjeski AK. Lack of effectiveness of tramadol hydrochloride for the treatment of pain and joint dysfunction in dogs with chronic osteoarthritis. J Am Vet Med Assoc. 2018;252(4):427–32.

184. Stevens BJ, Frantz EM, Orlando JM, et al. Efficacy of a single dose of trazodone hydrochloride given to cats prior to veterinary visits to reduce signs of transport- and examination-related anxiety. J Am Vet Med Assoc. 2016;249(2):202–7.

185. Gruen ME, Sherman BL. Use of trazodone as an adjunctive agent in the treatment of canine anxiety disorders: 56 cases (1995–2007). J Am Vet Med Assoc. 2008;233(12):1902–7.

186. Gruen ME, Roe SC, Griffith E, Hamilton A, Sherman BL. Use of trazodone to facilitate postsurgical confinement in dogs. J Am Vet Med Assoc. 2014;245(3):296–301.

187. Schwasinger-Schmidt TE, Macaluso M. Other antidepressants. Handb Exp Pharmacol. 2019; 250:325–55.

188. O'Donnell EM, Press SA, Karriker MJ, Istvan SA. Pharmacokinetics and efficacy of trazodone following rectal administration of a single dose to healthy dogs. Am J Vet Res. 2020;81(9):739–46.

189. Fox AW, May RE, Mitch WE. Comparison of peptide and nonpeptide receptor-mediated responses in rat tail artery. J Cardiovasc Pharmacol. 1992;20(2):282–9.

190. Wenzel V, Lindner KH, Prengel AW, Lurie KG, Strohmenger HU. Endobronchial vasopressin improves survival during cardiopulmonary resuscitation in pigs. Anesthesiology. 1997;86(6):1375–81.

191. Thies M, Bracker K, Sinnott V. Retrospective evaluation of the effectiveness of xylazine for inducing emesis in cats: 48 cats (2011–2015). J Vet Emerg Crit Care. 2017;27(6):658–61.

192. Dunn RW, Corbett R. Yohimbine-induced seizures involve NMDA and GABAergic transmission. Neuropharmacology. 1992;31(4):389–95.

193. Lagos-Carvajal A, Queiroz-Williams P, da Cunha A, Liu CC. Determination of midazolam dose for co-induction with alfaxalone in sedated cats. Vet Anaesth Analg. 2019;46(3):299–307.

194. Court MH, Greenblatt DJ. Pharmacokinetics and preliminary observations of behavioral changes following administration of midazolam to dogs. J Vet Pharmacol Ther. 1992;15(4):343–50.

195. Visser M, Zaya MJ, Locuson CW, Boothe DM, Merritt DA. Comparison of predicted intrinsic hepatic clearance of 30 pharmaceuticals in canine and feline liver microsomes. Xenobiotica. 2019;49(2):177–86.

196. Dholakia U, Seddighi R, Cox SK, Sun X, Pypendop BH. Pharmacokinetics of midazolam in sevoflurane-anesthetized cats. Vet Anaesth Analg. 2020;47(2):200–9.

197. Ambros B, Duke-Novakovski T, Pasloske KS. Comparison of the anesthetic efficacy and cardiopulmonary effects of continuous rate infusions of alfaxalone-2-hydroxypropyl-beta-cyclodextrin and propofol in dogs. Am J Vet Res. 2008;69(11):1391–8.

198. Herbert GL, Bowlt KL, Ford-Fennah V, Covey-Crump GL, Murrell JC. Alfaxalone for total intravenous anaesthesia in dogs undergoing ovariohysterectomy: a comparison of premedication with acepromazine or dexmedetomidine. Vet Anaesth Analg. 2013;40(2):124–33.

199. Ferré PJ, Pasloske K, Whittem T, Ranasinghe MG, Li Q, Lefebvre HP. Plasma pharmacokinetics of alfaxalone in dogs after an intravenous bolus of Alfaxan-CD RTU. Vet Anaesth Analg. 2006;33(4):229–36.

200. Pypendop BH, Ranasinghe MG, Pasloske K. Pharmacokinetics of alfaxalone infusions, context-sensitive half-time and recovery times in male neutered cats. Vet Anaesth Analg. 2018;45(5):630–9.

201. Correa Mdo A, Aguiar AJ, Neto FJ, Mendes Gda M, Steagall PV, Lima AF. Effects of remifentanil infusion regimens on cardiovascular function and responses to noxious stimulation in propofol-anesthetized cats. Am J Vet Res. 2007;68(9):932–40.

202. Rawlings CA, Kolata RJ. Cardiopulmonary effects of thiopental/lidocaine combination during anesthetic induction in the dog. Am J Vet Res. 1983;44(1):144–9.

203. Wilson SH, Wolf BJ, Bingham K, et al. Labor analgesia onset with dural puncture epidural versus traditional epidural using a 26-gauge Whitacre needle and 0.125% bupivacaine bolus: a randomized clinical trial. Anesth Analg. 2018;126(2):545–51.

204. Apseloff G, Onel E, Patou G. Time to onset of analgesia following local infiltration of liposome bupivacaine in healthy volunteers: a randomized, single-blind, sequential cohort, crossover study. Int J Clin Pharmacol Ther. 2013;51(5):367–73.

205. Thomasy SM, Pypendop BH, Ilkiw JE, Stanley SD. Pharmacokinetics of lidocaine and its active metabolite, monoethylglycinexylidide, after intravenous administration of lidocaine to awake and isoflurane-anesthetized cats. Am J Vet Res. 2005;66(7):1162–6.

206. Binder DR, Herring IP. Duration of corneal anesthesia following topical administration of 0.5% proparacaine hydrochloride solution in clinically normal cats. Am J Vet Res. 2006;67(10):1780–2.

207. Watanabe R, Marcoux J, Evangelista MC, Dumais Y, Steagall PV. The analgesic effects of buprenorphine (Vetergesic or Simbadol) in cats undergoing dental extractions: a randomized, blinded, clinical trial. PLoS One. 2020;15(3):e0230079.

208. Doodnaught GM, Monteiro BP, Benito J, et al. Pharmacokinetic and pharmacodynamic modelling after subcutaneous, intravenous and buccal administration of a high-concentration formulation of buprenorphine in conscious cats. PLoS One. 2017;12(4):e0176443.

209. Barletta M, Ostenkamp SM, Taylor AC, Quandt J, Lascelles BDX, Messenger KM. The pharmacokinetics and analgesic effects of extended-release buprenorphine administered subcutaneously in healthy dogs. J Vet Pharmacol Ther. 2018;41(4):502–12.

210. Nunamaker EA, Stolarik DF, Ma J, Wilsey AS, Jenkins GJ, Medina CL. Clinical efficacy of sustained-release buprenorphine with meloxicam for postoperative analgesia in beagle dogs undergoing ovariohysterectomy. J Am Assoc Lab Anim Sci. 2014;53(5):494–501.

211. Steagall PV, Monteiro-Steagall BP, Taylor PM. A review of the studies using buprenorphine in cats. J Vet Intern Med. 2014;28(3):762–70.

212. Houghton KJ, Rech RH, Sawyer DC, et al. Dose-response of intravenous butorphanol to increase visceral nociceptive threshold in dogs. Proc Soc Exp Biol Med. 1991;197(3):290–6.

213. Wells S, Glerum L, Papich M. Pharmacokinetics of butorphanol in cats after intramuscular and buccal transmucosal administration. Am J Vet Res. 2008;69(12):1548–54.

214. Kukanich B, Clark TP. The history and pharmacology of fentanyl: relevance to a novel, long-acting transdermal fentanyl solution newly approved for use in dogs. J Vet Pharmacol Ther. 2012;35 Suppl 2:3–19.

215. Machado ML, Soares JHN, Kuster de Albuquerque Gress MA, et al. Dose-finding study comparing three treatments of remifentanil in cats anesthetized with isoflurane undergoing ovariohysterectomy. J Feline Med Surg. 2018;20(2):164–71.

216. De Monte V, Staffieri F, Caivano D, Bufalari A. Anaesthetic management for balloon dilation of cor triatriatum dexter in a dog. Acta Vet Scand. 2015;57:29.

217. Van Wijnsberghe AS, Marolf V, Claeys S, Sandersen C, Ida KK. Effects of fentanyl-lidocaine-ketamine versus sufentanil-lidocaine-ketamine on the isoflurane requirements in dogs undergoing total ear canal ablation and lateral bulla osteotomy. Vet Anaesth Analg. 2020;47(5):595–603.

218. Scott JC, Cooke JE, Stanski DR. Electroencephalographic quantitation of opioid effect: comparative pharmacodynamics of fentanyl and sufentanil. Anesthesiology. 1991;74(1):34–42.

219. Lebkowska-Wieruszewska B, De Vito V, Owen H, Poapholatep A, Giorgi M. Pharmacokinetics of grapiprant, a selective EP4 prostaglandin PGE2 receptor antagonist, after 2 mg/kg oral and i.v. administrations in cats. J Vet Pharmacol Ther. 2017;40(6):e11–e5.

220. Rausch-Derra LC, Rhodes L. Safety and toxicokinetic profiles associated with daily oral administration of grapiprant, a selective antagonist of the prostaglandin E2 EP4 receptor, to cats. Am J Vet Res. 2016;77(7):688–92.

221. Dretchen KL, Mesa Z, Robben M, et al. Intranasal epinephrine in dogs: pharmacokinetic and heart rate effects. Pharmacol Res Perspect. 2020;8(2):e00587.

222. Grubb T, Sager J, Gaynor JS, et al. 2020 AAHA Anesthesia and Monitoring Guidelines for Dogs and Cats. J Am Anim Hosp Assoc. 2020;56(2):59–82.

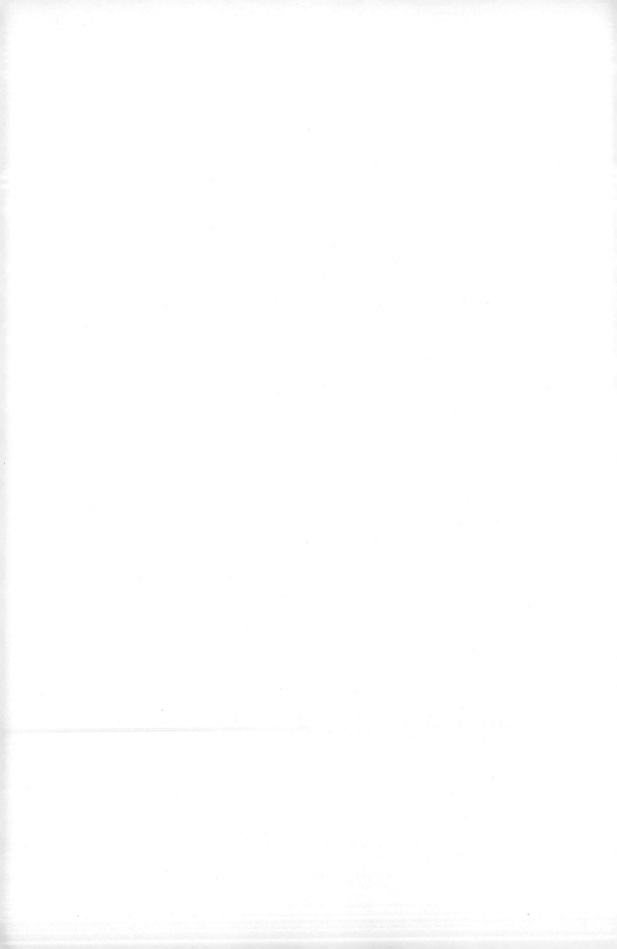

Appendices

Appendix A: Pain scale options

Please note, this Appendix is not designed to provide all pain scale options available, but to present the user with options that may assist in incorporating a pain scale into their practice.

Glasgow Composite Pain Scale (Canine)

INTERVENTION STUDY
SHORT FORM OF THE GLASGOW COMPOSITE PAIN SCALE

Dog's name _____

Hospital Number _____ **Date** / / **Time**

Surgery Yes/No (delete as appropriate)

Routine analgesic intervention Yes /No

Procedure or Condition_____

_____

| Name of assessor: |
| _____ |

Do you think this animal requires Analgesia? Y / N
In the sections below please circle the appropriate score in each list and sum these to give the total score.

A. Look at dog in Kennel

Is the dog?

(i)

Quiet	0
Crying or whimpering	1
Groaning	2
Screaming	3

(ii)

Ignoring any wound or painful area	0
Looking at wound or painful area	1
Licking wound or painful area	2
Rubbing wound or painful area	3
Chewing wound or painful area	4

> In the case of spinal, pelvic or multiple limb fractures, or where assistance is required to aid locomotion do not carry out section **B** and proceed to **C**
> *Please tick if this is the case* ☐ then proceed to C.

Figure A.1 Glasgow Composite Pain Scale (Canine). Please follow instructions listed to execute pain scale appropriately. *Source:* Reprinted with permission from Jacky Reid.

Small Animal Anesthesia Techniques, Second Edition. Edited by Amanda M. Shelby and Carolyn M. McKune.
© 2023 John Wiley & Sons, Inc. Published 2023 by John Wiley & Sons, Inc.
Companion website: www.wiley.com/go/shelby/anesthesia2

Appendices

B. Put lead on dog and lead out of the kennel.

When the dog rises/walks is it?

(iii)

Normal	0
Lame	1
Slow or reluctant	2
Stiff	3
It refuses to move	4

C. If it has a wound or painful area including abdomen, apply gentle pressure 2 inches round the site.

Does it?

(iv)

Do nothing	0
Look round	1
Flinch	2
Growl or guard area	3
Snap	4
Cry	5

D. Overall

Is the dog?

(v)

Happy and content or happy and bouncy	0
Quiet	1
Indifferent or non-responsive to surroundings	2
Nervous or anxious or fearful	3
Depressed or non-responsive to stimulation	4

Is the dog?

(vi)

Comfortable	0
Unsettled	1
Restless	2
Hunched or tense	3
Rigid	4

© University of Glasgow 2002

Total Score (i+ii+iii+iv+v+vi) = _____

Figure A.1   (continued)

Glasgow Composite Pain Scale (Feline)

Glasgow Composite Measure Pain Scale: CMPS - Feline

Guidance for use

The Glasgow Feline Composite Measure Pain Scale (CMPS-Feline), which can be applied quickly and reliably in a clinical setting, has been designed as a clinical decision making tool for use in cats in acute pain. It includes 28 descriptor options within 7 behavioral categories. Within each category, the descriptors are ranked numerically according to their associated pain severity and the person carrying out the assessment chooses the descriptor within each category which best fits the cat's behavior/condition. It is important to carry out the assessment procedure as described on the questionnaire, following the protocol closely. The pain score is the sum of the rank scores. The maximum score for the 7 categories is 20. The total CMPS-Feline score has been shown to be a useful indicator of analgesic requirement and the recommended analgesic intervention level is 5/20.

Figure A.2   Glasgow Composite Pain Scale (Feline). Please follow instructions listed to execute pain scale appropriately. *Source:* Reprinted with permission from Jacky Reid.

Glasgow Feline Composite Measure Pain Scale: CMPS - Feline

Choose the most appropriate expression from each section and total the scores to calculate the pain score for the cat. If more than one expression applies choose the higher score

LOOK AT THE CAT IN ITS CAGE:

Is it?
Question 1
    Silent / purring / meowing   0
    Crying/growling / groaning   1

Question 2
    Relaxed   0
    Licking lips   1
    Restless/cowering at back of cage   2
    Tense/crouched   3
    Rigid/hunched   4

Question 3
    Ignoring any wound or painful area   0
    Attention to wound   1

Question 4
    a) Look at the following caricatures. Circle the drawing which best depicts the cat's ear
        position?

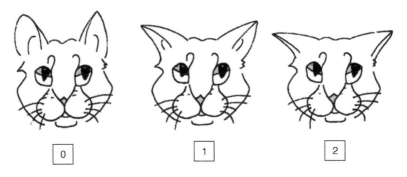

0	1	2

    b) Look at the shape of the muzzle in the following caricatures. Circle the drawing which
       appears most like that of the cat?

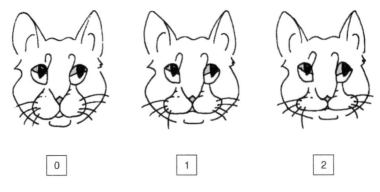

0	1	2

Figure A.2   (continued)

APPROACH THE CAGE, CALL THE CAT BY NAME & STROKE ALONG ITS BACK FROM HEAD TO TAIL

Question 5
Does it?

Respond to stroking	0

Is it?

Unresponsive	1
Aggressive	2

IF IT HAS A WOUND OR PAINFUL AREA, APPLY GENTLE PRESSURE 5 CM AROUND THE SITE. IN THE ABSENCE OF ANY PAINFUL AREA APPLY SIMILAR PRESSURE AROUND THE HIND LEG ABOVE THE KNEE

Question 6
Does it?

Do nothing	0
Swish tail/flatten ears	1
Cry/hiss	2
Growl	3
Bite/lash out	4

Question 7
General impression
Is the cat?

Happy and content	0
Disinterested/quiet	1
Anxious/fearful	2
Dull	3
Depressed/grumpy	4

Pain Score ... /20

Figure A.2   (continued)

Colorado State University (CSU) Acute Pain Scale

Instructions for using the CSU Acute Pain Scale for dogs and cats

The Colorado State University Acute Pain Scale is intended primarily as a teaching tool and to guide observation of clinical patients. The scale does not meet validation criteria [1] and should not be used as a definitive pain score, although its user-friendly nature makes it an appropriate introduction to pain scaling. Use of the scale employs both an observational period and a hands-on evaluation of the patient. In general, the assessment begins with quiet observation of the patient in its cage at a relatively unobstructive distance. Afterward, the patient as a whole (wound as well as the entire body) is approached to assess reaction to gentle palpation, indicators of muscle tension and heat, response to interaction, and so on.

1. The scale utilizes a generic 0–4 scale with quarter marks as its base, along with a color scale as a visual cue for progression along the five-point scale.
2. Realistic artist's renderings of animals at various levels of pain add further visual cues. Additional drawings provide space for recording pain, warmth, and muscle tension; this allows documentation of specific areas of concern in the medical record. A further advantage of these drawings is that the observer is encouraged to assess the overall pain of the patient in addition to focusing on the primary lesion.
3. The scale includes psychologic and behavioral signs of pain as well as palpation responses. Further, the scale uses body tension as an evaluation tool, a parameter not addressed in other scales.
4. There is provision for nonassessment in the resting patient. To the author's knowledge, this is the only scale that emphasizes the importance of delaying assessment in a sleeping patient while prompting the observer to recognize patients that may be inappropriately obtunded by medication or a more serious health concern.
5. Advantages of this scale include ease of use with minimal interpretation required. Specific descriptors for individual behaviors are provided, which decreases interobserver variability. Additionally, a scale is provided for both the dog and cat.
6. A disadvantage of this scale is a lack of validation by clinical studies comparing it with other scales. While interrater reliability (when used by veterinarians) was moderate to good, validity could not meet correlation coefficients [1]. Further, its use is largely limited to and is intended for use in acute pain.

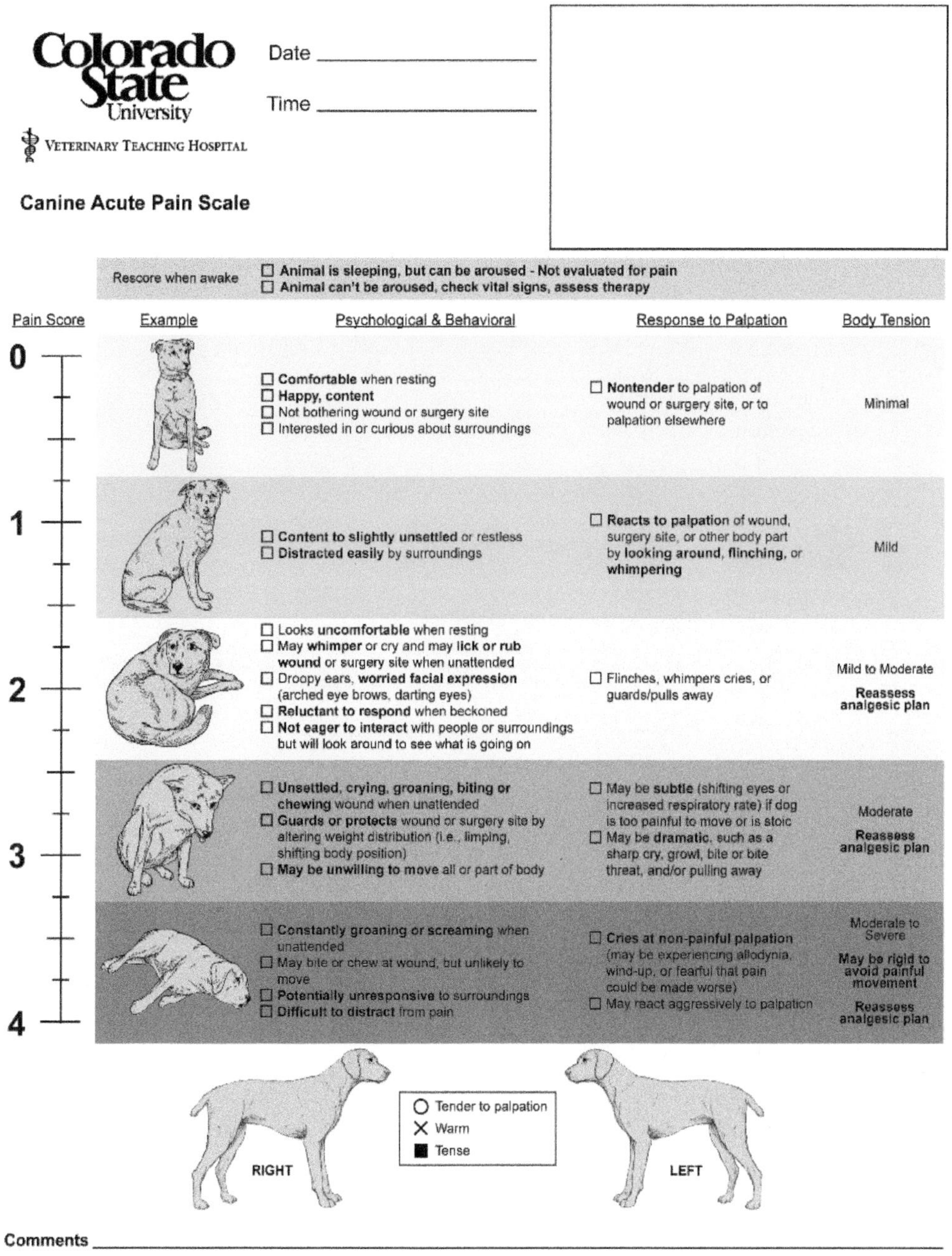

Figure A.3 Subjective and objective pain scoring sheet in dogs. *Source:* Reprinted with permission from Dr Robinson and Dr Hellyer at Colorado State University.

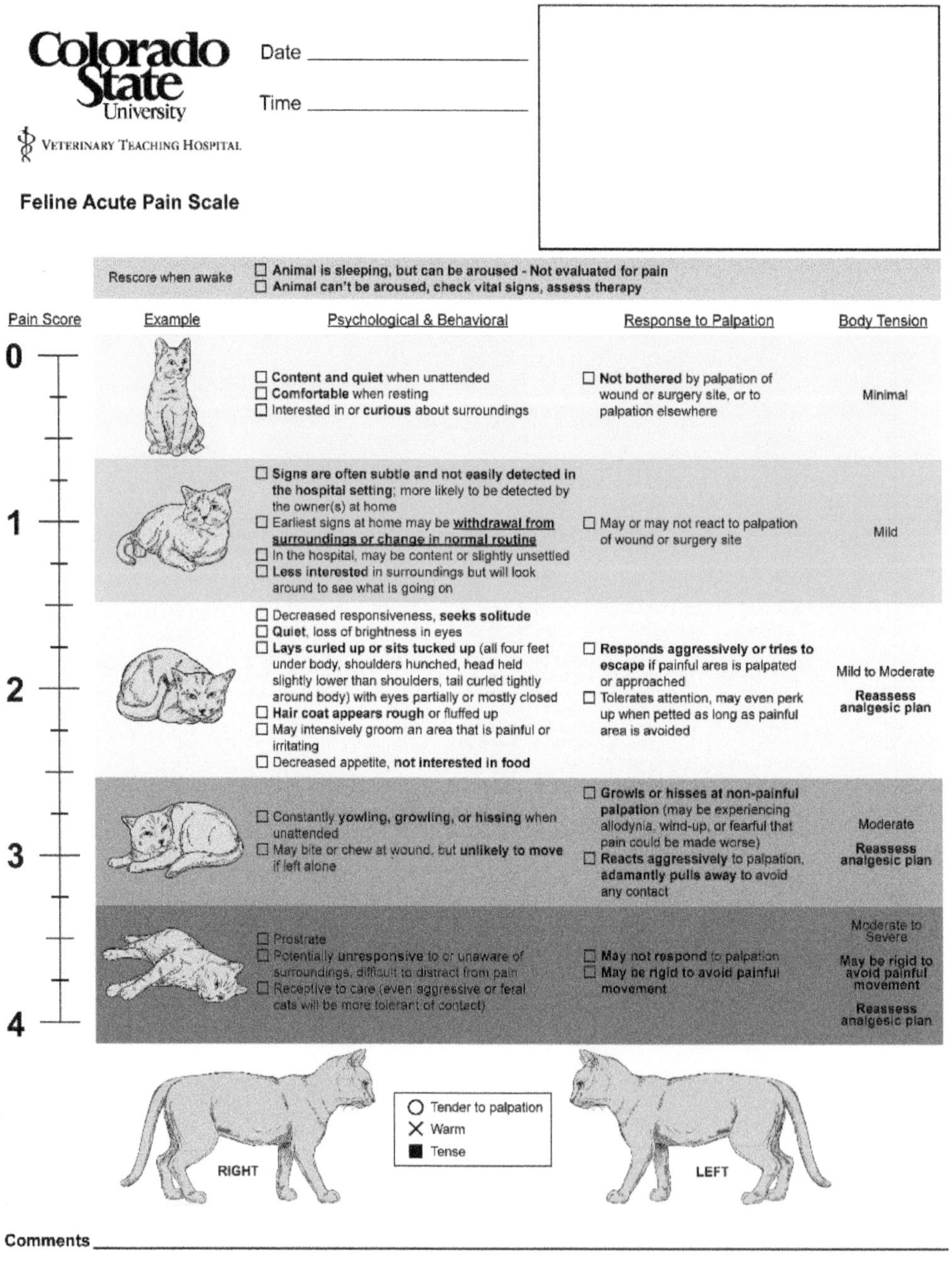

Colorado State University
VETERINARY TEACHING HOSPITAL

Date _____

Time _____

Feline Acute Pain Scale

| Rescore when awake | ☐ Animal is sleeping, but can be aroused - Not evaluated for pain
☐ Animal can't be aroused, check vital signs, assess therapy |

Pain Score	Example	Psychological & Behavioral	Response to Palpation	Body Tension
0		☐ **Content and quiet** when unattended ☐ **Comfortable** when resting ☐ Interested in or **curious** about surroundings	☐ **Not bothered** by palpation of wound or surgery site, or to palpation elsewhere	Minimal
1		☐ **Signs are often subtle and not easily detected in the hospital setting**; more likely to be detected by the owner(s) at home ☐ Earliest signs at home may be <u>withdrawal from surroundings or change in normal routine</u> ☐ In the hospital, may be content or slightly unsettled ☐ **Less interested** in surroundings but will look around to see what is going on	☐ May or may not react to palpation of wound or surgery site	Mild
2		☐ Decreased responsiveness, **seeks solitude** ☐ **Quiet**, loss of brightness in eyes ☐ **Lays curled up or sits tucked up** (all four feet under body, shoulders hunched, head held slightly lower than shoulders, tail curled tightly around body) with eyes partially or mostly closed ☐ **Hair coat appears rough** or fluffed up ☐ May intensively groom an area that is painful or irritating ☐ Decreased appetite, **not interested in food**	☐ **Responds aggressively or tries to escape** if painful area is palpated or approached ☐ Tolerates attention, may even perk up when petted as long as painful area is avoided	Mild to Moderate **Reassess analgesic plan**
3		☐ Constantly yowling, growling, or hissing when unattended ☐ May bite or chew at wound, but **unlikely to move if left alone**	☐ **Growls or hisses at non-painful palpation** (may be experiencing allodynia, wind-up, or fearful that pain could be made worse) ☐ Reacts aggressively to palpation, adamantly pulls away to avoid any contact	Moderate **Reassess analgesic plan**
4		☐ Prostrate ☐ Potentially unresponsive to or unaware of surroundings, difficult to distract from pain ☐ Receptive to care (even aggressive or feral cats will be more tolerant of contact)	☐ May not respond to palpation ☐ May be rigid to avoid painful movement	Moderate to Severe May be rigid to avoid painful movement **Reassess analgesic plan**

○ Tender to palpation
✕ Warm
■ Tense

RIGHT   LEFT

Comments _____

Figure A.4 Subjective and objective pain scoring sheet in cats. *Source:* Reprinted with permission from Dr Robinson and Dr Hellyer at Colorado State University.

Appendix B: Cardiopulmonary resuscitation

A key goal in anesthesia is preventing the necessity for cardiopulmonary resuscitation (CPR), when possible. However, even in relatively healthy animals, cardiopulmonary arrest occurs [2]. CPR is most successful when the team is prepared, the crisis is recognized early, and CPR is started immediately. Anesthetized patients that experience cardiac arrest have better survival rates because of early recognition, established patent airway, and IV catheter. It is important during a crisis to remain systematic in your approach to resuscitation.

1. Perform a rapid airway, breathing, and circulation (ABC) assessment, taking no longer than 5–10 sec. If ABC assessment suggests cardiopulmonary arrest (CPA) or leaves doubt as to the presence of circulation, go to Step 2.

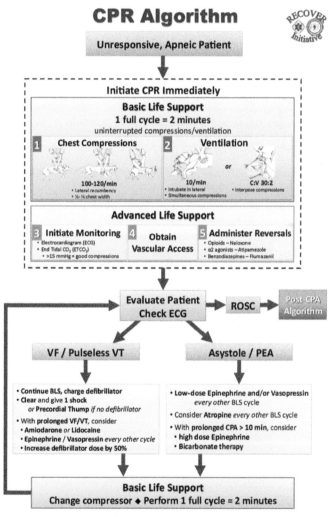

Figure A.5 CPR algorithm. CPR, cardiopulmonary resuscitation; PEA, pulseless electrical activity; VF, ventricular fibrillation; VT, ventricular tachycardia. *Source:* Reprinted from Fletcher DJ, Boller M, Brainard BM, et al. RECOVER evidence and knowledge gap analysis on veterinary CPR. Part 7: Clinical guidelines. J Vet Emerg Crit Care. 2012;22 Suppl 1:S102–31, with permission from John Wiley and Sons.

2. Discontinue anesthesia (turn off vaporizer, CRIs, etc.).
3. Begin basic life support with "CAB."
   - *C = compressions.* Compressions are started immediately, even before securing an airway in an unintubated patient, as the lack of forward blood flow makes ventilation a moot point. Keel chest patients are placed in lateral recumbency; compressions are targeted at 100–120 bpm. Barrel chest patients (e.g., English bulldogs) can be placed in dorsal recumbency. Compress one-third of the circumference of the patient's chest. It is important to allow complete recoil of the chest before the next set of compressions. Once begun, it is imperative to minimize interruption of chest compressions. The compressor is rotated every 2 minutes; the next compressor will place their hands over the current compressor's hands, and there is communication regarding the hand-off to new compressor, so transition is as seamless as possible. Use of appropriate compressor posture delivers effective compressions and reduces fatigue. Appropriate compressor posture includes elevation over the animal (using a stool if necessary), locking the elbows, interlocking the hands, and bending at the waist to utilize the entire upper body to deliver effective compressions.
   - *A = airway.* Compressions provide some ventilation. A second person obtains supplies to intubate the patient (ET tube, laryngoscope, oxygen and a securing tie). Again, interruption of compressions should be minimal. It is important for the most experienced and confident team member to quickly intubate the patient while compressions are occurring, if possible. If this is not possible, compressions are continued immediately once the ET tube is secured.
   - *B = breathing.* Once intubated, ventilate the patient at 10 breaths per minute with either room air or 100% oxygen. If a manometer is available, the PIP should be 20 cmH_2O per breath. Targeted tidal volume is 10 mL/kg.

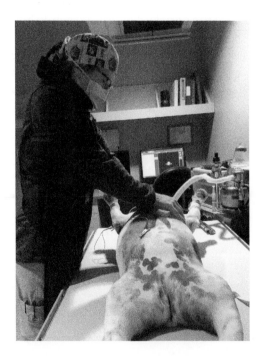

4. Monitoring during CPR.
   - Place monitoring equipment. A capnograph is now considered standard of care for use during CPR, with a target goal of 12–15 mmHg $EtCO_2$ or greater. Place ECG on patient; assessment of the rhythm is made during chest recoils, if possible, although a sudden rise in $EtCO_2$ may suggest a return of circulation and warrants an ECG assessment.
   - Assess for pulse either by palpation of the femoral artery or by placing a gelled Doppler over the eye between compressor swaps.
5. Administer drugs via IV access closest to the heart (i.e., jugular catheter when available) (Table A.1). Delivery of drugs is followed with a sufficient saline bolus, especially if a peripheral catheter is used.
   - Epinephrine (0.01 mg/kg IV/IO or 0.02–0.1 mg/kg diluted 1:1 with saline; IT if no IV access is available) is administered for asystole or PEA; this is repeated every 4 min. High-dose epinephrine (0.1 mg/kg IV) is considered after prolonged CPR.
   - Vasopressin (0.8 IU/kg IV/IO) is an alternative for interchangeable use with the first dose of epinephrine.
   - Atropine (0.04 mg/kg IV/IO) is still recommended for use in the small animal, especially if high vagal tone is suspected, although it has lost favor for routine use in human CPR [3].
   - Reverse any anesthetics or drugs administered for analgesia (reversal agents include naloxone, flumazenil, and atipamezole; see Table 3, p.288).
   - Fluids during CPR: use of IV fluids is reserved for patients considered hypovolemic prior to arrest.
   - Sodium bicarbonate (1 mEq/kg, diluted 1:4, once) is considered for administration in cases of prolonged CPR (>10–15 min).
6. Electrical defibrillation is delivered if it can be performed safely (i.e., without putting the CPR team members at risk) at 2–4 J/kg for a biphasic defibrillator, 4–6 J/kg for a monophasic defibrillator (biphasic preferred). Chest compressions are begun immediately post defibrillation. In human CPR, there is a prevalence of ventricular fibrillation as the arrest rhythm and thus time to defibrillation is a major determinant of survival [4]. In animals, it is still prudent to defibrillate early when possible and applicable. If the first defibrillation attempt is unsuccessful, a 50% increase is deemed reasonable; however, there is no evidence of increased success in dogs and cats with this methodology.

Table A.1   Primary emergency drugs.

Drug	Intravenous	Intrathecal[a] (max. dose)
Epinephrine	0.01 (mg/kg)	0.1 (mg/kg)
Atropine	0.04 (mg/kg)	0.4 (mg/kg)
Vasopressin	0.8 (unit/kg)	0.8 (units/kg)

[a]When IV/IO access is not available, IT doses up to 10 × the IV doses are administered, and are often diluted 1:1 with saline. A long red rubber catheter is placed down the endotracheal tube to facilitate administration.

If return of spontaneous circulation occurs, the veterinary team begins postresuscitative care. The reader is directed to a more thorough review of CPR and postresuscitative care in the companion animal, as this Appendix's target goal is that of an overview [3].

Appendix C: Constant-rate infusion calculations

Constant-rate infusions (CRIs) are extremely beneficial for balancing the anesthetic technique. Often, they are used to provide multimodal analgesia, minimum alveolar concentration (MAC) reduction, and supportive therapies (e.g., paralysis, inotropic support, electrolyte supplementation). The purpose of a CRI is to maintain a constant plasma level of the administered drug. In most situations, a loading dose is used to fill the plasma compartment, followed by the start of the CRI to maintain the target plasma concentration. Depending on the availability of equipment (e.g., syringe or fluid pumps), CRIs are routine practices in many clinics. Equation A.1 assists in calculating and administering CRIs from a bag of fluids. Steps in Table A.2 are followed when calculating CRIs.

$$\frac{\text{Dose (mg/kg/h)}}{\text{Rate (mL/kg/h)}} \times \text{Total Volume (mL)} = \text{mg of drug to add} \qquad (A.1)$$

As with any calculation, accuracy of the mathematics is assured when the units "cross-cancel" and the answer is delivered in the units desired.

Example: Hydromorphone, lidocaine and ketamine (HLK) CRI in a 20 kg dog

This CRI is a combination of opioid, sodium channel blocker, and n-methyl-D-aspartate (NMDA) antagonist for painful procedures when locoregional blocks cannot be performed or (e.g., orthopedic procedures, median sternotomy, total ear canal ablation and ventral bulla osteotomy [TECABO]), or fail. Hydromorphone is a common opioid administered but other opioids are also suitable.

- Step 1. For this example, the patient will receive HLK during the procedure in the anesthetic maintenance fluids. Total volume: 1000 mL LRS (1 L bag).
- Step 2. Hydromorphone at 0.03 mg/kg/h, lidocaine at 3 mg/kg/h, and ketamine at 0.6 mg/kg/h intraoperatively will be used in fluids given at anesthetic maintenance of 5 mL/kg/h.

Table A.2   Steps for calculating CRIs.

Step 1: Determine what total volume is desired (dependent on dose, duration, and size of patient).
Step 2: Select drug or drugs.
Step 3: Calculate (see Equation A.1).
Step 4: Create solution.

- Step 3. Separate calculations are performed for each drug used.

$$\text{Hydromorphone: } \frac{0.03 \text{ mg/kg/h}}{5 \text{ mL/kg/h}} \times 1000 \text{ mL} = 6 \text{ mg of drug to add}$$

$$\text{Lidocaine: } \frac{3 \text{ mg/kg/h}}{5 \text{ mL/kg/h}} \times 1000 \text{ mL} = 600 \text{ mg of drug to add} \qquad \text{(A.2)}$$

$$\text{Ketamine: } \frac{0.6 \text{ mg/kg/h}}{5 \text{ mL/kg/h}} \times 1000 \text{ mL} = 120 \text{ mg of drug to add}$$

The answers to the calculations are in milligrams. The anesthetist divides by the concentration of the drugs used to determine the volume of each drug to be added to the bag of fluids.

$$\text{Hydromorphone: } 6 \text{ mg} \times \frac{\text{mL}}{2 \text{ mg}} = 3 \text{ mL}$$

$$\text{Lidocaine: } 600 \text{ mg} \times \frac{\text{mL}}{20 \text{ mg}} = 30 \text{ mL} \qquad \text{(A.3)}$$

$$\text{Ketamine: } 120 \text{ mg} \times \frac{\text{mL}}{100 \text{ mg}} = 1.2 \text{ mL}$$

- Step 4. Creating: The total volume of drugs calculated is removed from the bag of LRS first. Then the drugs are added.

When this bag of LRS (now containing HLK) is administered to the 20 kg canine patient at the rate of 5 mL/kg/h, the patient receives 100 mL/h LRS with hydromorphone at 0.03 mg/kg/h, lidocaine at 3 mg/kg/h, and ketamine 1.2 mg/kg/h. Loading doses of these drugs are administered prior to starting the CRI, often as part of the patient's premedication and induction agents. A fluid pump is recommended to accurately deliver the 100 mL/h or additional fluid drip rate calculations are used to determine drop/sec for administration (see Appendix G).

Appendix D: Creating dilutions and reconstituting solutions

$$C_1 V_1 = C_2 V_2 \qquad \text{(A.4)}$$

Dilutions

Making diflutions is completed using the simple equation above. C_1 and C_2 are concentrations and V_1 and V_2 are volumes. C_1 represents what the anesthetist would like to obtain for the final concentration. V_1 is the volume available to work with. C_2 is the concentration the anesthetist has available. V_2 is the unknown volume the equation will solve, to then add and create the desired concentration. This equation is beneficial in that units are irrelevant if they are the "same" on both sides of the equation.

Example 1: Dextrose dilution

An anesthetist wants to make 5% dextrose in a 1000 mL bag of saline. Dextrose is available as a 50% solution.

C_1 = 5% dextrose
V_1 = 1000 mL bag of saline
C_2 = 50% dextrose
V_2 = volume of 50% dextrose needed

$$(5\%)(1000 \text{ mL}) = (50\%)(V_2) \qquad \text{(A.5)}$$

By solving the equation for V_2 (multiply 5% times 1000 mL then divide by 50%), the anesthetist determines that 100 mL of the 50% dextrose solution needs to be added to the 1000 mL bag of 0.9% saline. One should first remove 100 mL from the saline bag then add the 100 mL of 50% dextrose, thus creating 1000 mL of 5% dextrose in 0.9% saline.

Example 2: Diluting dopamine

Dopamine is available as a very concentrated solution (40 mg/mL) and is diluted prior to administration. The anesthetist would like 20 mL of a 1 mg/mL dilution. See equation A.6 and solve for the unknown volume (V_2).

$$(1 \text{ mg/mL})(20 \text{ mL}) = (40 \text{ mg/mL})(V_2) \qquad \text{(A.6)}$$

C_1 = 1 mg/mL
V_1 = 20 mL
C_2 = 40 mg/mL
V_2 = Unknown volume of dopamine

By solving the equation for V_2 (multiply 1 mg/mL times 20 mL, then divide by 40 mg/mL), the anesthetist determines that 0.5 mL of the 40 mg/mL dopamine needs to be added to 19.5 mL of saline.

Reconstituting a solution

$$\text{Concentration of powder (mg)} \div \text{concentration of desired solution (mg/mL)} \\ = \text{volume to add (mL)} \qquad \text{(A.7)}$$

Some drugs (i.e., remifentanil) come as concentrated powders that reconstitute into a solution for administration. Equation A.7 is used to determine how much diluent is added to create a desired concentration in solution. It is important to recognize that the "math" of any calculation is only correct when the units cross-cancel and the answer is in the units desired (see Example 1).

Example: Reconstituting remifentanil

Remifentanil is available in 2 mg of powder per vial. Assume the desired concentration for administration is 50 µg/mL. For this example, one needs to calculate how much diluent (V_1) to add to 2 mg powder (C_1) to get a concentration of 50 µg/mL (C_2). It is important to convert units to equal powers (i.e., mg to µg or µg to mg). The desired concentration involves micrograms when the originating powder is in milligrams. First convert 2 mg into 2000 µg (see Appendix I).

$$2000 \text{ mg} \div 50 \text{ mg/mL} = 40 \text{ mL} \tag{A.8}$$

Dissolving 2 µg mg powder into 40 mls creates the desired 50 µg/mL solution.

Appendix E: Abdominal tap

Table A.3

Materials: Clippers, aseptic scrub, 16 G catheter, three-way stopcock, extension set, sterile gloves, 60 mL syringe, large container with volume markings, +/– ultrasound
Techniques:
1. The patient is premedicated according to the anesthetic plan.
2. Maintain the patient in sternal recumbency or standing, if the patient tolerates it. Clip and prep the patient ventral medially on the right side of the abdomen (to avoid the spleen).
3. Open sterile gloves and, without contaminating the catheter, drop the catheter onto the gloves, along with one extension set.
4. In a sterile manner, carefully glove, taking care not to contact the sterile catheter and extension set.
5. Palpate the fluid wave in the abdomen in the context of the clipped and prepped location. Grasp the catheter approximately 0.5–1.0 inch from the tip. Insert the catheter and stylet slowly through the skin and abdominal wall, watching for fluid flow from the catheter. The fluid should be of the expected composition (e.g., serosanguinous); if unexpected fluid is encountered (e.g., frank hemorrhage), pull out needle and apply direct pressure. Alternatively, an ultrasound probe is used to guide the needle into the fluid pocket.
6. When expected fluid flows back through the stylet, feed the catheter off the stylet. Minimal resistance is felt if the location is correct.
7. Attach the sterile extension tubing to the catheter hub; the other end is handed to an individual operating the syringe.
8. The individual operating the syringe attaches the three-way stopcock to the extension set and a 60 mL syringe to the three-way stopcock.
9. The stopcock is turned off to the environment, and the fluid is drained from the abdomen by pulling back on the syringe. When the syringe is full, the stopcock is turned off to the patient and emptied into the container.
10. Steps 8 and 9 are repeated until no more fluid is withdrawn; final volume is measured and recorded.

Appendix F: Drugs to withhold or continue in the perianesthetic period (see drug formulary, Section II)

Table A.4

Medication	Administer or withhold?	Dose and timing of administration	Reason for administration/ withholding	Other notes
ACE inhibitors	Withhold	Withhold 24 h before anesthesia	Avoid refractory hypotension during anesthesia [5]	Resume dosing interval post anesthesia
Anticoagulants	Withhold	Withhold 10–14 days prior to anesthesia	Avoid excessive hemorrhage	This includes aspirin
Behavioral modifiers	Pending drug	As prescribed	Careful evaluation of which drug an animal is on assists with whether or not it is prudent to administer or withhold this medication	While abruptly withdrawing behavioral medications is not desirable, this category of drugs has significant potential for drug interaction. Consult a drug handbook for more information on drug interactions
Famotidine	Administer	1 mg/kg IV or PO 12–24 h before anesthesia	Neutralization of stomach pH should regurgitation occur	Few evidence based studies exist [6,7]
Furosemide	Administer	As prescribed	This drug helps to reduce complications from congestive heart failure	Patients receiving furosemide often have considerable cardiovascular instability; consider consultation with a boarded anesthesiologist prior to anesthesia
Gabapentin	Administer	10 mg/kg PO	Sedation	This may facilitate handling of stressed animals when they arrive at the clinic

Table A.4 *(Continued)*

Medication	Administer or withhold?	Dose and timing of administration	Reason for administration/ withholding	Other notes
Glucose supplementation	Administer	0.5–1 g/kg IV bolus (diluted 1:4 with saline); 2.5–5% additive to maintenance fluids	Treatment of hypoglycemia, maintain serum glucose	Bolus is administered if serum glucose is less than 60 g/dL
Insulin	Administer	Dosing depends on patient serum glucose; ½ dose considered in patient fasted 2–4 h [8]	Assist with serum glucose regulation in diabetic patients	Frequent serum glucose checks recommended
Intraoperative antibiotics (cefazolin, ampicillin sulbactam)	Administer	Administered 30–60 min before surgical approach; q 90 min intraoperatively	Minimize infection	Routine dosing: Cefazolin 22 mg/kg IV ampicillin sulbactam 30 mg/kg IV
Maropitant	Administer	2 mg/kg PO 2 h before premedication; 1 mg/kg SC 1 h before premedication, 1 mg/kg IV 10 min before premedication	Reduce incidence of vomiting associated with opioid administration [9–11]	Wide margin of safety, as the published dose for motion sickness is up to 8 mg/kg
Metoclopramide	Administer	1 mg/kg bolus IV followed by 0.08–1 mg/kg/h CRI [12]	Reduce incidence of gastroesophageal reflux	Most studies demonstrate this does not considerably reduce the incidence of regurgitation and subsequent aspiration pneumonia [13]
Pantoprazole	Administer	0.7–1 mg/kg IV SID or 1 mg/kg omeprazole PO BID; must be started 36 h prior to anesthesia to have the desired effect	Neutralization of stomach pH should regurgitation occur [14,15]	Recommended for patients with history of regurgitation and brachycephalic breeds [16]

(Continued)

Table A.4 *(Continued)*

Medication	Administer or withhold?	Dose and timing of administration	Reason for administration/ withholding	Other notes
Pimobendan	Administer	0.2–0.3 mg/kg BID PO	Improve cardiac sensitization, and thus contractility	While injectable pimobendan is incredibly difficult to obtain at the time of writing, this drug simply cannot be duplicated by other injectable agents and warrants administration preoperatively, if the patient is currently receiving this medication
Steroids	Administer	Prior to anesthesia as prescribed	Abrupt withdrawal may result in an Addisonian crisis under anesthesia	An injectable steroid equiva- lent may be administered to patients who did not receive oral medication
Thyroid medication	Administer	As prescribed	Thyroid hormone is important for many of the metabolic functions that are critical to normal physio- logic function	These pills are usually small and easy to administer orally on the same day as anesthesia
Trazadone	Administer	8 mg/kg PO	Antianxiety	Especially when coupled with gabapentin, this may help increase handlability of patients presenting on the same day of surgery

ACE, angiotensin converting enzyme; BID, bis in die (twice a day); IV, intravenous; PO, per os (by mouth); SC, subcutaneous; SID, semel in die (once a day).

Appendix G: Calculating fluid drip rates

$$\text{Body Weight (kg)} \times \text{Fluid Rate}\left(\frac{\text{mL}}{\text{kg/h}}\right) \times \text{conversion factor}\left(\frac{\text{h}}{3600 \text{ sec}}\right)$$

$$\times \text{Drip Set}\left(\frac{\text{drops}}{\text{mL}}\right) = \frac{\text{drops}}{\text{sec}} \tag{A.9}$$

Example

A 36 kg dog is undergoing anesthesia with a maintenance fluid rate of 5 mL/kg/h using a 10 drop/mL drip set. At how many drops/sec should the drip set be set?

$$36 \text{ kg} \times \frac{5 \text{ mL}}{\text{kg/h}} \times \frac{\text{h}}{3600 \text{ sec}} \times \frac{10 \text{ drops}}{\text{mL}} = \frac{0.5 \text{ drop}}{\text{sec}} \tag{A.10}$$

Appendix H: Epidural calculations

$$\text{Body weight (kg)} \times \frac{0.2 \text{ mL}}{\text{kg}} = \text{Total volume for epidural} \tag{A.11}$$

First, calculate total volume desired for the epidural. A common total volume is 0.2 mL/kg. This will typically provide enough cranial migration of epidural solution to provide analgesia for hindlimb, abdominal, or thoracic procedures. Lower volumes (0.1 mL/kg) may be used for exclusively hindlimb procedures. Morphine is dosed at 0.1 mg/kg and bupivacaine at 0.5–1 mg/kg. Once these doses have been calculated and drawn, sterile saline is added to the drug solutions to equal the remaining volume from equation A.11.

Appendix I: Conversions

Table A.5

1 kg = 2.2 lb
1 kg = 1000 g
1 g = 1000 mg
1 mg = 1000 µg
1 L = 1000 mL
°C × 9/5 + 32 = °F
(°F − 32) × 5/9 = °C
1.36 cmH$_2$O = 1 mmHg
PSI × 0.3 = estimate of liters in oxygen tank
% = 1 g/100 mL

References

1. Shipley H, Guedes A, Graham L, Goudie-DeAngelis E, Wendt-Hornickle E. Preliminary appraisal of the reliability and validity of the Colorado State University Feline Acute Pain Scale. J Feline Med Surg. 2019;21(4):335–9.
2. Brodbelt D. Perioperative mortality in small animal anaesthesia. Vet J. 2009;182(2):152–61.
3. Fletcher DJ, Boller M. Updates in small animal cardiopulmonary resuscitation. Vet Clin North Am Small Anim Pract. 2013;43(4):971–87.
4. Stokes NA, Scapigliati A, Trammell AR, Parish DC. The effect of the AED and AED programs on survival of individuals, groups and populations. Prehosp Disaster Med. 2012;27(5):419–24.
5. Coleman AE, Shepard MK, Schmiedt CW, Hofmeister EH, Brown SA. Effects of orally administered enalapril on blood pressure and hemodynamic response to vasopressors during isoflurane anesthesia in healthy dogs. Vet Anaesth Analg. 2016;43(5):482–94.
6. Costa RS, Abelson AL, Lindsey JC, Wetmore LA. Postoperative regurgitation and respiratory complications in brachycephalic dogs undergoing airway surgery before and after implementation of a standardized perianesthetic protocol. J Am Vet Med Assoc. 2020;256(8):899–905.
7. Marks SL, Kook PH, Papich MG, Tolbert MK, Willard MD. ACVIM consensus statement: Support for rational administration of gastrointestinal protectants to dogs and cats. J Vet Intern Med. 2018;32(6):1823–40.
8. Grubb T, Sager J, Gaynor JS, et al. 2020 AAHA Anesthesia and Monitoring Guidelines for Dogs and Cats. J Am Anim Hosp Assoc. 2020;56(2):59–82.
9. Hay Kraus BL. Spotlight on the perioperative use of maropitant citrate. Vet Med. 2017;8:41–51.
10. Hay Kraus BL. Effect of dosing interval on efficacy of maropitant for prevention of hydromorphone-induced vomiting and signs of nausea in dogs. J Am Vet Med Assoc. 2014;245(9):1015–20.
11. Hay Kraus BL. Efficacy of orally administered maropitant citrate in preventing vomiting associated with hydromorphone administration in dogs. J Am Vet Med Assoc. 2014;244(10):1164–9.
12. Favarato ES, Souza MV, Costa PR, et al. Evaluation of metoclopramide and ranitidine on the prevention of gastroesophageal reflux episodes in anesthetized dogs. Res Vet Sci. 2012;93(1):466–7.
13. Milovancev M, Townsend K, Spina J, et al. Effect of Metoclopramide on the incidence of early postoperative aspiration pneumonia in dogs with acquired idiopathic laryngeal paralysis. Vet Surg. 2016;45(5):577–81.
14. Tolbert MK, Odunayo A, Howell RS, Peters EE, Reed A. Efficacy of intravenous administration of combined acid suppressants in healthy dogs. J Vet Intern Med. 2015;29(2):556–60.
15. Zacuto AC, Marks SL, Osborn J, et al. The influence of esomeprazole and cisapride on gastroesophageal reflux during anesthesia in dogs. J Vet Intern Med. 2012;26(3):518–25.
16. Downing F, Gibson S. Anaesthesia of brachycephalic dogs. J Small Anim Pract. 2018;59(12):725–33.

Index

Small Animal Anesthesia Techniques, Second Edition. Edited by Amanda M. Shelby and Carolyn M. McKune.
© 2023 John Wiley & Sons, Inc. Published 2023 by John Wiley & Sons, Inc.
Companion website: www.wiley.com/go/shelby/anesthesia2